MW00780238

THE
STRESS
PARADOX

THE
STRESS
PARADOX

Why You Need Stress to Live Longer,
Healthier, and Happier

◆

Sharon Horesh Bergquist, MD

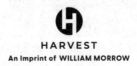

HARVEST
An Imprint of WILLIAM MORROW

This book contains advice and information relating to health care. It should be used to supplement rather than replace the advice of your doctor or another trained health professional. If you know or suspect you have a health problem, it is recommended that you seek your physician's advice before embarking on any medical program or treatment. All efforts have been made to assure the accuracy of the information contained in this book as of the date of publication. This publisher and the author disclaim liability for any medical outcomes that may occur as a result of applying the methods suggested in this book.

I have changed the names of some individuals, and modified identifying features, including physical descriptions and occupations, of other individuals in order to preserve their anonymity. In some cases, composite characters have been created or timelines have been compressed, in order to further preserve privacy and to maintain narrative flow. The goal in all cases was to protect people's privacy without damaging the integrity of the story.

HarperCollins books may be purchased for educational, business, or sales promotional use. For information, please email the Special Markets Department at SPsales@harpercollins.com.

FIRST EDITION

Designed by Renata DiBiase
Graphics by James Harrill and Nitya Bellani
Spot art by Nitya Bellani

Library of Congress Cataloging-in-Publication Data has been applied for.

ISBN 978-0-06-334596-6

24 25 26 27 28 LBC 5 4 3 2 1

In loving memory of my father

Contents

Author's Note

This book is based on hundreds of studies on the science of how stress can defend our health, longevity, and well-being. The hardest part of translating this knowledge into meaningful messages and actionable steps is ensuring that it preserves the integrity of the science. I've done my best to present the information without overstating or extrapolating the findings and striking a balance between simplicity and complexity. My goal is to empower you with a new mindset and approach to living a longer, more vibrant, and happier life and spark the conversation about trusting our natural ability to build our disease defenses and human potential through stress. The science of good stress is an exciting area of research; there's more than enough information for us to implement it into our lives, but there is also still much to learn. I invite you to join me in this conversation and welcome and look forward to continuing an open dialogue as the science invariably advances.

THE
STRESS
PARADOX

Introduction

One evening in late 2011, I found myself sitting alone in my office after a long day of seeing patients, sifting through dozens of charts and labs, at a crossroads. Despite how quickly I could move from room to room or how many patients I could see, I didn't feel I was making a real impact on their health. We were having the same conversations every six months or so about the same problems, just escalating their medications. Their numbers looked good, and we were reducing their risk of complications, but I knew that the underlying process of their disease would progress. I had all this knowledge about physiology and the pathways in our body that lead to disease, but I wasn't applying that knowledge to prevent disease.

Like most doctors, I had the skills to confidently diagnose and treat a wide range of diseases, but my help was intervening far downstream from the mouth of the problem. I spent my time trying my best to slow the flow of symptoms when what they really needed was for me to fix the dam. I knew I was capable of offering more.

At the time, I had been practicing internal medicine for more than a decade and had worked really hard to be the best physician I could possibly be. I was leaning into the skills I had learned in residency at Harvard's Brigham and Women's Hospital and my training by incredible mentors at Harvard Medical School. I was proud of the outcomes I was achieving for my patients. I consistently ranked as having among the highest percentage of patients who achieved quality metrics for measures like blood sugar and blood pressure control. And year after year, I received awards for excellence in patient care based on being in the top percentile in national rankings. My peers consecutively voted me as one of the top doctors in Atlanta. However, I was so busy working long days and weekends that I didn't have time to think about how we were measuring and defining "excellence." That evening, all these thoughts overwhelmed me with frustration and helplessness.

So I stepped back and asked myself what was most meaningful to me in my job. I had chosen to specialize in internal medicine because I wanted to help people live better, healthier, and longer lives. I had a natural ability for seeing the forest for the trees, to see the whole body as a function of its many parts. I also valued the relationships I built with my patients and the privilege of being entrusted with their care, a responsibility I take very earnestly. I realized that these thoughts combined could fuel a renewed sense of purpose for me. I could think differently about my role as a physician, using my energy and knowledge for reimagining how we provide care.

From that day forward I set out to learn everything about health and longevity. I got up early most mornings before seeing patients at the clinic and spent weekends diving into all the information I could get my hands on: research on nutrition, resilience, stress management, and all things related to wellness. I relied on my undergraduate studies in molecular biophysics and biochemistry at Yale University, along with the two years I spent there working on pre-messenger RNA splicing in a world-renowned lab, to understand pathways that are disrupted by disease and aging. I delved into thousands of clinical studies and became obsessed with how to optimize those pathways using nutrition, exercise, sleep, and other lifestyle habits.

What I found was that many of the diseases we consider "adult-onset" such as heart disease, dementia, and diabetes, take root early in life. They evolve over a runway of decades before they are manifest, which means we have ample opportunity to change their course. And I found that we could prevent many of those diseases through lifestyle changes like a whole-food plant-based diet, exercise, sleep, stress management, and social connection. The logical decision for me was to approach medicine differently by bringing these practices and this information to my patients.

I began talking to my patients about their diet and taught an open-access course on nutrition and weight loss. I navigated a complex healthcare system to introduce a teaching kitchen, an innovative model for offering culinary medicine and other healthy living skills developed by one of my mentors, Dr. David Eisenberg at Harvard. Working with dietitians and experts in exercise physiology and mindfulness, we developed an award-winning worksite wellness program for our healthcare and university employees. I also collaborated with like-minded experts across the globe to advance a healthier culture through advisory boards, committees, and nonprofit organizations. With the support of generous philanthropy, we led my institution to being recognized as one of the pioneering centers across the country using lifestyle as medicine. I ran clinical trials and received grants for using cutting-edge technologies to find early disease biomarkers and measure the effects of our interventions; we conducted studies and published papers. I was well on my mission to help my patients live more fulfilling lives.

As my research went deeper, I was surprised to find something else, some-thing really fresh and new—and very paradoxical: the science of how our bodies need stress to thrive. This new science showed that stress can repair and regenerate upstream factors in our cells that lead to disease, which we can't fully access through the traditional pillars of lifestyle I was using as medicine. This new science also uncovered what makes it difficult for people to stick with the healthy habits I had begun recommending in my practice: our bodies are designed to become healthier through intermittent stress. Instead of striving for continuous habit change (which we often fail at!), it is more natural for us to alternate between challenging ourselves and then strategically recovering over time. This natural rhythm has been programmed in our cells and has been honed over the course of two million years of our species' history.

It turns out that the scientific community is in the midst of a health revolution aimed at powering up and regenerating our cells, the trillions of building blocks that make our tissues, organs, systems, and body. Our cells control how we think, feel, and function. For our bodies to perform their best, our cells must function their best. Our cellular health is a micro-version of our overall health. The new science of using stress to improve cellular health is at the heart of this revolution in medicine—it lives at the intersection of regenera-tive medicine, natural, holistic health, and longevity.

As a physician, I have always been fascinated by the ability of the human body to heal itself. As a scientist, my interest is being at the forefront of apply-ing, with precision, simple behaviors that can improve our health in a way no pill could. This cellular stress research was exactly what I had dreamed of that night in my office—it is the next frontier in a lifestyle that optimizes human resilience, health, and aging. It is the convergence of how we could use mo-lecular technology to develop regenerative therapies to heal our organs and tissues and restore function through our daily habits and behaviors. This is science that needs to be shared and implemented.

◆

When you think of stress, you probably think of chronic stressors, like work stress, family-related stress, or financial stress. That's the type that is the most common in our lives. You've probably also read about its potential harm and have come across a lot of advice on how to manage it.

This book is about a different kind of stress: brief, intermittent bursts of stress, rather than chronic, continuous stress.

While chronic stress can indeed be damaging, this type of brief, intermittent stress paradoxically heals, repairs, and regenerates us.

Our need for this type of stress is so deeply hardwired in our genes that my goal is to convince you that you can't achieve optimal health, longevity, and vitality without it.

Some of these stressors can be emotional and mental challenges, but they can also be physical. The most widely known is the brief, controlled stress of fasting intermittently, but we are going to cover many others to which our genome has adapted, like phytochemicals found in plant food and deliberate exposure to cold and heat.

These "good" stressors activate our natural healing defenses through what's called hormesis. From the Greek meaning "to excite," hormesis is using certain kinds of stress to trigger recently discovered cellular stress responses that make us stronger. When we experience hormetic stress, our cells switch to a stress-resistance state where they turn on repair and renewal mechanisms that are the biological equivalent of housecleaning. They repair DNA and proteins, increase antioxidant and anti-inflammatory defenses, turn on genes for producing new mitochondria, and remove and recycle old and damaged parts. These changes set us up so that when we recover from hormetic stress, we grow healthier, new cells and remodel existing pathways and circuits so that we are better prepared to handle future stress.

The pathways that are activated by hormetic stress counter the common pathways that lead to a wide range of chronic diseases and aging, which is my fascination about the science of "good" stress. Hormesis uses our cells' own ability to heal, regenerate tissues and organs, and restore function lost due to damage, disease, and aging, and it does so in a counterintuitive way: by using stress to build stress resilience.

Resilience usually refers to the ability to "bounce back" from stress. However, recent research shows that we don't ever truly go "back to normal" after encountering any stressor. Instead, we are somehow changed, down to the level of our cells, and we emerge with a new baseline. Improving our resilience really means reaching a new baseline where we are less susceptible to future chronic and harmful stressors. We can improve our mental, emotional, and physical resilience through hormesis, where physical challenges build emotional and mental resilience and vice versa. Stress is necessary to cultivate our *resilience*—that, in a word, encapsulates our capacity for living longer, healthier, and more vibrantly.

This distinction is important because it redefines our strategy toward wellness. In a world of chronic stress, we do want to find ways to reduce stress and draw boundaries around it. However, the insight from the new science of good stress is that not enough stress can be just as bad for us as too much (and the wrong kind). It can lower our resilience to combat mental and physical illnesses. Scientists even have a new term for this called sustress (inadequate stress) and have revised the entire framework of stress into three types: sustress (inadequate stress), eustress (good stress), and distress (bad stress). This updated framework requires us to make a shift in our approach to wellness by redirecting part of our energy from eliminating stress to learning to use the right kind to build our resilience to emotional, mental, and physical stress and become better prepared at handling life's inevitable challenges in the future.

If, like most of us, you are already overwhelmed and stressed out, the idea of taking on more stress may seem nonsensical. But choosing stress as a health solution seems like a paradox only because we stress ourselves out the wrong way. We either take on too much and burn out, or retreat and avoid it. My aim is to show you that you can incorporate mild to moderate hormetic ("good") stress even if you are feeling mentally and physically overwhelmed. It can help you feel calmer, more joyful, energetic, and resilient to emotional and physical illness. It's a new paradigm for becoming a healthier, happier, and stronger version of yourself by adding new behaviors that push you out of your comfort zone. While that may seem daunting, I can reassure you that all the good stressors are very practical and accessible. They are a new set of tools that will help you approach your health entirely differently—by regenerating your body from the level of your cells—and will give you a new mindset about stress.

Simply put, this book is about stressing yourself the right way, with brief bursts of specific kinds of stress, at the right intensity, followed by the right kind of recovery.

THE SCIENCE AND ART OF CELLULAR RESILIENCE

The notion of growth through adversity is not new; it has long been a part of the teachings of numerous religions and philosophical works. And since the 1990s, it's been embraced by positive psychology advocates and used as a mantra by psychologists, fitness trainers, and coaches.

For me, the ability to grow from stress has felt enticing and intuitive since childhood. As someone who at a very young age experienced political and civil unrest and then had to flee from my home and my birth country with my family during the Iranian Revolution in the late 1970s, then navigate learning a new culture, a new language, and new opportunities I had never imagined in the United States, I became fascinated by how we deal (or don't) with challenges and uncertainty. As human beings, we have all invariably encountered and sought to turn around adverse events in our own lives. It's how we make meaning out of our experience.

Yet the concept of stress-induced growth has mainly been conceptualized and explored thus far from a psychological perspective. As a result, we have only a partial understanding of what helps us flourish under adversity, traits such as realistic optimism, gratitude, and altruism. Hormesis expands our knowledge from the psychological aspect to a biological one. It explains the molecular and cellular mechanisms that underlie our long-felt knowing that we can grow stronger under stress. It connects our body with our mind and shows how each profoundly influences the other. Hormesis brings together everything I know about our biology to reevaluate our relationship with stress, to gain a better understanding of it, to measure it, and ultimately, to *use it to our advantage*.

The science of good stress teaches us that, unlike Nietzsche's maxim "That which doesn't kill us makes us stronger," stress doesn't have to come close to killing us to make us stronger. In fact, it *shouldn't* come anywhere near that. It's ordinary rather than seismic stress that activates our healing defenses. A mild to moderate amount is just enough to knock our body out of balance and force it to reestablish balance at a new baseline that makes us more resilient. It's the repetition of everyday stressors that leads to transformation.

In my clinical trials on stress and health, I have found that hormetic stress is associated with a biological age—an age determined by biological and health markers instead of your birth year—that is lower than a person's chronological age, suggesting it's an important tool for healthy aging. Beyond the science, I have applied hormesis in my personal life and experienced an immediate increase in my energy, creativity, happiness, and productivity. It has raised my lifelong quest for resilience to a new level, and I emerged stronger and healthier from stressful periods. I have taught hundreds of patients with conditions like diabetes, obesity, and heart disease to use hormetic stress. I have seen it help them drop or reduce the dosages of their medications and even reverse their disease. The most rewarding part for me is seeing them feel better and live the life they want. They feel joy and renewed optimism that they are in control of their health. I work with executives from all over the world, including CEOs of Fortune 500 companies, professional athletes, and industry leaders, and help them use hormetic habits to reach their personal and professional goals. I have seen how dramatically it improves their performance and optimizes their health and human potential, while slowing their rate of aging. Now, it's your turn.

MODERN SCIENCE, ANCIENT GENES

Before the discovery of hormesis and the powerful cellular stress response it triggers, the most common way people tried to tap into our evolutionary past for optimal modern-day health was through the Paleo diet and fitness movement. The premise was that since humans evolved during the Stone Age, re-creating the hunter-gatherer lifestyle is the best match for our genes. Most health professionals agree that we aren't adapted to a world of processed foods, desk jobs, and chronic stress. However, there is much debate about the best way to cope with our modern reality.

The scientific limitations of the Paleo movement are twofold. First, *many* Paleo diets and lifestyles originated from the diverse range of habitats in which our hunter-gatherer ancestors lived, so there is no one way to re-create the diet and lifestyle. Second, natural selection is driven by reproductive fitness rather than health, so not all ancestral habits are healthy, and conversely, not all components of our modern lifestyle are unhealthy.

The discovery of cellular stress response genes has revolutionized our understanding of our evolutionary past and its impact on our present-day health. These genes provide the physiological basis for what our bodies truly need for good health. We can activate our ancestral survival responses—by activating these inherited genes—in specific ways to achieve measurable changes, support cellular regeneration, and cultivate a science-backed lifestyle for health and happiness. The science of good stress provides the road map.

I wrote this book because I believe the more you know about how your body works, the better you can understand the practices that work *with* your inherited biology, rather than *against* it, and feel motivated to make sustainable choices that improve how you feel and function. I want you to understand why hormesis matters and how it works in your body. I won't just tell you about how good stressors will transform your health, though; I'll also teach you how to use them. I'll give you examples of what they are, help you determine which ones and what doses are right for you, explain how to best recover from stress for maximum growth and healing, and give you a framework to choose everything from food, to exercise, to ways to mentally challenge yourself that inspire possibility.

In Part I, I'll explain the science of good stress, how we worked these ancient challenges out of modern life and why you need to work them back in to optimize your health and longevity. We'll go through the importance of cellular health for reducing your risk of disease and slowing your rate of aging, and how hormesis regenerates, repairs, recycles, and renews your cells.

In Part II, I'll teach you the key good stressors and how to choose the right kind, at the right dose, for the right duration.

Part III explains how to use hormetic stress to age better, prevent and manage disease, and improve your energy, mental clarity, mood, pain, and other symptoms that may be compromising your well-being. Hormesis provides an alternative way to improve your health habits if you feel stuck in your current efforts. You will understand how to use good stressors to complement your existing methods for improving your health and vitality.

Part IV includes the Stress Paradox Protocol, your comprehensive guide to making this all happen in your day-to-day life. There you will find detailed protocols with easy-to-follow steps for implementing and recovering from each good stress, such as fasting, exercise, and heat and cold exposure. The steps explain how to assess your starting point, find the amount of stress that is right for you, and adequately recover for growth. The protocols are blueprints that you can personalize based on your needs and preferences. They are designed to be a self-paced approach that empowers you to continually challenge yourself outside your comfort zone through repeat cycles of stress and recovery while honoring your body.

Additionally, I have included delicious recipes that will stress your cells (in a good way!) with plant "toxins" based on a point system that reflects their phytochemical load. You will also find recipe templates that teach you how to make endless variations of meals that will transform your kitchen into a hormetic kitchen. Ultimately, the beauty of hormesis is how powerful, flexible, and simple it is to incorporate into your daily life.

My intent is to give you a different approach to thinking about your health. By shifting your energy toward embracing good stressors rather than resisting bad stressors, I want to provide you with a new set of tools for accessing your natural ability to heal and grow and build your health on a strong foundation of healthier cells.

PART I

HARDWIRED
FOR
STRESS

Our Body's Natural Regenerative Systems

If "too much of a good thing is a bad thing,"
a little bad thing can be good.

—Xin Li

The science of good stress isn't exactly new. Hormesis dates back to the late 1880s in a historic city in northern Germany. Like many scientific discoveries, it was found serendipitously. And because hormesis was counter to the prevailing viewpoint of the time, it was fiercely discredited until years later.

The story of the science of hormesis begins with Hugo Schulz, a bright and promising young professor at the University of Greifswald, who was at the start of his career. By the 1880s, microbiologists had already identified and cultured disease-causing organisms. Schulz became occupied with finding an effective dose or concentration of disinfectant to eliminate these organisms that was safe for human use. He tested nearly a dozen disinfectants on yeast, making a similar observation: at higher doses, they were toxic, but at low doses, they actually *enhanced* the growth and survival of yeast. This observation was so counter to his education and training in toxicology and pharmacology that Schulz believed this nonlinear response was simply a mistake. As any well-trained scientist would do, he repeated his experiments over and over with a discerning eye. But each time, he got the same result. "First, I did not know how to deal with it," he reflected, "and in any event at that time still did not realize that I had experimentally proved [a] fundamental law of biology."

During this time, Schulz attracted the attention of a German physician, Rudolf Arndt. Together, they combined their research into the Arndt-Schulz law, claiming that for every substance, high doses kill while low doses stimulate. There are so many obvious exceptions to this rule—some toxins like cyanide are so poisonous that they can paralyze with the smallest dose—that this speculative, broad-reaching generalization cast doubt on Schulz's credibility. They then went one step further to claim that all homeopathic drugs worked in this same manner and that they had discovered the principle explaining how homeopathy works.

Let me back up. At the time, homeopathy was a school of thought vehemently in conflict with traditional medicine. Thus, rather than launching him into a prosperous career, Schulz's unsubstantiated generalization of his law and the association of his observations with homeopathy quickly brought him under attack by his colleagues. His very traditional university distanced itself from him. His once-supportive work environment became hostile and stymied his opportunities for advancement. For nearly a century, the science of good stress was excluded from research funding. Anyone who supported or even was curious about Schulz's observation was intimidated or defunded by those in power, essentially preventing others from exploring their own experiments to test his model. Some called it the academic equivalent of a death sentence. Instead of a long and influential research career, Schulz spent most of his fifty-year professional life being shunned and ridiculed by his colleagues.

Along with the decline of his career, the extraordinary promise of his discovery became a casualty of the backlash toward the researcher who first observed it. This bizarre historical circumstance is why this fundamental biological principle, that cells can *acquire* resilience when exposed to a particular dose of challenge, has been overlooked by the mainstream scientific community for more than a century.

DOSE AND RESPONSE

When I was in medical school during the 1990s, we were taught that drugs, vitamins, supplements, and even some environmental exposures each have a threshold dose where they transition from being safe to hazardous. The overarching and widely accepted principle was that the response was linearly proportional to the dose. Germ theory is a good example of this. Ever since the realization that microorganisms like bacteria and viruses are major contributors to infections, both medicine and public health have doubled down on sanitation, hand hygiene, antibiotics, and vaccines, aiming to keep their exposure below the threshold of harm. The thinking has been that if eliminating these bugs is good, then the smaller the exposure, and the more we eradicate them, the better.

All doctors and scientists were educated since the twentieth century in this model, which owes its roots to the aftermath of the Schulz controversy. In the process of discrediting Schulz and with him, homeopathy, traditional medicine proposed this rival model that response is always proportional to dose. As a result, Schulz's accurate observation that low doses of certain exposures can stimulate a paradoxical benefit was not to be found in any of the leading textbooks. In the case of germs, it was only later that we learned that low exposure to some microorganisms is necessary to train our immune system and develop a diverse gut microbiome.

It's not that the concept put forth by traditional medicine isn't correct. It does indeed apply to a wide variety of medications, toxins, pollutants, and environmental exposures. But it shuts out an equally valid concept that originally emerged from Schulz's research: we not only tolerate but thrive from low doses of some challenges.

This may seem like a small, "inside baseball" distinction. But understanding the differences in your body's responses is more than a scientific curiosity. It's a path for closely connecting your health to how your body responds to your environment and choices. In effect, Schulz's discovery has become the scientific blueprint for how you can biologically build your most powerful innate defenses against disease and aging.

THE REDISCOVERY OF HORMESIS

Nearly half a century later, two forestry researchers from the University of Idaho, Chester Southam and John Ehrlich, were deep in the woods when they stumbled on a peculiar property of toxic red cedar heartwood extract. They tested this extract on certain wood-decaying fungi and were surprised to find that in certain doses, it wasn't just *not lethal* but, in fact, *stimulating* to the fungi's metabolism. Many fungi even adapted to progressively higher concentrations and overcame its toxicity. They published their findings in 1943, for the first time naming this observation "hormesis" from the Greek "to excite."

Scientists in other fields were making this same curious observation. Botanists and microbiologists were observing how this concept could improve crop yields. Researchers in agriculture (investigating the growth of germ-free birds fed antibiotics), ionizing radiation, toxicology, and pharmacology were noticing similar patterns. By the 1970s and 1980s, scientists from diverse disciplines were documenting hormetic effects. Some were directly using the term "hormesis," while others more broadly observed a stimulating response to low doses of various exposures. The biggest leap forward came from the impressive contributions of University of Massachusetts at Amherst physiologist and toxicologist Edward J. Calabrese, who has championed a complete rethinking of the scientific foundation of our risk assessment and environmental and medical regulations based on hormetic principles.

Although Schulz didn't live to see it, hormesis has come full circle to traditional medicine and public health. Over the past three decades, leading scientists in these fields have revived and are exploring the potential of hormesis to transform health, longevity, and the very depths of our human potential. In the Web of Science database, the term "hormesis" was cited only an average of seventeen times per year in the 1980s. By the 2010s, there were, on average, 7,627 citations. In 2019, that number reached 12,400, and in 2020 rose exponentially to 93,762. Hormesis is now solidly established as an alternate biological model to the one that dominated the twentieth century.

THE SCIENCE OF GOOD STRESS

Hormesis is not a rare occurrence. It is commonplace. It's not limited to just yeast and fungi; it applies to all forms of life, including animals and humans. First and foremost, it explains how we respond—*and can actually benefit*—from stress.

Hormesis is the science of how certain stressors—the right kind, at the right intensity, and for the right duration—activate built-in defenses that protect, repair, and regenerate our bodies. This hardwired process is vital to how we, and all living beings, survive and thrive. It is, in fact, so fundamental to our biology that the mechanisms by which it works have been honed for millennia, conserved evolutionarily, and passed down for generations from our hunter-gatherer ancestors. They are inextricably intertwined with our ability to adapt to new environments and expand the limits of our human potential.

Your body has sensors that identify different types of good stress. In response, the sensors send signals throughout the body to reallocate internal resources away from growth and proliferation and, instead, toward protection and repair. Good stressors essentially reprogram your cells by changing the genes you express when your body is in survival or energy-conserving mode. And these changes set you up to emerge stronger and fitter when you recover from the stress.

When you think about stress, what comes to mind is probably the fight-or-flight response. Yet, we have another stress response system that works at the cellular level. Rather than an "alarm system" that prepares us within a split second to deal with an imminent threat by mobilizing our energy, increasing our heart rate, and heightening our awareness, cellular stress responses have a different purpose and operate on a different timescale. They help us survive by adapting to stress. They divert our resources to repair and maintenance processes that make our bodies operate more efficiently. While the brain senses threats and activates the sympathetic nervous system and adrenal glands to release hormones, neurotransmitters, and cytokines as part of our fight-or-flight response, threats are also sensed by molecular sensors that switch on cellular stress response pathways, such as DNA repair, autophagy, and heat shock proteins. In the days to weeks after the stress passes, they rewire our bodies to better handle future stress. You can think of the two levels of our stress systems as stressing fast and slow. The latter is how we can not only get good at stress but also thrive from it.

How the two stress response systems work together may sound seductively simple. And at a big-picture level, it is. Close up, stress responses are more like complex electrical circuits with tens of thousands of wires communicating between and inside your cells and molecules, each rapidly firing like a series of dominoes set into motion by different stressors. To scientists and physicians like me, it's amazingly cool. And many ongoing studies are working on understanding the master controls, their downstream signals, the myriad connection points, and, ultimately, the benefit of good stress on your health and vitality. Most importantly, we are learning that there are daily habits and choices you can make to stress your body toward health, longevity, and vitality.

The pivotal insight underlying the science of good stress is that your stress responses are not directly proportional to the "dose" of stress in the traditional manner we have come to expect. Instead, your response to good stressors follows the pattern Schulz observed over a century ago. This opens the door to thinking about challenges in an entirely new way. A Goldilocks amount accesses your innate potential for forestalling disease, slowing aging, and optimizing human performance. By repeatedly taking on small challenges, you can counter and increase your resilience to damage in a world where adverse stress abounds.

CHAPTER 1

The Stress Dilemma

Trends show we are getting fatter, sicker, and more medicated than ever. In 1994, shortly after I started medical school, only two states had an obesity rate greater than 18 percent, and only one state had a rate of diabetes of 6 percent or higher. By 2015, these rates of obesity and diabetes had spread to all fifty states. Paralleling the increase in chronic disease has been a dramatic rise in prescription drugs—a whopping 85 percent between 1997 and 2016. Now, 55 percent of Americans regularly take a prescription medication; those who use prescription drugs take four, on average. Perhaps most alarming are projections about our life expectancy. In a sobering study published in the *New England Journal of Medicine* nearly two decades ago, the authors forecasted that despite all the technological advances in medical interventions, public health, and overall living conditions, our life expectancy is likely to drop in the early part of this century, for the first time in nearly two hundred years, based on the rise in obesity and its impact on longevity. Our children may face a poorer health fate than us.

The most common explanation for these health trends is that our lives today differ vastly from the lives of our Paleolithic hunter-gatherer ancestors. This is often referred to as "mismatch theory" or an "evolutionary mismatch"—when previously advantageous traits become maladaptive in our rapidly changing environment. This mismatch explains how with the invention of agriculture, food preservation, and technology, we introduced processed foods and a sedentary, socially isolated lifestyle that clashes with our biology. We have surrounded ourselves with limitless fast-food options laden with fat and sugar, we can get virtually anything delivered to our doorstep without needing to move, and we have become constantly vigilant by watching endless streams of headlines and "social" updates. Because these behaviors activate our immune and nervous systems, leading to chronic, smoldering inflammation that is detrimental to our physical well-being and mental health, we can consider them as "bad" or toxic stressors.

Part of the problem is indeed that the rapid pace of our technological advances has ushered in these bad stressors at a rate that far outpaces our ability to adapt genetically. Since the latter part of the nineteenth century, industrial food processing technology has markedly altered the nutritional characteristics of our food, making it more calorie dense, less nutrient dense, and devoid of fiber. We invented mechanized roller mills that produce highly refined grain flour. We developed chromatographic fructose enrichment technology that produces high-fructose corn syrup, which is the added sugar in a startling number of food labels. Mechanized steel expellers have mass-produced refined vegetable oil, which has substantially increased in our American diet. As a result, about 60 percent of the calories on our plates are now from ultra-processed foods. Mechanization has also drastically decreased the need for physical labor. And in the last century, television and screens have displaced social interactions with family and friends.

In addition to these harmful stressors being ever present, they're also hard to resist because we are programmed to seek them out. Built into our hard-wired biology is a reward system for eating energy-dense foods. It developed to entice our ancestors to leave the safety of their caves, forage potentially hazardous terrain, and risk encounters with predators to avoid starvation. When they ate sugar and fat, which they would get only from a few concentrated sugars like seasonal honey and wild-roaming, lean animals, they would experience a surge of dopamine—the same energizing and feel-good neurotransmitter released from gambling, drugs, and sex. In our modern environment of ultra-processed foods high in fat and sugar, we continually activate our reward systems. That is why we find ultra-processed foods so irresistible. They are designed to overwhelm the amount of reward we are genetically adapted to handle.

Another safeguard we developed to buffer the threat of starvation is to conserve energy. This is why we may have a tendency or inclination to sit for long periods of time. Plus, our bodies cleverly adapted to match capacity to demand—by ramping up metabolism, cardiac endurance, and mental acuity with activity and, like an inactive computer screen in power-saving mode, power down metabolically expensive functions during rest. Protecting against staying powered down for hours at a time and days in a row wasn't necessary—our ancestors didn't have the luxury of eating Seamless meals while binge-watching the latest Netflix hit. Because of this, there was never strong selection pressure to avoid harm from the extreme physical inactivity that is common in our lives today. In other words, we evolved for a world that isn't quite so comfy, and our genetic code has yet to catch up with the conveniences of our modern world. Our ancestors also developed an instinct to stay vigilant against predators. In our present-day world of round-the-clock headline-grabbing news, this makes it hard to avoid seeking updates and continually feeling anxious and on high alert.

So yes, our modern environment has in many ways engineered "bad" stressors that make us sick by taxing our ancient survival genes. You can find this mismatch story in lots of health books, and the solution is usually about avoiding or overcoming these bad stressors in some way. Yet I see an additional mismatch in the development of the contemporary world. It's one that was lost for a time in the siloing of the science of hormesis from medicine but is just as important—possibly even more so—to our health and longevity: it's the story of how we engineered "good" stress *out* of our lives.

THE COMFORT CONUNDRUM

If we view our lives in the broader context of evolutionary history, our human story is one of overcoming stress. From the inception of our genus, *Homo*, approximately 2.4 million years ago, until the agricultural revolution 10,000 years ago, our Paleolithic hunter-gatherer ancestors lived in often harsh and stressful environments. Under the canopy of the sub-Saharan African sky, as the climate became more arid and lush tropical rainforests turned to deforested land, they roamed long distances in the natural world, foraging in search of food. They continually faced climate extremes and an environment that threatened their survival.

As a result, all Paleolithic dietary patterns, which differed greatly depending on the latitude and season, included periods of relative plenty and others of shortage. If they were not hunting, our ancestors would explore their diverse and sometimes toxic plant world for uncultivated edible berries and fruit. By necessity, the *Homo sapiens* diet of our ancestors included over three thousand plant species. And, as part of the hunter-gatherer way of life, our prehistoric ancestors—men and women, young and old—had to be able to sustain bursts of physical movement to endure intense periods of hunting prey and escaping predators.

Early hunter-gatherers were nomads, moving as nature dictated. They traveled in bands of thirty to fifty and depended on their tribe for survival. In these early communities, evenings brought everyone together around the embers of fire to share stories, learn from each other, think imaginatively, envision their future, and develop ideas that transpired into innovation and "culture"—the very high-order "big picture" thinking that makes us distinctly human. Our late Stone Age ancestors slept in impermanent shelters or, at times, open-air settlements, with their eating synchronized with their sleep-wake cycle, which was dependent on the setting and dawning of the sun to repeat and reinforce a daily pattern that became the natural rhythm of our body.

Over time, our hunter-gatherer ancestors developed adaptive mechanisms to cope with the unique stressors in their environment. Their genes evolved to retain traits well suited for surviving stress. Those whose bodies and brains worked well hunting in the fasted state were likelier to outlive their peers. Those who adapted to eating a broader range of plants without succumbing to their potential toxicity consumed more calories. Nomadic ancestors who could adjust to a wider range of temperatures could migrate farther distances. Those who shouldered pro-social, generative pursuits were valued in their community. The ones who could endure periods of high-intensity running could better capture and avoid predators. And those who challenged themselves to explore beyond the horizon and innovate tools that leveraged strength and subsistence were able to conquer their environment. The obligatory need for episodic fasting, running, consuming sublethal toxins, enduring sweltering and frigid temperatures, doing generative work that benefited their tribe, and exploring and thinking creatively in their daily lives made our ancestors stronger and smarter. Their lives were far from idyllic, yet our prehistoric ancestors didn't just survive—they became the most successful species to inhabit the Earth.

That all began to change around ten thousand years ago when some independent groups of people in the ancient Middle East, living in the semi-arid and humid region of the Fertile Crescent, had this idea of planting seeds in the area's unusually rich soil. After cultivating wild grains and cereals, the domestication of animals followed—and with that, our ancestors made the shift from foraging to farming, from roaming for subsistence to having a more stable food supply. About two hundred years ago, we made another big shift: the technological advances developed during the Industrial Revolution transformed agrarian societies into ones dominated by industry and machine manufacturing. Along with food processing came food preservation techniques. These techniques, coupled with the advent of refrigeration, made food more widely available at all times, further removing us from the intermittent stress of food scarcity and the diverse range of sublethal plant toxins with which we coevolved. We currently cultivate only approximately 150 of the roughly 30,000 edible plants worldwide, and only about 30 of those plants make their way into a typical modern diet over a whole year.

Infrastructure, transportation, and communication developments, including the automobile, airplane, radio, telephone, and computers, progressively reduced the need for intense intervals of human energy expenditure. They also diminished the importance of family and community, replacing them with the promise of individualism. Furnaces, radiators, and air conditioners added to our modern indoor comforts. Additionally, the Information Age has introduced an unprecedented amount of new bits of incoming information that is changing how we think and problem-solve.

All these advances were intended to make our lives more comfortable—and they have. They have alleviated food shortages, reduced arduous physical labor, and improved efficiency and productivity. Improvements in housing, sanitation, and medical care have lessened the impact of infection and trauma, the chief causes of death from the Paleolithic era until 1909. As a result, average life expectancy is now approximately double that of preagricultural humans. However, the rapid cultural transformation has brought along unintended consequences, creating new survival challenges. These changes have engineered important forms of discomfort *out* of our lives: periods of food scarcity, intervals of moderately intense activity, diverse sources of plant chemical toxins, climate extremes, deep, creative thinking, and episodic psychologically challenging activities.

The advent of ease over the past ten thousand years has disrupted a critical part of our primordial hardwiring for health—it has silenced genes that enable us to heal and grow. Without the science of good stress in our toolbox, we have overlooked that a deficiency in activating these types of good stress—and their resulting housekeeping and growth effects—is just as destructive to us as is too much "bad" stress. This is not to convey a moral judgment about stress in your life; it's a way to see that stress can have vastly divergent effects on your health and longevity.

Comfort is a Trojan horse. We have willingly let it into our body's fortress. And it is fighting our defenses within. We need to win the war. We can't go back to living in a prehistoric world, but we can learn lessons about our biology and apply them to our modern lives. Lack of good stress is a new risk factor that threatens our health.

NAVIGATING HEALTH IN THE TWENTY-FIRST CENTURY

Using stress to build stress resilience is a paradigm shift in medicine. Unprocessed foods, movement, sleep, and meditative and mindfulness practices effectively prevent and treat disease. But fighting our cravings for sugar and fat and our predisposition toward inactivity and chronic mental stress is also incredibly hard to do. Embracing good stress is a solution to our modern-day dilemma that doesn't require constantly fighting our instincts. It works *with* rather than *against* the biology inherited from our ancestors. If you feel stuck in a pattern of hard-to-break habits, you have choices—powerful, natural ones that are instinctive and remarkably easy to adopt and sustain.

CHAPTER 2

Cellular Resilience

Getting at the Big Picture by Understanding the Small

To understand how good stress remodels your body and transforms challenges into better health, we need to step into the world of our cells. That's where we begin to see how our cellular responses to good stress aren't simply a reaction to adversity but a proactive step toward nurturing our bodies.

In the late 1600s, an English physicist and distinguished microscopist, Robert Hooke, looked down his self-designed microscope at a piece of cork; what he saw was bewildering. The cork appeared to be made of tiny units. He called them "cells" because they resembled cells in a monastery. Over the following two centuries, his glimpse into a previously invisible world rippled through science and medicine and became solidified as the cell theory. This biological tenet, which is so commonplace today that we take it for granted, is that each and every living being is made of cells. All our tissues and organs are made of these basic functional building blocks. In fact, it's hard to fathom the astounding number of cells we have in our body—a whopping thirty trillion.

Our cells are home to all the biological machinery we need for everything that happens inside our bodies. For example, the cell's nucleus houses our genetic blueprint or DNA. Cells have power plants called mitochondria, which can convert energy from food to the body's primary fuel source, adenosine triphosphate (ATP). They have recycling centers, called lysosomes, that can break down and dispose of waste material and salvage reusable parts in a process called autophagy. And they even have manufacturing plants to make proteins called ribosomes.

Although all cells contain the same machinery, they each serve distinct functions within our bodies. Immune cells fight invaders and help us heal wounds. Heart cells maintain circulation. And brain cells help us think and feel. With nearly two hundred different cell types, each specialized to perform a unique function, our cells work together to keep us healthy. Yet, when any aspect of our cells becomes compromised—leading to genes not getting expressed properly, proteins malfunctioning, waste building up, or inefficient energy production—it can lead to disease. While we've long recognized inflammation and oxidative damage as disease triggers, modern science is homing in on a critical facet: impaired cellular function. Damaged DNA, protein abnormalities, mitochondrial dysfunction, and autophagy breakdown play a substantial role in this. Common conditions such as heart disease, diabetes, Alzheimer's dementia, cancer, and even our aging rate can stem from cellular malfunction. As a result, if you want to understand health and disease, you need to understand your marvelous cells. Everything that affects the way your body functions unfolds at the cellular level.

This discovery not only helped us conceive of the human body as an intricate network of cells but has also birthed a game-changing kind of medicine, called regenerative medicine, based on manipulating cells for therapeutic purposes. If heart disease, cancer, Alzheimer's disease, diabetes, arthritis, and emphysema result from cells not functioning correctly, this type of medicine posits they can all be targets for cell-based therapies. This new approach borders on sounding like science fiction, yet it is already a reality. It harnesses the body's natural capacity to repair itself, to *regenerate* lost or damaged cells. For example, T cells are immune cells that are part of your body's natural defense against cancer. However, certain cancers can hide from T cells. In a type of cell-based therapy called immunotherapy, scientists have learned how to remove cancer-fighting T cells from the body, engineer them to recognize and target cancer cells, and then return them to the body where they home in on cancer cells with the precision of heat-seeking missiles. Stem cells are another part of your body's natural defense system. They quietly regenerate our organs by multiplying and differentiating into different types of cells and tissues. Stem cells are now being injected in areas where there is disease or damage to reconstruct healthy, new tissue. Scientists are even looking into ways to regenerate entire organs from stem cells as one would construct an object from a 3D printer! The aim of regenerative medicine is to go beyond just treating symptoms to discovering therapies that get at the root cause of disease.

You might be wondering: This is all great, but what does it have to do with me? The exciting news is that we don't have to rely on advanced technologies such as immunotherapy or stem cell treatments to take advantage of these scientific advancements. Each of us has the power to activate our cells' regenerative potential using simple, everyday habits. That is precisely what we achieve when we challenge our cells with good stress. Good stressors trigger our cells' innate capacity to resist, repair, recycle, and recharge: they resist inflammation and oxidative damage, repair DNA and proteins, recycle damaged and old components, and recharge mitochondrial energy production—forming a defense against the common denominators leading to chronic disease and aging. This remarkable regenerative capability resides in our cellular stress responses.

CELLULAR STRESS RESPONSES

You can think of your cellular stress responses as your natural defense against disease and aging, like a personal army protecting you around the clock. Your army is made of seven specialized units that work together:

- **DNA damage response** detects damaged DNA and temporarily stops cell division to allow time to make repairs.
- **Antioxidant response** patrols for harmful free radicals and protects cells from oxidative stress by ramping up antioxidant enzymes that neutralize free radicals and detoxification enzymes that disarm and eliminate toxic substances from the body.
- **Autophagy response** identifies damaged or old parts, breaks them down into basic building blocks like amino acids and fats, and uses them to make new parts or produce energy.
- **Inflammatory response** ensures that the body responds to a threat with the right level of inflammation and immune activity, which it resolves after the threat passes to prevent unnecessary damage to healthy tissues.
- **Heat shock protein response** activates a group of proteins that help fix or remove damaged proteins in the cell's cytosol, or matrix.
- **Unfolded protein response** maintains the balance of properly folded proteins in a specific part of the cell where many proteins are assembled called the endoplasmic reticulum.

- **Sirtuin response** involves the actions of a family of enzymes known as sirtuins that protect and repair cells by regulating energy metabolism, enhancing DNA repair, controlling inflammation, and extending cellular lifespan.

Each specialized unit is trained to respond to different threats. Multiple stressors activate each of the response units, and not all specialized troops get activated by each threat.

Our cellular stress responses are encoded in genes that are so essential for fitness and survival they have been conserved for millions of years and across all species. These genes form the ancient defense system that helped our ancestors survive and adapt to new environments, and they are shared by all living things, from simple unicellular organisms like bacteria and yeast to complex multicellular organisms such as plants and animals. They are part of our "vitagenes," short for "vitality genes"—a powerful gene network that carries the instructions for protecting us when times are hard and making us stress resistant. Yet they do more than increase our resilience—they help us live longer and healthier. They are the ancient genes we need to activate in modern times to access our regenerative capabilities.

Good stressors activate our vitagenes in two main ways: by mobilizing special proteins called transcription factors and by making epigenetic changes to our DNA. When cells sense stress, through either receptors on their surface or cascades of cell signaling pathways, they activate transcription factors that are inactive under normal conditions. Once activated, they move into the cell's nucleus and attach to specific parts of DNA, acting as on-off switches that directly target expression of stress response genes. They work with precision, making sure the cell rapidly responds the right way and for the right amount of time.

Good stress also helps determine what genes you express over longer periods. You may have heard that your genes aren't your destiny. Your lifestyle choices and environment ultimately play a larger role in determining your health. This mainly happens through epigenetic changes, which are long-lasting modifications to DNA or histone proteins around which DNA is wrapped that help cells remember past exposures and environmental conditions. This process doesn't change the actual DNA code but changes how the DNA is read.

Reintroducing good stress reprograms gene expression, turning on powerful cell-protective processes that increase your longevity, health, and happiness. On the other hand, living in your comfort zone leaves these stress defense genes dormant, making you more susceptible to disease, frailty, and rapid aging. Having dynamic and overlapping ways of detecting and responding to stress is nature's way of ensuring we're equipped to handle many diverse challenges.

Through activating transcription factors and modifying gene expression, good stressors turn on your vitagenes, or your cellular stress response pathways, which bolsters your troops and reinforces your entire army of defenses. Good stressors are pleiotropic, meaning each switches on multiple stress response pathways. If you picture your cellular stress responses as regenerative machinery, good stressors are the levers that maximally amplify your innate responses. By doing so, they repair and rejuvenate critical cellular functions— the very foundations of disease. Since cells are the building blocks of organs, such as your heart and brain, hormesis is a "systems biology," or whole-body way to radically transform your physical, cognitive, and emotional health from your cells on up.

THE FOUR Rs OF GOOD STRESS: RESIST, REPAIR, RECYCLE, RECHARGE

How does activating your cellular stress responses through good stress add healthy years to your life? Through the Four Rs:

Resist: Defending Against Damage

Resisting damage caused by inflammation and oxidative stress is a well-established way of combating disease and aging. You can use various strategies, like avoiding pro-inflammatory processed food, ensuring sufficient sleep, and nurturing social connections, to mitigate such damage. Using good stressors to activate your cellular stress responses, however, is a distinctly different approach: they strengthen your body's inherent antioxidant and anti-inflammatory capabilities. They achieve this by increasing the activity of specific genes responsible for producing proteins that bolster these defense mechanisms. In essence, these responses enhance your body's natural ability to fend off the harmful effects of inflammation and oxidative stress.

Repair: DNA and Protein Maintenance

Through activating your cellular stress responses, you have the capability to repair DNA and protein damage to keep your cells healthy and functional.

Each day, your cells' DNA accumulates over ten thousand injuries, which is more than seven times per minute! If this damage isn't repaired, your DNA code can't be read correctly, and that can lead to diseases like heart disease and cancer, and even speed up aging. Your DNA damage response has multiple mechanisms to repair DNA and keep your genetic code intact. If the damage is too extensive, the same response is so sophisticated that it either initiates cell senescence, retiring a cell to prevent it from dividing further, or programmed cell death, called apoptosis. The DNA damage response collaborates with your immune response to remove damaged cells that could turn into cancer.

Inside your cells, there are between twenty thousand and more than one hundred thousand different proteins, each performing a different job. These proteins are like the workers in a factory, doing most of the tasks. To keep your cells healthy, the right amount of proteins needs to be produced, folded, assembled, and broken down correctly. A breakdown in protein quality control—when proteins either can't perform their task or, worse yet, clump together and make a mess inside your cells—increases vulnerability to disease and aging. That's why you have an elaborate network of stress response mechanisms that can detect and repair disruptions in protein balance. Heat shock proteins (HSPs) are part of this defense team. They help with protein folding, assembly, and transport. HSPs even act as "molecular chaperones," escorting damaged proteins to the correct cell compartments where they can be repaired or degraded. Yes, proteins are that important! Despite their name, HSPs are triggered not only by heat (think hot sauna); cold, exercise, and fasting can activate them, too. Another way the cellular stress response safeguards protein is through the unfolded protein response (UPR), which helps maintain the right balance of unfolded proteins that are necessary for cell health.

Recycle: Cellular Housecleaning

By now, you are aware that cells are prone to accumulating various forms of damage that can eventually lead to illness. If your body can't resist or repair this damage, cells rely on a clever process called autophagy, which is like cellular housecleaning. Derived from the Greek words "auto," meaning self, and "phagy," meaning eating, it is your body's way of recycling old or damaged parts to rejuvenate itself and use its energy efficiently. Imagine a car in a junkyard; the usable parts are salvaged, while the scraps get discarded. Similarly, when a cell faces good stress, it ushers damaged components to its lysosome, where they're broken down and repurposed. This cellular cleanup function holds significant potential for fighting cancer, neurodegenerative disease, heart disease, and other illnesses.

Recharge: Maximizing Cellular Energy and Mitochondrial Health

Here is the most critical benefit of good stress: optimizing cellular energy. Cells require energy to carry out repair and growth tasks. The amount and efficiency of this energy production are determined by the health of mitochondria—the powerhouses within cells. Think of mitochondria as the life force responsible for converting food energy into usable cellular energy. They orchestrate metabolism, which underpins every bodily function. When mitochondria lose their ability to function properly or decrease in number, the cells' energy output falters. This particularly impacts energy-intensive cells like those in the heart and nervous system. Energy impairment is found in nearly all chronic diseases, including metabolic syndrome, diabetes mellitus and insulin resistance, heart disease, stroke, and metabolic dysfunction-associated steatotic liver disease (MASLD). Even neurological conditions such as dementia, Parkinson's, and mental illness trace back to mitochondrial dysfunction.

Good stressors activate sirtuins, which are remarkable molecules that support mitochondria, among their many roles. Within cells, they act as energy and nutrient detectors, linking the cell's nutrient supply with its metabolism and mitochondrial balance. In response to stress arising from a fall in energy or nutrients, the sirtuin response, along with other molecules, triggers mitochondrial biogenesis—a fascinating process where existing mitochondria generate new ones. Moreover, sirtuins aid in eliminating damaged mitochondria. By improving mitochondrial quantity and efficiency, cellular stress responses elevate energy levels and bolster our cellular defenses against diseases and the aging process.

HORMETINS: THE GOOD STRESSORS

We call good stressors that trigger these beneficial cellular stress responses "hormetins." Hormetins can be metabolic, physical, and cognitive, as well as psychological. They can encompass everything from when and what we eat to how we move, think, and feel. Collectively, hormetic stressors form the foundation of a holistic, integrated lifestyle for feeling stronger, happier, and more energetic by making our cells healthier.

In the following chapters, I'll provide more information on how and why hormetic stressors work, along with the various ways you can use this science in your daily life. We are living in an exciting era of medicine. Along with the progress in cell-based therapies like immunotherapy and stem cell treatments, scientists are rapidly deciphering how we can use good stress and hormetins to maximize our cellular defenses to reach our full human potential for health and well-being. We have long recognized that our lifestyle choices are paramount in preventing disease, slowing aging, and improving our well-being. Because hormetins reverse root causes of disease and aging through intricate pathways involved in improving cellular health and resilience, they make us healthier and younger in a foundational way that can't be replicated by medications or supplements. Resisting, repairing, recycling, and recharging our thirty trillion cells through the science of good stress may be our most powerful tool yet for longer, healthier, and more enjoyable lives.

CHAPTER 3

The Stress Solution

Ancient Stress as a Modern Cure

You have a gift embedded in the DNA you inherited from your ancestors: hundreds of genes designed to withstand times of scarcity and challenge and build resilience in the face of it. Your genome wasn't designed for abundance or comfort; it was built to thrive on challenge. Yet we don't need to re-create our Stone Age past or turn back the clock on all the incredible advances we've made in medicine, technology, food and crop production, communication, and more. We can take the good of all that progress and apply it to our physiology to find solutions that are in sync with our body's natural rhythms.

Your body has innate wisdom. It is wondrously designed to protect your health and ensure your survival naturally. It does this by continually striving to maintain a state of inner balance, known as homeostasis. This fundamental principle is one of the most unifying concepts in biology. It was formulated in 1926 by Harvard physiologist Walter Cannon and brought to the forefront in his book *The Wisdom of the Body*. This wisdom is hardwired through feedback loops that work together to sustain a stable, consistent internal environment despite the ever-changing conditions of the external world. Essentially, your body comes equipped with a natural mechanism to cope with the multitude of stressors you encounter. When we make choices that support our intrinsic equilibrium, our bodies are remarkably adept at safeguarding our well-being. This underlying aspect of your nature—your biological hardwiring for health—is the basis for understanding how to nurture your body and work in harmony with it to amplify your capacity for health, rather than wear down and overwhelm it.

While the idea of homeostasis continues to be a core concept in scientific studies, we rarely talk about balance in the practice of modern Western medicine. However, many symptoms and diseases arise because we are not living in harmony with our biology and our environment. Common issues like fatigue, bloating, mental fog, diarrhea, sleep disturbances, and many more indicate a disruption in the balance among cells and the hormones and neurotransmitters that facilitate communication between them. This balance ensures that our body systems function in a coordinated manner. Therefore, restoring it is crucial for well-being, disease prevention, and slowing the aging process.

Stress, whether harmful or beneficial, throws our bodies off-balance. Our body's natural response is to restore inner harmony. However, we've learned that we don't always return to our original state after recovering from stress. Instead, we adapt to stress by establishing a new equilibrium, or "set point," much like selecting a new temperature setting on a thermostat. Harmful stress can reset this balance to a setting that causes internal "wear and tear," leading to symptoms and diseases over time. Good stress also prompts our body to adapt by counteracting the stress. However, the insight from the science of good stress is that our body overcompensates and resets the balance at a setting that nets growth and resilience. In other words, good stress uses our body's wisdom to steer us toward a state that enhances overall well-being.

Central to the science of good stress is the idea that your body has a kind of plasticity: it is constantly being shaped and molded. Stressors are the inputs, and your physical and mental health are the outputs. For better or worse, stress changes us. As a result, your health is constantly evolving. I don't want you to think of good stress and bad stress as black and white, like opposing binary forces balancing each other out as if on a seesaw. Rather, I want you to envision stressors as architects of a dynamic and interconnected three-dimensional network. By deliberately experiencing good stress, you can configure your body to its healthiest state.

THE NEW WISDOM OF YOUR BODY

Hormesis has peeled back a new layer in understanding our body's capabilities. It reveals how we can reset and rejuvenate ourselves through a wisdom far more extraordinary than Walter Cannon imagined a century ago. A pioneer in the field of hormesis, Suresh Rattan, PhD, has updated the traditional concept of homeostasis with the idea of a "homeodynamic space," which takes into account the dynamic, ever-changing ways stress impacts us. Your homeodynamic space records all the stressors you have experienced over your lifetime—the "bad" stressors that have caused damage and the "good" stressors that have nudged you toward regeneration and healing. It's a real-time narrative of your health and vitality that measures your resilience, or ability to handle and bounce back from physical, mental, and emotional stressors. Through the lens of homeodynamic space, we can perceive our health as an ongoing balance of life's stressors rather than a static state.

I think of homeodynamic space like a bank account. When you are born, you have a certain amount of funds—let's call it your resilience fund—that you spend as you age. Bad stressors are like bills that drain your account and decrease your ability to buffer unexpected hardship. When your funds start to dry up, that's when you notice something is off—maybe you feel tired more often or just out of sorts. If your account gets depleted, the next hardship could push you into debt or, in our case, to the onset of illness. The quicker you spend down your resilience fund, the more you increase your risk of disease and the faster you age. At a molecular level, as your account dwindles, you are accumulating damage. Gene expression goes haywire, unrepaired mutations gather, cells lose their ability to divide, and they don't talk to each other as well as before. Eventually, tissues become disorganized, and organs don't function properly, making you more prone to serious health problems.

One way to help preserve your resilience fund is by staying away from bad stressors such as processed foods and a sedentary lifestyle. On the flip side, when you embrace good stressors, it's like you are depositing bonus money that pays interest into your account. They expand your homeodynamic space, shielding you against disease and slowing the aging clock. They make you feel and literally become younger. In our culture of comfort, we aren't making enough of these wise investments, especially compared to our ancestors. We're trying to preserve our resilience fund with healthy habits, stress-reduction practices, and lifestyle changes, but we aren't putting enough money into it to fully activate our body's built-in defenses and thrive. This shortfall makes us more vulnerable to disease, shortens our life expectancy, and hinders us from reaching our full potential. The most important thing to remember about your homeodynamic space is that even though your genes play a part in shaping it, you have most of the control. By reintroducing certain challenges like plant toxins, bursts of exercise, heat and cold exposure, fasting intermittently, and facing mental and psychological hurdles, you can actually grow your resilience fund and expand your homeodynamic space.

USING HORMETIC STRESS
TO INCREASE YOUR RESILIENCE

Our cells and biochemical pathways coevolved with the natural stressors of our ancestors' environments. For most of humankind, those stresses were injury, infection, food scarcity, temperature extremes, and mental challenges. Our ancestors evolved mechanisms to survive all of these—every one of these stresses sends a danger signal, and the body responds by activating stress response pathways to reestablish balance. If you cut yourself, you will mount just enough inflammation to heal. If you face food deprivation, you metabolize energy more efficiently. If you go out in the cold, your body kicks on an internal heater to restore your body temperature. If you eat a sublethal toxic plant, your body activates detoxification systems. Encoded in our genome are built-in programs that get switched on by these stressors, unique defensive responses that get activated through transcription factors and epigenetic changes to our DNA, as described in Chapter 2. They protect our cells by restoring harmony and leaving a molecular fingerprint that makes them more resilient to injury. We need to reintroduce these challenges and their adaptations to build our homeodynamic space and thrive in our modern world.

This may sound like very high-level science, but it's actually very simple and easy to do this in your daily life. We can focus on the five hormetic stressors that are known to make a meaningful impact on our health. Here's a brief overview of each, along with an explanation as to why we evolved to thrive with these particular stressors.

Eat a Variety of Plant Toxins

The limited food supply available to our ancestors necessitated exploring and consuming newly discovered plant species. While some were invariably fatally toxic, others had lower levels of toxins to which they could gradually adapt. Our ancestors developed two main ways to prevent noxious chemicals from damaging them. One was to metabolize and detoxify the plant toxin rapidly. The other was to gradually build tolerance to the toxin by activating an adaptive cellular stress response—just like the yeast in Schulz's experiments. Their bodies learned to sense the toxin, develop a complex cell signaling network, and select for genes that enhanced the resilience of their cells and organs. Over time, the toxins began to protect their cells—they turned on genes that made survival proteins, antioxidant enzymes, and immune system chemicals that block excessive, harmful inflammation. The variety of plants, with their respective toxins, paradoxically helped them build resistance against injury and survive.

What this means for you: By increasing the diversity of plants you consume—and being adventurous and going beyond your comfort zone when it comes to new foods—you can activate different stress responses that work together to maximize healing, repair, and growth. In Chapter 4, we will cover which plant toxins activate hormesis and their respective food sources. Through the Stress Paradox Protocol in Chapter 13 and the recipes and build-your-own recipe templates in Chapter 14, you will learn how to increase your toxin intake and turn foods that contain them into delicious meals.

Practice Intermittent Bursts of Movement

A prototypic challenge required as part of the hunter-gatherer way of life was episodes of running—for hunting and for escaping predators. Running takes energy, imposing a heavy metabolic stress on muscles and the cardiovascular system, and milder stress on other body parts. Muscles respond by secreting messengers, including hormones and growth factors, that send signals between cells and organs throughout the body and brain that bolster their ability to withstand injury and disease. One of the primary adaptations our ancestors developed to moderate to high-intensity exercise is increasing the number of mitochondria in our muscles and brain cells, which increases their energy capacity. Intense bouts of physical activity can also activate our immune cells in ways that reduce chronic inflammation and improve immunity.

Like plant chemical toxins, a Goldilocks amount of exercise works through hormesis: the type, intensity, and duration matter. Paleontologists and anthropologists have found that preagricultural humans had more strength and muscularity than all their descendants—not just us, their sedentary ancestors, but also their succeeding agriculturalists, who physically worked much longer hours. From a biological standpoint, this suggests that the intensity of intermittent peak demand—not continuous physical activity, but sporadic bursts of high-intensity movement—is uniquely important for developing muscle mass and strength.

What this means for you: You can gain the greatest benefits from physical activity by including short intervals of high-intensity exercise in your weekly routine. Chapter 5 will explain how exercise works through hormesis to improve your energy, metabolism, and overall health. Regardless of your starting point, the protocol will teach you how to create a tailored hormetic exercise program that's just right for you.

Experience Extremes of Heat and Cold

Living in impermanent shelters, our nomadic ancestors were exposed to the elements and vulnerable to unpredictable conditions. Our human body thus adapted mechanisms to endure extremes of heat and cold, which can be turned on by deliberate exposure. At a cellular level, heat stress activates a master regulator of our vast network of vitagenes, which tightly controls functions that protect cells, such as upregulating antioxidant and anti-inflammatory capability, cleaning out damaged parts through autophagy, and maintaining protein integrity. Deliberate cold stress similarly switches on a suite of protective mechanisms that boost the immune system and metabolism, reduce inflammation, activate antioxidant enzymes, and build resilience to stress.

What this means for you: Intentionally exposing yourself to uncomfortable cold and heat can improve your health and longevity. Chapter 6 explains the science behind its hormetic benefits and the proven kinds, dose, and duration. Spoiler alert: you don't have to take an ice plunge! Then in the protocol, I will guide you in incorporating thermal stress into your life.

Endure Periods of Food Scarcity

The universal feature of the nomadic hunter-gatherer diet is that it included periods of food deprivation. As a result, there was a survival advantage for those who could tolerate and adapt during these periods. They mainly did this by metabolically switching from using carbohydrates to fat for energy. Once their stores of carbohydrates in liver and muscle cells, called glycogen, got depleted, they acquired the ability to convert adipose, or fat, stores to ketones as an alternate form of energy. In addition to being an energy source, ketones have downstream effects that activate master regulators in cells, which ramp up anti-oxidative and anti-inflammatory activities, improve mitochondrial function and growth, repair DNA, and trigger autophagy.

What this means for you: By extending your daily overnight fast to trigger a switch in fuel source, you can activate your innate healing and regenerative capabilities. Chapter 7 explains the eating pattern that aligns with our natural biorhythm, which developed over generations. We will go through the steps from getting started to reaching your personal goal in the protocol in Chapter 13.

Engage in Deliberate Psychological Challenges

Our ancestors had obligatory periods of acute stress navigating uncharted terrain and outsmarting their prey for survival. Their brains acquired the ability to grow pathways after dealing with stress, which made them better at handling subsequent similar situations. Since their survival depended on cooperation within a tribe, their genes protected them from sensing adversity during pursuits that benefited others. Early humans also had to stay one step ahead of their environment, adapt to climate changes and varying availability of food and other resources, and cope with increased complexity among their social groups. During the Paleolithic period, the human brain doubled in size and increased in complexity. We developed the neocortex, the brain area responsible for higher-order activities such as language, abstract thinking, and problem-solving. The psychological and mental challenges our ancestors faced created beneficial adaptive responses.

What this means for you: Engaging in purposeful and creative activities that require critical thinking builds pathways in your brain that make you better at handling future challenges. We will delve into the remarkable science behind how good psychological stress changes your brain chemistry and reconfigures your nervous system in Chapter 8. Additionally, the Stress Paradox Protocol presents a challenge that will help you gradually build from tiny good stressors followed by strategic recovery to ultimately live the life you envision.

◆

When we nurture these adaptations, we build our resilience to stress and make it possible to live with less pain, disability, and suffering. Regardless of where you are starting from, remember that your body is remarkably adaptable. You aren't set in stone. Even if you don't think you can handle physical exercise, specific foods, or stress well, you can train your body to cope better over time. This adaptability follows a "use it or lose it" principle. Gradually exposing yourself to longer fasting periods, higher exercise intensities, extreme temperatures, a variety of plant toxins, and more challenging mental and emotional stressors encourages your body to remodel at every level—from your cells to entire organ systems. This remodeling enhances your resilience, making you fitter, stronger, and sharper. Be aware that the opposite also happens: indiscriminately avoiding stress leads your body in the opposite direction. You gradually remodel it to be less tolerant of stress and more vulnerable to illness.

Nearly two millennia ago, Hippocrates, hailed as the father of medicine, said, "The natural healing force within each one of us is the greatest force in getting well." State-of-the-art modern science is now validating this time-honored teaching and is showing us how to honor our body's ancient wisdom. Whether you are healthy and want to optimize your performance and longevity or have a condition like diabetes or heart disease that you want to manage with less reliance on medication, you can use your ancient cellular defense systems to become vastly healthier, younger, and more energized. Your natural healing power can be medicine. Sometimes it's the best medicine.

PART II

GOOD HORMETIC STRESSORS

The Right Kind, Dose, and Duration

If the idea of voluntarily choosing to add stress still feels daunting, I don't blame you. The word "stress" instinctively makes most people—including most scientists—think of a threat to their health! It is no wonder that we spend so much time figuring out how to avoid stress, draw boundaries around it, and develop techniques to tame it. But we are here to change this common misconception about stress and give it an upgrade to keep pace with the decades of advances in research.

To get started, you need to think of stress more broadly, to include the good and the bad. You don't have to abandon everything you know about stress—excess stress can certainly lead to burnout and fatigue, and wreak havoc on the metabolism; but you need to trust that deliberately taking on stress, that doing hard things, opens you to a life of more meaning, joy, and strength.

When we think of changing our habits, we often think of it as overhauling our lifestyle, which can feel exhausting and unsustainable. It can trap you in an all-or-nothing mentality where you keep waiting for the "right" time to prioritize your health. The types of good stress I am talking about are simple, flexible steps. They don't involve extreme undertakings such as a multiday fast or rigid protocol. Rather, they are small changes that we can all make, no matter our age or fitness level, because they are natural exposures our body has adapted to handle over hundreds of generations. You can think of good stressors as micro-habits. They are bite-size changes that compound to big results. *Trust that you were made for this.* We all have the ability to take on good stress and build our resilience. Most of us just don't yet know how to summon our natural capability.

THE THREE PILLARS OF GOOD STRESS

The principle behind "good" stress is that it needs to be the right kind, at the right intensity, and for the right duration, followed by recovery. Let's break this down.

Choosing the right kind of stress. How can you know when stress is good? At a biological level, the criterion for stress to be good is that it has to activate your inherited stress response pathways in a way that promotes stress resilience, repair, and growth. We will go through the specific types of stress that meet this criterion. I will guide you, for example, through the kinds of workouts and psychological challenges you should choose. As a rule of thumb, you will know when stress is good based on how you feel afterward. Unlike the uncomfortable, overburdened feeling you may associate with the concept of stress, good stress doesn't leave you feeling fatigued, drained, and over-whelmed. Instead, you can expect to feel energized, clearer in your thinking, and stronger. You will feel you can take on more, not less.

Let me clarify that you don't need to take on all the good stressors. In fact, there may be some that you simply can't do based on your current health. One of the coolest things about hormetic stress is a phenomenon called "cross-adaptation," which is that exposure to one type of stress increases your toler-ance to other types. It's a different way of thinking about how to overcome life's biggest challenges. For example, if you want to get better at handling psychological stress, you aren't limited to techniques that calm your mind, like meditation. You can use cold stress to improve your resilience to psycholog-ical stress. So, you can start with any of the good stressors. And you can pick different tools from your toolbox at different times. While you don't have to do all of them to be more vibrant and healthier, each builds on and reinforces the other.

"Dosing" good stress. Every medicine is ideally dosed high enough to be effective but not too high where it causes side effects. The same holds for good stress. You want to reach a level of stress sufficient to stimulate your body's natural defenses and promote a beneficial response but not a level that overwhelms your body's ability to cope and causes harm. Hormesis research-ers call this optimal dose your "hormetic zone." They describe it as the sweet spot along a dose-response curve that is shaped like an inverted U. At either end of the U—where there is not enough or too high a dose of stress—there is harm. Stress that is in the middle falls under the part of the inverted U curve where the response is optimal.

With this in mind, you want to dose stress to where you are pushing past your comfort zone and feeling a little discomfort but not much beyond where you feel uncomfortable.

Keeping the stress episodic. The third dimension of good stress is the duration. Good stressors are short-lived. The stressors our ancestors faced were intermittent—bursts of moderate to high-intensity running, intervals of time without food, and moments of fear outsmarting predators. Our stress biology is designed for episodic stress. Prolonged stress causes a very different outcome than acute stress. If you went too long without food, you would starve. If you were immersed in cold water for an extended period, you would get hypothermia. So, you want to press the brakes periodically rather than keep your foot full throttle on the gas pedal.

The episodic nature of good stress harmonizes with the rhythmic pattern of our biology. Activities in our cells occur cyclically, according to our circadian rest-wake cycles. Genes in cells predictably turn on or off to optimize our body's processes, such as digestion, hormone levels, daily performance, and sleep. Because good stressors honor our biorhythms, they can feel more natural and viable as a long-term strategy for health.

Inherent in keeping stress episodic is the need for recovery. During stress, your body switches to an energy-conserving, stress-resisting mode where it uses energy more efficiently and turns on protective functions, such as moderating inflammation and upregulating antioxidant genes. It sets you up so that when you recover, you can grow in ways that help you adapt to subsequent stress. In stress mode, we prepare for damage, reallocate and conserve resources, and recycle. During recovery, we repair, remodel, and regenerate. Both stress *and* recovery are critical. Ultimately, repeated cycles of stress and recovery are how we optimally rewire our networks, enhance our function, and become more resistant to disease.

◆

The following chapters dive deeper into five key hormetic stressors that we know build resilience and longevity—plant "toxins," exercise, thermal stress, fasting, and psychological stress—with an eye to these three principles as well as the mechanisms through which they work. You will learn how they benefit you and how to incorporate them into your life.

CHAPTER 4

Food "Toxins" as Medicine

You probably know eating your veggies or an apple a day is good for you. Fruits, vegetables, and other plant-based foods are full of vitamins, minerals, and fiber, which can prevent and reverse disease and extend longevity.

But did you know that the secret weapon of plant foods is that they all contain plant chemicals called phytochemicals? More than five thousand phytochemicals have been found in fruits, vegetables, legumes, grains, nuts, seeds, and spices; many others have been identified, but we don't yet know much about them. They are nonnutritive, meaning they don't provide nutrition like protein, fats, or carbs, but they are molecular powerhouses with antioxidant, anti-inflammatory, and anticancer properties that work like tiny little bites of medicine.

Phytochemicals concentrate in the skin of plants, giving them their vibrant colors. In fact, the bright colors of fruits and vegetables like blueberries, strawberries, and carrots *are* their antioxidants and anti-inflammatories. Phytochemicals also give plants their distinctive taste and smell. The bigger the burst of flavor and aroma from a strawberry, the more phytochemicals it contains.

You'll often hear health advocates recommend "eating the rainbow," or focusing on getting lots of color on your plate. That's because the mix of phytochemicals varies among plant foods, and they work through mechanisms that complement each other. Therefore, you get the maximum health benefit from eating more colors. Thousands of studies show that high consumption of fruits and vegetables and plant-based diets rich in phytochemicals, such as the Mediterranean diet, can reduce the risk of chronic diseases, including heart disease, stroke, cancer, and Alzheimer's disease, and improve longevity. However, recent evidence suggests there is far more to how these magical chemicals interact with us.

Most of the thinking in phytochemical research over the past fifty years has been that fruits and vegetables have antioxidant chemicals that directly neutralize harmful oxygen-derived free radicals. These free radicals are notorious for damaging DNA, proteins, and cell membrane lipids. The idea is that antioxidants in plant foods scavenge destructive free radicals, essentially squelching them, like throwing a wet blanket on a fire, before they cause damage.

While it's true that certain phytochemicals, especially phenolics, can work this way, some scientists have recently noted a flaw in this theory: it would take incredibly higher concentrations of phytochemicals to put out the fire from free radicals than we typically get from eating plant foods. Phytochemicals are poorly absorbed from our intestines, and only a small fraction enters our circulation. A typical diet with fruits, vegetables, and other plants doesn't come close to the amount of antioxidants you would need for them to work solely at neutralizing free radicals in a tit-for-tat way. Nor are supplements the answer. Even megadose antioxidant supplements have not been shown to prevent cancer, cardiovascular diseases, or mortality.

If the antioxidants in phytochemicals aren't *directly* responsible for the health benefits we attribute to eating plant foods, how do they work? Around two decades ago, renowned experts like neuroscientist Dr. Mark P. Mattson, who was head of the Laboratory of Neurosciences at the National Institute on Aging, began reporting that some of the chemicals in plants activate our cells' adaptive stress responses. In other words, they optimize our health and longevity by hormesis.

The pieces of the puzzle began to fit together. While we absorb only tiny amounts of phytochemicals from plant foods—not enough to eliminate free radicals on their own—these amounts are just enough to trigger a hormetic response. Our cells sense certain phytochemicals as potentially dangerous (the reasons for which we will come back to shortly). As a result, instead of directly supplying us with disease-fighting chemicals, some phytochemicals mildly stress our cells. This stress prompts our cells to activate their own defense mechanisms against damage, disease, and aging.

Yes, we need phytochemicals—not so much to supplement something our bodies lack, but more because they activate our inherent antioxidant capacity for scavenging and neutralizing oxidative damage. They also stimulate other maintenance and repair responses that improve energy metabolism, reduce inflammation, protect the integrity of DNA and protein, and stimulate growth factors that make us stronger. Different phytochemicals activate different stress response pathways. Eating foods with a blend of specific phytochemicals amplifies their benefit, creating a cascade in our body that is like fireworks.

Plant chemicals are part of the ancient secret code that unlocks our most powerful defense systems. They are a vital part of how we can use stress to reprogram our body to heal, repair, and grow.

IF YOU CAN'T OUTRUN THEM, POISON THEM

You may be wondering why our bodies perceive phytochemicals as good stress. To understand this, it's helpful to look at why plants have phytochemicals in the first place and how our complex relationship with plants evolved over time. Plants are a major food source not just for us but also for insects, birds, and mammals. Since they can't flee their predators, plants developed an elaborate array of chemical defenses—phytochemicals—to protect themselves. These phytochemicals act as natural pesticides and are often concentrated in parts of the plant most vulnerable to attack, like the skin and buds, to deter insects and other creatures, including us, from eating them. The bitter taste of many phytochemical pesticides may be nature's way of making sure we don't overconsume them, since in high doses, they may be toxic (this might explain our tendency to peel fruits and vegetables and pass on a second helping of brussels sprouts!).

Because our ancestors' survival depended on consuming plants, they coevolved with them by developing detoxification enzymes that degrade, metabolize, and efficiently eliminate potentially harmful phytochemicals. This allowed them to safely consume plants while protecting their cells from prolonged exposure. The bitter taste and our natural detoxification system reduce our risk of toxicity from these natural compounds. Lucky for us, another way our ancestors adapted is by activating stress responses to low doses of these plant chemicals so that they could gradually build resistance to consuming higher amounts and a wider variety of plant food. Moreover, these phytochemicals, through hormesis, helped them become more resilient to other stressors in their ever-changing environment. In other words, they grew to *depend* on these plant toxins to function optimally—a trait we have inherited. Our modern genes are shaped by our ancient food past.

We coevolved not only with plants but also the microorganisms living within them. These tiny life-forms are a crucial yet often underappreciated part of the ecosystem that enables us to hormetically thrive from plants. Plants, like humans, have their own microbiome, consisting of bacteria and fungi. These microorganisms protect plants by producing many of their phytochemicals. Since they reside inside plants, these microorganisms have a vested interest in ensuring the plant survives. Therefore, the phytochemicals they produce not only protect plants from getting consumed but also build their resilience to other environmental stressors like drought, nutrient scarcity, and temperature extremes. Just as phytochemicals enhance our innate defenses, they do the same in plants. This is part of the interconnectedness between plants, microorganisms, and our health.

Eating these plant chemicals is one of the oldest and most natural ways to improve our fitness, health, and longevity. Plants have been perfecting their stress responses for nearly a billion years, and the complexity of their stress responses rivals and perhaps surpasses ours. So, the next time you are browsing the produce aisle, think about the health benefit you are gaining from the culmination of an eon of plants' highly sophisticated adaptive survival strategies!

Another Theory of How We Benefit from Eating Stressed Plants

Some scientists, including Konrad T. Howitz and David A. Sinclair, believe that we benefit from phytochemicals in a different way: their theory proposes that when we eat a stressed plant, instead of being gently stressed out of balance by the toxicity of phytochemicals, we absorb its stress tolerance. They use the term "xenohormesis" to describe this cross-species hormesis, with the prefix "xeno" coming from the Greek word for foreigner. Essentially, we piggyback off plants: they (and their resident bugs) form phytochemicals to build their resistance to stressors like drought, heat, and predation—and when we consume phytochemicals, they activate our own stress response pathways by working on enzymes and receptors at various steps involved in these processes.

But why would plants bother to make chemicals that enhance our survival? Well, they don't exactly. The premise is that back when our ancestors lived near their food sources, phytochemicals may have been a way for plants to communicate an impending downturn in the environment. Animals that evolved to pick up on these signals had a survival advantage since they could prepare while the conditions were still favorable.

Whether the benefits come through hormesis or xenohormesis doesn't matter much; more than likely, it's through both. Chemicals often work in more than one way, and the mechanisms are usually synergistic. What is clear is that we benefit from eating stressed plants—and the more of them we consume, the better our health and longevity.

EATING FOR RESILIENCE

Plants' stress response builds our stress response. Plants' adaptation to their environment builds our ability to adapt to our modern environment. Once you see food through the lens of hormesis, it can fundamentally change your approach to eating. Phytochemicals activate your stress biology at a molecular level to improve your well-being, health, and longevity. They increase your energy by supporting mitochondrial function. They enhance mental clarity by repairing damaged and misshapen proteins that clump together and impair neurons, and they uplift your mood by reducing harmful inflammation, countering oxidative damage, and increasing your detoxification capacity. The truly empowering part is they help you feel better using your own cellular machinery, which is remarkably efficient at keeping your body in balance.

Beyond making you feel better, phytochemicals ramp up your disease defenses and slow down your rate of aging. As discussed in Chapter 2, many chronic diseases and the aging process itself are driven by the same mechanisms that our adaptive stress responses counteract—inflammation, oxidative damage, DNA damage, mitochondrial dysfunction, protein degradation, and insufficient autophagy. That means that phytochemicals build resilience against the very factors that cause illness and are associated with premature aging. They are essential to a proactive strategy for living a long and healthy life. Phytochemicals leverage your innate biological plasticity to help you reach your full potential in ways you couldn't achieve without them.

Lab studies show that phytochemicals work similar to other hormetins, such as nutrient restriction and exercise. And like other hormetic stressors, they are pleiotropic, meaning the same phytochemical can activate multiple disease resistance pathways and have reinforcing health benefits. They are a phenomenal tool for repairing and healing the damage we inevitably accumulate over time. Harnessing their power maximizes the medicinal properties of food. It's like getting the most health and longevity benefit with every bite we take.

While more hormetic phytochemicals are sure to be discovered, let me share some of the ones known to be powerful. I make it a priority to eat as many of them as I can. It's easy to do because the plant chemicals that optimize our stress biology are abundant in a variety of foods, including fruits, vegetables, legumes, grains, nuts, seeds, herbs, and spices.

Need some help figuring out how to incorporate these phytochemicals into your daily diet? Turn to Chapter 14 (page 219) for some delicious recipes and ideas! They include a point system for calculating and increasing your phytochemical intake.

Marlissa's Story

When I first met Marlissa, she was taking part in my Healthy Kitchen program, a hands-on group course designed to teach nutrition and culinary skills. Marlissa was struggling with intense cravings, energy slumps, brain fog, hunger, and fluctuations in her mental health. She had tried to alleviate these symptoms by cutting out foods that she thought might be the cause, such as sugar and gluten. At the beginning of the program, her diet primarily consisted of chicken, broccoli, plain yogurt, and avocados. However, nothing had helped her feel better. Marlissa confided in me, "I've removed every-thing, but I still don't feel well." She was frustrated and exhausted, unsure of what else to eliminate to control her symptoms.

I was more concerned about what she wasn't getting enough of rather than what she was eating. More symptoms and health problems arise from a shortage of primarily plant-based nutrients than from an excess of pro-cessed sugary foods and drinks. I guessed that she wasn't giving her body enough good stress from plant toxins, which was causing her resilience to be low. Each week of the program spotlights different plant foods, such as whole grains and legumes, and as Marlissa worked with our chef to learn cooking tips and prepare meals from ingredients she had never tried before, her hunger and cravings eased, and her energy began to increase.

After several months, she told me she was feeling better than she had in years—her brain fog was gone, her mental health improved, and her sleep was more restful. One day a coworker brought in a chocolate cake. She put her new way of eating to the test and had a small slice after lunch. She was expecting an afternoon crash, but it never came. Increasingly, she felt con-fident adding phytochemical-rich plants that helped her mood and hunger. Most of all, she was excited that instead of struggling at every meal with off-limits foods, she was able to shift her focus to getting an abundance of foods that nourished her body.

Resveratrol

The connection between phytochemicals and hormesis started in the late 1990s with resveratrol, a chemical compound you have probably heard a lot about because of its potent antioxidant properties. At the time, investigators noticed a peculiar phenomenon known as the French Paradox: despite a diet relatively high in saturated fat, people in southern France had surprisingly lower rates of mortality from coronary arterial disease compared to other industrialized countries. This anomaly was attributed to their daily habit of consuming mod-erate amounts of red wine. It ignited interest in resveratrol, which is abundant in red wine, as the active agent because of its rich antioxidant concentration. However, like most phytochemicals, resveratrol is rapidly absorbed in the gastrointestinal tract and quickly metabolized. Only nanomolar amounts are left in the blood, which makes it nearly impossible for it to work as an antioxidant in the traditional sense—that is, like a missile shooting down invaders. This led to the hypothesis that resveratrol benefits health through hormesis.

In plants, resveratrol is a natural fungicide and antibiotic that protects plants from getting destroyed by fungi and bacteria. The more stressed a plant is by predators, the more resveratrol it produces. When we consume this natural pesticide, it mildly stresses our cells, activating energy sensing and other stress response pathways. Its functions are more complex than a directly neutralizing antioxidant.

Resveratrol activates sirtuin 1 (SIRT1), part of the seven-member family of proteins known as sirtuins, which are one of the cellular stress response pathways mentioned in Chapter 2. Sirtuin 1 then stimulates a transcription factor called FOXO to express genes that counteract oxidative stress. In other words, resveratrol is potent because it activates powerful cellular machinery that amplifies its antioxidant effects in our cells. Resveratrol also stimulates stress circuits that induce autophagy, DNA repair, regulation of inflammation, and the creation of new mitochondria.

The best part is you can stress your cells with this natural pesticide and build your resilience through many delicious options. In addition to getting high amounts from grapes and red wine, you can get lots of resveratrol from eating berries (blueberries, cranberries), nuts (pistachios, peanuts), and dark chocolate (my favorite!).

Resveratrol is the prototypic plant toxin that builds our healing and housekeeping systems through hormesis. It was the impetus behind discovering the other hormetic plant toxins on this list, each a superstar in its own right in helping us survive and thrive in a stressful and rapidly changing world.

Sulforaphane

Sulforaphane is a phytochemical found exclusively in cruciferous vegetables, such as broccoli, cabbage, cauliflower, brussels sprouts, kale, and arugula.

These vegetables have evolved a clever defense mechanism involving an enzyme called myrosinase. This enzyme converts sulfur-containing compounds, known as glucosinolates, into "toxic" phytochemicals to protect the plant. Normally, myrosinase and glucosinolates are stored in separate parts of the plant, but when predators—like us—take a bite, myrosinase is released. This triggers a chemical reaction that produces isothiocyanate toxins, such as sulforaphane. (Cooking tip: Chop or blend cruciferous vegetables before cooking them because heat destroys the myrosinase enzyme. By chopping or blending the vegetables first, you release the enzyme and give it time to work before cooking, which preserves more of the vegetables' phytotoxin. The enzyme is also deactivated in frozen cruciferous vegetables, so you have to mix them with a small amount of fresh chopped or blended cruciferous vegetable to add the enzyme.)

So, what happens when this toxin is released in our body? It activates a master regulator of our antioxidant stress response called nuclear factor erythroid 2-related factor 2 (Nrf2). Nrf2 is a transcription factor that controls the expression of our vitagenes, the highly conserved circuit of survival genes that promote health and longevity by building cellular stress tolerance. Vitagenes encode the antioxidant enzymes glutathione, catalase, and superoxide dismutase, and phase II detoxification enzymes. These enzymes ramp up our antioxidant and detoxification capacity far more effectively than the amount of antioxidant defense we get from absorbing antioxidants from food.

This is a perfect example of how a plant's sophisticated defense works as our defense. Many plant "toxins" activate the master regulator Nrf2, which makes it a common mechanism by which phytochemicals stress our body just enough to help prevent the onset and progression of numerous chronic diseases.

Allicin

Allicin, the phytochemical in garlic, onions, shallots, and leeks, stresses cells by opening pores in their membrane lining that allow calcium to flow in. The influx of calcium activates a transcription factor that turns on genes responsible for making growth factors, which are natural compounds that prompt our body to remodel and regenerate after handling good stress. Plants and humans have developed mechanisms to control how much calcium gets inside cells because in excess amounts, calcium is a harmful toxin, but in low doses, it works hormetically. So, after billions of years of evolution, plants and other organisms, including us, have evolved channels and gates to allow in just the right amount to signal cells hormetically. Allicin is also a natural pesticide, forming part of plants' defense against fungi and bacteria. Like sulforaphane, a precursor of allicin is stored in a different plant part than the enzyme that activates it. Allicin also upregulates antioxidant enzymes, stimulates DNA repair, and modulates inflammation.

Quercetin

You can ingest the toxin quercetin from many fruits, vegetables, and teas, with good sources including apples, onions, kale, berries, broccoli, tomatoes, grapes, and both green and black tea. You may notice that many of these plant foods have already been mentioned. This is important to note because each plant food has not one but an array of phytochemicals. If a single chemical can activate multiple stress response pathways, think about the burst of defenses you set off from a blend of phytochemicals every time you eat just a single plant food!

Quercetin is another phytochemical with a hormetic dose-response effect on cells: at the low concentrations typically obtained from food, quercetin works as an antioxidant; at high doses, it can be a pro-oxidant. Antioxidants protect us from developing many chronic diseases, including cancer, which many people fear the most. Cancer arises from DNA mutations that cause cells to grow uncontrollably. These mutations commonly result from free radicals damaging DNA. Therefore, by ramping up antioxidant defenses, quercetin protects DNA from damage and plays a role in cancer prevention. Like sulforaphane, quercetin turns on antioxidant genes by activating the Nrf2 pathway. It also has anti-inflammatory effects by inhibiting a different transcription factor called nuclear factor-κB (NF-κB). And like resveratrol, quercetin can also activate the sirtuin stress response, which, in turn, can upregulate other cellular stress responses, including heat shock proteins, DNA repair, anti-inflammation, and growth factors. The greater the variety of plants you eat, the more toxins you get, and the more you activate your natural ability to stay healthy and vibrant.

Capsaicin

If you have ever put an entire chili pepper in your mouth at once, you have experienced firsthand how effective capsaicin is at deterring us from consuming this plant! Capsaicin is the chemical that sets your mouth on fire when you eat spicy peppers, such as serrano or cayenne. This toxin mainly builds cellular defenses by activating the anti-inflammatory stress response pathway. Capsaicin can also open pores in cell membranes to allow calcium in, which turns on genes that produce growth factors and enhance regeneration.

Curcumin

Curcumin is the bioactive toxin in turmeric, one of the main spices in curry powder. As a culinary spice, it is bitter with a bright yellow color. Additionally, it has also been valued as a medicinal substance for four thousand years. For plants, the benefit of making curcumin is clear: it is a strong antibacterial and antiviral chemical. Decades of research has shown that it doubles as our defense by acting as a hormetin with anti-inflammatory, antioxidant, anticarcinogenic, and other healing abilities. In lab studies, curcumin can induce autophagy, and through its interactions with other cellular components, it has been shown to be effective against various cancers.

Ferulic Acid

Ferulic acid is in oranges, apples, grapefruit, tomatoes, beets, carrots, sweet corn, spices, peanuts, avocado, whole grain rolled oats, chocolate, coffee, and other plant-based foods. It's another protective chemical in plant cells that has hormetic anti-inflammatory and antioxidant benefits. If you recall, one of the most amazing things about hormesis is that it stimulates cross-adaptation— hormetic phytochemicals not only build physical resilience but they also cross over to fortify psychological resilience. Most of what we know about ferulic acid's antidepressant-like effects is from animal studies. This toxin has been shown to reduce neuroinflammation in mice exposed to chronic unpredictable mild stress. One way ferulic acid may work as an antidepressant is by mitigating inflammation. Another is that it can raise serotonin and norepinephrine levels in mice. Ferulic acid has also been shown to have antidepressant-like effects in rats exposed to stress in utero, attributed partly to its anti-inflammatory properties and its impact on the pathway that produces cortisol.

Epigallocatechin Gallate (EGCG)

Matcha tea, anyone? Matcha differs from traditional green tea in that it's made from ground whole leaves rather than brewed from tea leaves that are discarded. Mixing the ground powder with hot water creates a creamy, frothy, and delightful tea. Green tea contains less caffeine than coffee, but it's still wise to limit yourself to one or two cups. Both green tea and dark chocolate are excellent sources of epigallocatechin gallate (EGCG), another phytochemical that can build psychological and cognitive resiliency. A review of twenty-one studies on green tea found that it can reduce anxiety while improving attention and memory. EGCG works by activating multiple stress response pathways, including the Nrf2 antioxidant pathway, sirtuin 1, and autophagy responses.

Genistein

Genistein was originally found in the plant dyer's broom, *Genista tinctoria*, from which it gets its name. It is a naturally occurring plant chemical from the isoflavone family that protects against UV damage. Soybeans are a cholesterol-free and high-protein major source of genistein. You can also find genistein in soy milk, tofu, and edamame, but it is even more concentrated in fermented soy products like miso and natto. In humans, genistein acts as an anti-estrogen, reducing the risk of breast and prostate cancers. If that's not enough reason to incorporate more soy foods, genistein also activates stress responses that stimulate autophagy and inhibit harmful inflammation and oxidative damage.

Luteolin

Luteolin is another plant defense against insects, microbes, and UV light that is present in many fruits, vegetables, and herbs, including carrots, fennel, peppers, celery, rosemary, thyme, oregano, peppermint, and chamomile. Despite its presence in these commonly available foods, most typical diets don't contain enough of this phytochemical to reap its benefits. As a result, we often miss out on luteolin's anti-inflammatory, antioxidant, and sirtuin response activating effects.

Plant Toxins, Their Food Sources, and the Main Stress Response Pathways They Activate

Plant Toxin	Food Sources	Stress Response Pathway
Resveratrol	Red grapes, red wine, peanuts, pistachios, dark chocolate, blueberries, cranberries	Antioxidant response; sirtuin response; autophagy response; DNA damage response; inflammatory response
Sulforaphane	Broccoli, cabbage, cauliflower, brussels sprouts, kale, arugula	Antioxidant response
Allicin	Garlic, onions, shallots, leeks	Stimulates growth factors; antioxidant response; DNA damage response; inflammatory response
Quercetin	Green and black tea, apples, onions, capers, kale, spinach, elderberries, blueberries, broccoli, tomatoes, grapes, plums	Sirtuin response; DNA damage response; heat shock protein response; antioxidant response; inflammatory response; stimulates growth factors
Capsaicin	Chili peppers, such as cayenne, serrano, and jalapeño	Inflammatory response; stimulates growth factors
Curcumin	Turmeric, curry powder	Autophagy response; inflammatory response; antioxidant response

Ferulic acid	Oranges, tomatoes, carrots, sweet corn, ginger, thyme, oregano, apples, chocolate, grapefruit, coffee	Antioxidant response; inflammatory response
Epigallocatechin gallate (EGCG)	Green tea, dark chocolate	Sirtuin response; autophagy response; antioxidant response
Genistein	Soy products (soy milk, tofu); fermented soy (miso, natto)	Sirtuin response; antioxidant response; inflammatory response
Luteolin	Many fruits, vegetables, and herbs, including carrots, fennel, peppers, celery	Inflammatory response; antioxidant response; sirtuin response

HOW TO EAT PLANT TOXINS FOR HORMESIS

Now that we have our list of foods rich in phytochemicals that help us heal and regenerate, let's talk about how to incorporate the right kind, in the right dose, followed by the right recovery into your routine for building resilience. In the Stress Paradox Protocol in Chapter 13 and the recipes that follow, I worked with plant-based nutritionist and chef Ashley Madden to bring you lots of delicious options to get more plant toxins, but first let me show you what to keep in mind when determining how to eat plant chemicals for hormesis.

Choosing the Right Kind

Phytochemicals are food's superpower. All plant foods have phytochemicals. Yet the type and amount of hormetic phytochemicals vary widely among different fruits, vegetables, legumes, and other plant foods. Since phytochemicals work more effectively as a team and reinforce each other in activating your healing and defense systems, you maximize their health and longevity benefit when you consume a variety of plant foods. As with all hormetins, you should personalize your choices to find what makes you feel best and fits your preferences, taking into consideration your culture, medical condition, and allergies. At the same time, don't be afraid to experiment with ones that you haven't yet tried. Of the more than fifty thousand edible plants worldwide, 90 percent of calories come from just fifteen plants—with more than half from rice, corn, and wheat. What that means is that you have to be intentional about getting diverse phytochemicals.

Getting a variety of fruits, vegetables, and other plant food in your diet is a big step in the right direction. However, another factor to consider is that crops today are cultivated for calories rather than phytochemicals. They are grown under controlled conditions that maximize their carbohydrate yield and protect them from stressors such as drought and predators. Because plants make a higher concentration of phytochemicals under stress, plants grown under controlled conditions have fewer phytochemicals than ones grown in the wild. You can tell the phytochemical content in a plant food by following the flavor. The richer the taste, the higher the concentration of phytochemicals. The order goes like this: wild plants are richest in phytochemicals, followed by organic produce, which are estimated to have 10 to 50 percent higher levels of phytochemicals than produce obtained from conventional farming. If you don't have access to wild or organic, you can increase the amount of plant food in your diet to get more phytochemicals—which brings us to the next pillar, the dose.

Dosing Phytochemical Stress

Based on the average intake of fruits and vegetables, only about one out of ten Americans gets the recommended amount. While we worry about protein and vitamins, our biggest dietary deficiency is in phytochemicals. One of the largest epidemiological studies, which included 195 countries and spanned over twenty-seven years, found that a diet deficient in phytochemical-containing plants is the biggest risk factor for mortality worldwide, accounting for one out of five deaths. Not getting enough good stress from fruits, vegetables, legumes, whole grains, nuts, and seeds accounted for more deaths globally than consumption of "bad" dietary stressors such as red meat, processed meats, and sugar-sweetened beverages. It wasn't even close. Inadequate intake of whole grains alone was attributed to thirty-fold more deaths globally than from the latter. Now, I completely support eliminating ultra-processed foods with refined sugars and grains. But the point I want you to remember is that *adding* plant food will do far more for your health and longevity than *removing* vilified foods. Start with adding a small dose of your favorite plant food. Then, gradually increase the dose by eating different plant foods. The more you add, the more you turn on your stress response genes, and the stronger, healthier, and happier you will feel. Eventually, you will have less room for the foods you should limit. For nearly three decades, I've worked with thousands of patients struggling with their health and nutrition and have seen them succeed with this approach.

Of course, too much of even a good thing can be harmful, and that applies to food. You don't want to get into a superfood mentality by picking one plant food and having it all day. Take what happens with green tea consumption as an example. One to two cups daily places you in the hormetic zone of the phytochemical epigallocatechin gallate (EGCG). However, consuming six cups per day for four months could lead to liver toxicity. It's best to get your doses of phytochemicals through moderate amounts of an assortment of plants. As long as you eat typical servings, your body does all the homework of figuring out the hormetic dose for you. That's the reason phytochemicals have low bioavailability and are rapidly detoxified in our body. It's to ensure we get only optimal doses. For example, only 16 percent of resveratrol is absorbed into the blood from dietary sources, while the values for EGCG and quercetin are even lower, at 2 and 5 percent, respectively. In other words, in the low concentrations we get from food, phytochemicals are toxins, but they are not toxic. After millions of years of coevolution with plants, you can trust that you will get an optimal dose of phytochemicals by eating plenty of different plant foods without needing to worry about safety.

When It Comes to Plant Toxins, Choose Food First

You may be wondering if you should increase your dose of phytochemicals by taking supplements. Let me tell you why you should take a food-first approach.

When you isolate a phytochemical in pure form as a dietary supplement, it may not work the same as it does in whole food form. Distinctive phytochemicals differ in their molecular size, bioavailability, and the metabolic pathways by which they are digested. These factors affect the distribution and concentrations of each phytochemical in different parts of your body, including your organs, tissues, and cells. Whole foods contain multiple phytochemicals and other nutrients such as vitamins and fiber that interact with each other and work in cooperation with cellular stress response pathways. As a result, in the whole food matrix, natural proportions of phytochemicals work together in ways that can't be replicated or mimicked by dietary supplements. Think of phytochemicals as star quarterbacks in plant food, with other team members being vitamins, minerals, and fiber. Even if they are the MVPs, phytochemicals need the whole team to succeed at winning.

A food-first approach is also the simplest way to keep the dose of plant chemicals in the optimal range. When a phytochemical is taken out of the context of food and consumed as a supplement, it's hard to know whether the dose will be beneficial or harmful. There are infinite supplement preparations, each with different concentrations of phytochemicals.

When you give your body doses that disrupt the delicate interplay between us and plants, there is an even bigger concern: you may suppress your adaptive stress responses by potentially getting too much of these chemicals from a supplement. For example, certain antioxidant supplements may interfere with the body's natural signaling pathways, having a net effect that is counter to health. They may dampen your natural production of antioxidant enzymes and decrease immune protection, DNA damage repair, and cellular cleanup of damaged cells. In fact, beta-carotene, vitamin A, and vitamin E supplements may increase mortality. Given that we spend $12.8 billion out-of-pocket annually on natural product supplements in America, about one-quarter of what we spend on prescription drugs, we need to be aware of their potential interference with our innate healing and housekeeping systems.

High doses of antioxidant vitamins may even block the beneficial effects of other hormetins, such as exercise. In a groundbreaking study, German scientist Michael Ristow and his colleagues put thirty-nine healthy men on a monthlong exercise plan, giving half high doses of the antioxidant vitamins C and E. In men not taking antioxidant supplements, the oxidative stress from exercise increased their antioxidant defense capacity and sensitivity to insulin, a hormone that regulates blood sugar. But those taking supplements did not get the increase in their antioxidant defense and did not improve their insulin sensitivity. In other words, rather than counteracting oxidative stress, antioxidant supplements interfered with their natural cellular defenses.

Relying on food sources is the best way to keep your body in homeostatic balance.

Keep It Episodic

Phytochemical levels rapidly drop by half in minutes to hours. Therefore, the time interval between meals and an overnight fast are generally sufficient for your body to recover and grow from hormetic phytochemicals. Dietary patterns such as the Mediterranean diet, where hormetic foods are consumed at every meal, show health and longevity benefits. However, your gut microbiome composition and genetics influence the rate at which you absorb and detoxify phytochemicals. Think about these factors as well when finding your ideal recovery time. You may need to go more slowly with adding plant chemicals and work your way up to every meal.

◆

Phytochemicals are key in connecting food with health, acting like covert agents dismantling internal threats before they manifest as chronic disease and premature aging. They keep your body in balance by turning on your natural ability to heal, repair, and grow, making you stronger and happier. That may seem too remarkable to believe, but it's true. By consistently stressing your cells with plant chemicals, you can prevent and lessen the burden of disease *and* improve your energy, mental clarity, and mood. They nurture your nature, honoring the way your ancient past has programmed your body to rely on these molecules to adapt to our modern world and manage life's unavoidable challenges.

CHAPTER 5

Exercise Stress for Cellular Fitness

Give every individual the right amount of exercise,
not too little and not too much.
—Hippocrates

While you may not have used the term "hormesis" to describe how exercise builds muscle, it is a concept that is likely familiar: if you work out your muscles enough to cause a little breakdown but not too much to get injured, and then allow time for recovery, the muscle rebuilds stronger; over time, if you keep working out in this way, you develop the capacity to lift heavier weights. The same concept applies to building endurance, flexibility, power, and agility. Exercise is the quintessential hormetic stress. However, the changes we see and feel are just a small part of the resilience we build from the molecular adaptations triggered by exercise-induced stress.

In the last two decades, scientists have significantly advanced our understanding of how exercise affects us at a cellular level. The pathways triggered by exercise are complex and interdependent, yet they share a common theme: exercise disrupts our body's internal balance in various ways, inducing just enough stress to trigger cellular responses that enhance our overall fitness, which is our overarching ability to survive and thrive in our environment. Exercise isn't just for people who want to burn calories or sculpt their body, even though it will do that. It is essential for all of us. Exercise is the foundation for our ability to function effectively throughout our lives. By making our cells more efficient at energy production, exercise lays the groundwork for repair, growth, and renewal. Our capacity for resilience relies on exercise to such an extent that I have come to think of this good stress as the Fountain of Youth; it really is that powerful for living a healthy, long, and fulfilling life.

When we exercise, our bodies become chemical factories, releasing loads of chemicals into our circulation with far-reaching benefits beyond muscle. The roster of these chemicals is growing at a fast pace as more continue to be discovered. Referred to as exerkines, they include essential anti-inflammatory, anticancer, and growth factors, including a key brain growth hormone called brain-derived neurotrophic factor (BDNF) that repairs, maintains, and builds our brain circuits to protect us against the mental health and neurodegenerative diseases that are sweeping the globe. Exerkines send signals that communicate with every part of our bodies, enabling us to adapt to our environment with greater cognitive, physical, and emotional flexibility.

Exercise generates many kinds of good stress in your body. In addition to the mechanical stress it places on your muscles and joints, it creates heat stress, which we'll talk about more in the next chapter, and hypoxic stress, which is caused by oxygen shortage when you exert yourself to the point of breathlessness. Yet, the two forms of exercise-induced stress that I think are the most critical for our cells are oxidative and metabolic stress.

Oxidative stress is often understood as a harmful process where free radicals, a kind of reactive oxygen species, damage cellular components upon contact. The discovery that exercise, despite its well-established health benefit, generates oxidative stress by forming reactive oxygen species posed a long-standing conundrum to scientists. As with plant toxins, the pieces fell together when it was found that the type and amount of reactive oxygen species produced during exercise act hormetically, triggering our body's natural capacity for healing and growth. These reactive oxygen species primarily serve as signals switching on "master regulators" in cells that control genes responsible for antioxidant, anti-inflammatory, and DNA repair functions. As a result, the mild to moderate oxidative stress from exercise, being controlled and intermittent, actually enhances cellular resistance to oxidative damage over time. This contrasts with the chronic oxidative stress from poor diet and inactivity you may be familiar with, which contributes to disease and aging.

The metabolic stress imposed by exercise works hormetically in a similar way. By depleting energy reserves, exercise creates just enough stress to activate an enzyme that acts as an energy sensor, called AMP-activated protein kinase (AMPK). This enzyme tells your cells when the fuel gauge is in the red zone and nearing empty. (We'll come back to AMPK because it is also activated by fasting.) AMPK plays a crucial role in switching cells from energy storage mode to energy breakdown mode. This shift is particularly helpful for preventing and managing metabolic conditions, such as type 2 diabetes and obesity, where excess energy storage is an issue. As cells run low on fuel, they start to break down stored glucose and fats. They also use energy more efficiently by absorbing more glucose from the blood into cells, which lowers blood sugar. The health-promoting power of exercise-induced stress is so significant that people who are healthy but don't exercise have a higher risk of premature death from cardiovascular disease or other causes than people with metabolic diseases like type 2 diabetes and obesity who regularly exercise.

The foundation for the cellular resilience we gain from all these good stress pathways activated through exercise lies is our mitochondria—the little organelles commonly referred to as the powerhouse of the cell. Mitochondria actually do far more for us than power our cells. They communicate across cells as a command hub that is central to our health and longevity. The oxidative and metabolic stress induced by exercise are important because they activate stress response pathways that converge on mitochondria.

POWERING UP THE POWERHOUSE OF YOUR CELLS

While doctors hardly mention it, the health of our mitochondria may be the most important factor underlying our health. Our mitochondria determine how well our metabolism works. By metabolism, I don't mean if you are lucky enough to eat chocolate cake without gaining weight. Metabolism is a measure of how well we convert food into energy, and then use that energy for growth, repair, and maintenance. This energy flow is essential for our cells to work well. That's why mitochondria are key to our physical and mental performance, disease risk, and overall lifespan.

Mitochondrial dysfunction—not having enough mitochondria or mitochondria that are damaged and can't function properly—is incredibly common. Part of the reason is simply aging. The number of our mitochondria and how efficiently they function rapidly decline as we grow older. But the bigger problem is that many aspects of our modern lifestyle reduce and damage mitochondria. Bad stressors like a high-calorie, processed food diet, being sedentary, dealing with chronic stress, and loneliness can all cause mitochondrial dysfunction.

Some of the most common symptoms of mitochondrial dysfunction I see are fatigue and stubborn belly fat. Most of these patients have tried lots of different diets without much success and are desperate to know what they should eat to boost their energy and "metabolism." But when you have mitochondrial dysfunction, focusing on nutrition alone is like focusing on getting high-octane fuel when the problem is that the cellular engines—the mitochondria—are malfunctioning. If your body can't convert food to energy efficiently, you're going to tire easier and store the calories no matter what you eat.

Mitochondria make over 90 percent of the energy that fuels our cells' metabolism. Our tiny little cellular engines convert glucose and fat to adenosine triphosphate (ATP), our cellular energy currency, using oxygen in a process called oxidative phosphorylation. When mitochondria aren't healthy, we rely more on a less efficient energy generating system called glycolysis. By comparison, it generates only two ATP per glucose molecule compared to over thirty ATP generated by mitochondrial oxidative phosphorylation. You can begin to see why that's bad news.

We also need healthy mitochondria to burn fat. While both of our cellular energy systems can burn glucose, only mitochondria can burn fat. When mitochondria are healthy, we have "metabolic flexibility," meaning we can switch between using glucose or fats for energy (mainly relying on fats during low-intensity activities and on glucose for high-intensity activities like sprinting). When mitochondria aren't healthy, we can't access our fat stores to generate energy. Fat is by far our most abundant and efficient fuel source—we can make 106 ATP from one long-chain fatty acid like palmitate. When we can't access our fat stores, we deplete our glucose stores more quickly and tire more easily during energy-demanding activities. Yet even more troublesome, we can't burn the fat that leads to a bigger waistline and metabolic conditions such as obesity and diabetes.

There is a cruel irony here. Mitochondrial dysfunction makes our metabolism less efficient and can lead to metabolic conditions such as insulin resistance, type 2 diabetes, metabolic syndrome, and obesity. And in these conditions, mitochondria are impaired and less efficient at burning fat, which creates a vicious cycle of fat accumulation and a constant struggle to get rid of it.

Another common symptom I see from mitochondrial dysfunction is mental fogginess. Neurons rely almost entirely on mitochondria for their energy. So, when there is mitochondrial dysfunction, neurons face an energy deficit. The communication between neurons and the balance in the neurotransmitters they make gets disrupted, which makes cognitive processes like thinking, problem-solving, and concentration more difficult. Even more devastating, when mitochondria are damaged, they produce more free radicals when making energy, which further damages mitochondria. Like a rotten apple spoiling the bunch, damaged mitochondria in the brain can lead to a vicious cycle of oxidative stress and neuroinflammation. This can increase the likelihood of developing neurodegenerative illnesses such as Alzheimer's and Parkinson's disease. It's no wonder that, in the scientific literature, neuroscientists have started to advocate for preventing and slowing the progression of neurodegenerative diseases by improving mitochondrial health. And that's why I am advocating it for you.

You have the power to improve your mitochondrial health and reverse mitochondrial dysfunction simply by incorporating more good stress—particularly exercise—into your routine. Mitochondria have remarkable plasticity. When you challenge your cells with a mild to moderate amount of exercise-induced stress, a special type of hormesis occurs within your cells' mitochondria. It's called mitohormesis, which is short for mitochondrial hormesis. Mitohormesis repairs, regenerates, and grows new mitochondria, which can range from one to several thousand per cell. Exercise is the most potent way to stimulate mitohormesis, which is why it is so vital for living a long, healthy life.

Engaging in exercise depletes energy in our cells, which activates a "master regulator" called PGC-1α. This stimulates the growth of new mitochondria, a process known as mitochondrial biogenesis. Moreover, your mitochondria adapt to cellular stress not only by making new mitochondria but also by repairing existing ones. They do this by cleaving the damaged parts of mitochondria and fusing the healthy parts. In cases where mitochondria are irreparably damaged, they are removed through a specific type of autophagy called mitophagy.

If you think about the mitochondria throughout your body as a power grid, mitochondrial biogenesis essentially transforms your cells from a finite to a renewable energy source, enabling you to replenish your energy efficiently and naturally. Meanwhile, mitophagy reduces free radical emissions, leading to a cleaner, less polluted environment in your body. You are never too old or too unhealthy to make more mitochondria, increase your energy production, and regain metabolic flexibility. By reversing mitochondrial dysfunction, you essentially supercharge your body's engine so that you are running on a turbocharged, mega-horse-powered, efficient machine.

In recent years, we have learned that mitochondria do even more than just generate energy in cells: they also serve as crucial communication hubs. They form a network throughout the body, collaboratively cross-talking with one another to control the flow of energy, akin to the traditional East Asian concept of "chi," which represents vital energy or life force. Furthermore, mitochondria communicate with multiple bodily systems, including circadian rhythms, gut microbiota, and the immune system. They may even serve as key integrators of these interconnected systems, coordinating and exchanging information between them. Remarkably, mitochondria also produce hormones and essential neurotransmitters like noradrenaline and serotonin, which have significant impact on our stress responses and mood.

This means that mitochondrial dysfunction can lead to a range of issues beyond energy metabolism problems. Mitochondrial dysfunction can disrupt your body's circadian rhythm, alter gut bacterial balance, cause low-grade inflammation, and interfere with making crucial hormones and neurotransmitters. On the flip side, focusing on mitochondrial health can improve whole body health. The more we learn about mitochondria, the more apparent it becomes that their health underpins our overall well-being. The bottom line is that the benefit you get from improving your mitochondrial health has a ripple effect. Healthy mitochondria = healthy you.

Cheryl's Story

Cheryl was forty-six but felt decades older. She had zero energy and was struggling with weight gain. Desperate to lose a few pounds and shake off her sluggishness, she enrolled in an expensive meal delivery program with custom meals portioned and balanced by a nutritionist and sourced with fresh, locally grown organic ingredients. After several months, she added a daily women's vitamin, B complex vitamin, and several supplements that claimed to boost metabolism. Her weight didn't budge and neither did her energy. By the time she came to see me, she was losing hope. "I eat lots of greens and feel I am doing everything right with my diet," she said. "But I haven't lost an inch, and I'm still tired all the time."

When patients tell me they are struggling with fatigue—especially if they're eating well and getting enough sleep—my mind goes right to mitochondrial health. I worry about a mismatch between the amount of activity they are getting and the stress their body needs to maintain their metabolism. It turns out that while Cheryl was getting steps in when she could, she didn't have the time or energy to go to a gym, so she didn't make exercise a priority. I've seen this happen so many times: we focus on diet alone. I explained to Cheryl that just as you can't out-exercise a bad diet, you can't out-eat a lack of exercise. We could start slow. I gave her a fifteen-minute interval training routine she could do at home. She just had to push herself to the point where it felt hard but manageable and do the training twice a week.

Getting started wasn't easy, but a few weeks later, she was excited to share that she was doing it. She had gotten on the other side of what seemed impossible for her and for the first time in years felt energized and motivated to keep challenging herself.

USING EXERCISE AS GOOD STRESS

Our goal is to optimize the volume and efficiency of your mitochondria, and to do that we need something more tailored than the standard physical activity guidelines of getting 150 minutes of moderate-intensity activity, 75 minutes of vigorous-intensity activity, or some combination of moderate and vigorous activity, with two days of resistance exercise. Those are good guidelines for physical activity, but we are aiming higher.

We're going to focus on cardiorespiratory fitness. Cardiorespiratory fitness captures the adaptations you build when you exploit your marvelous stress physiology. It represents the efficiency of your metabolic system—the ability of muscle mitochondria to use oxygen to make ATP—and integrates it with the ability of your lungs to uptake oxygen and cardiovascular system to deliver oxygen to muscle. Cardiorespiratory fitness is often measured by a VO_2 max test, short for maximal oxygen uptake, which is the maximum amount of oxygen you can utilize during intense exercise. (We'll measure your VO_2 max in part IV when we put hormesis to work for you.) Since mitochondria burn glucose and fats in the presence of oxygen, your oxygen consumption is directly related to the efficiency of your mitochondria. The higher your VO_2 max, the more energy you have flowing through your power grid. Over nine thousand studies back the importance of VO_2 max.

Choosing the Right Kind

There are four primary forms of exercise—aerobic, strength training, stretching, and balance or stability training. The most potent kind of exercise for improving mitochondrial health is aerobic exercise, but keep in mind that these categories are interdependent. Aerobic fitness relies on muscle fitness because it works large muscle groups, and maintaining proper form and stability is essential in any exercise routine to prevent injury. Therefore, in addition to the aerobic exercises in the Stress Paradox Protocol, you should include strength training and stability exercises too.

Aerobic exercise, also called endurance exercise or cardio, includes a long list of activities from which you can choose, such as power walking, jogging, cycling, swimming, rowing, stair climbing, jumping rope, dancing, hiking, jumping jacks, high-intensity interval training, and team sports. They are called aerobic because they use oxygen to convert stored carbohydrates and fats to meet the energy demand of the exercise. In addition to increasing mitochondrial health, studies consistently show that endurance exercise raises antioxidant capacity by inducing a hormetic amount of oxidative stress. With endurance training, mitochondrial volume can expand by as much as 40 to 50 percent, and this increase is often accompanied by an improvement in each mitochondrion's oxidative capacity. An endurance training routine has the potential to double the amount of antioxidant enzymes in each gram of muscle.

To maximize improvement in aerobic metabolism, our exercise strategy is similar to using plant chemicals—we want a variety of different exercises at varying intensities. Different exercises engage different muscle groups, which is key to getting the most mitochondrial density on a per-muscle basis. For instance, if you do a lot of long-distance running, you will proportionately increase mitochondrial density in your legs, while rowers might have a higher concentration of mitochondria in their back and arm muscles. Alternating exercise intensity, such as switching between walking and jogging, recruits different muscle fiber types, which further enhances mitochondrial volume.

Dosing Exercise Stress

When thinking about the intensity, or "dose," of exercise, remember that it's not the specific activity that defines intensity, but rather the effort that you put into it—how challenging you find it and how much it increases your heart rate and breathlessness. For instance, a brisk walk might be high intensity for one person and low intensity for another. As you repeatedly extend beyond your comfort zone, you'll find yourself exercising with more force and power while maintaining the same level of perceived training intensity.

When dosing exercise stress, you need a Goldilocks amount that is not too little or too much. Simply moving at a leisurely pace for a minute or so around your home won't throw your body out of homeostasis. While it is true that any movement is better than none, you need to challenge yourself with at least moderate-intensity exercise to create enough oxidative and metabolic stress to trigger your body's stress responses. Remember that we optimize our bodies when we do hard things. The increase in energy demand leads to the growth of new mitochondria. The more sessions you do and the longer the duration of each session, the more you increase your mitochondrial volume.

Your power grid becomes better able to handle stress the next time you experience it. The process is pretty remarkable.

The optimal way to improve your mitochondrial health and cardiorespiratory fitness is to train at a combination of intensities. This creates different levels of stress, and your body responds by developing diverse stress adaptations. In addition to continuous moderate-intensity exercises like jogging at a steady pace, your mitochondria benefit from high-intensity interval training (HIIT), where you do cycles of higher intensity exercise followed by brief low-intensity periods. HIIT stresses your body at a faster rate, creating a quicker disturbance in homeostasis, which signals more robust and unique adaptations with particular benefit for the heart, brain, and liver. Higher intensity intervals also recruit and enhance mitochondrial development in more muscle fiber types. Intensity is key for maximizing our metabolic adaptations. Just as bouts of high-intensity exercise helped our ancestors survive and flourish, they protect us against modern-day diseases and threats to our well-being.

You can estimate your intensity zone fairly reliably by rating your perceived exertion, or RPE. On a scale of zero to ten, with one feeling like hardly any exertion and ten feeling like your maximum effort, you are at moderate intensity if you rate the difficulty between five and six—the activity feels somewhat hard and slightly uncomfortable. Another method is the "talk test": you are at a moderate intensity when you can speak in breathy sentences but aren't able to sing. If talking is easy, you are likely at a low intensity. On the other hand, if you can say a few words but not speak in complete sentences, you are likely in a vigorous intensity zone, which equates to an RPE of seven or higher. If you monitor your heart rate during exercise, moderate intensity typically corresponds to about 64 to 76 percent of your maximum heart rate, while vigorous, high-intensity exercises reach 77 percent or more of your maximum heart rate.

Keep It Episodic

Our body's built-in way of keeping the duration of each exercise session in hormetic range is by causing exhaustion. Exercise generates oxidative stress by producing reactive oxygen species. When reactive oxygen species build up to an optimal point for hormesis but where more would net harm, they cause muscle fatigue. Muscle fatigue is your internal barometer for knowing when you have maximized the benefit from each session. How long it takes you to get to this turning point, called the "breaking point," can vary based on the intensity of the exercise and from person to person. As you exercise regularly, it may take longer to get to your "breaking point"—but that is precisely what you want because it means you have built up your antioxidant capacity and mitochondrial health.

You should work up to doing 180 minutes or more of moderate-intensity exercise each week, such as four 45-to-60-minute sessions. You can achieve the same exercise volume in a shorter duration by replacing a moderate-intensity workout with HIIT. How much time you spend doing moderate-versus high-intensity training largely depends on the amount of time you allocate for exercise. Trained athletes often use the 80/20 rule, where 80 percent of their training is moderate intensity and 20 percent is HIIT, with the latter equating to several hours per week. For most of us who exercise less, the percentage of HIIT should be higher. You want at least one or two of your weekly aerobic sessions to be HIIT to get the greatest gains. Interestingly, our body is designed to respond optimally to stress with a routine that resembles the fitness patterns our ancestors probably followed. They would spend extended periods engaging in moderate-intensity endurance hunting for food, with occasional bursts of high-intensity activity when capturing prey or being pursued by predators.

Remember that your body makes all the adaptation gains from stress during recovery. If you don't give yourself time to fully recover, you may not get all the benefits of your workout. Excessive exercise or inadequate recovery can push you beyond your hormetic zone. The amount of time you need for recovery is different for each person and can depend on the intensity of the workout. As a general rule, more intense workouts require longer recovery periods. You can do moderate-intensity workouts most days, but allow yourself at least one day between HIIT sessions. Additionally, incorporate a rest day into your weekly routine.

Pairing Plant Toxins with Postexercise Recovery Can Be a Winning Strategy!

The timing and content of your meals significantly influence your recovery. High-quality carbohydrates are essential before or during long or intense workouts, and proteins are necessary post-workout for muscle repair and growth. An often overlooked aspect is the need for plant toxins! Phytochemicals, particularly polyphenols, play a key role in reducing post-workout inflammation, leading to faster recovery. For instance, fruits like bananas and dates offer carbohydrates and anti-inflammatory polyphenols. Phytochemical compounds like resveratrol, quercetin, and epigallocatechin gallate (EGCG) further enhance recovery by promoting mitochondrial biogenesis.

◆

Making our mitochondria healthy is at the heart of the cellular health revolution. So much of our health and resilience would improve if we made mitochondrial dysfunction a medical diagnosis; it's a common factor in most, if not all, chronic diseases and affects many aspects of our performance and quality of life, causing symptoms like fatigue, weight gain, and mental fog, and even affects the way we handle stress. Knowing about its role long before the onset of disease would empower so many of us to take action to support our health and well-being. Fortunately, you don't have to wait for medicine to catch up to the science—you can improve your mitochondrial health with exercise stress right now.

CHAPTER 6

Cold and Heat Therapy for Activating Thermogenesis

Long before I would have considered extreme cold or heat as "therapy," and a decade before an explosion of research on the hormetic effects of thermal stress, I inadvertently experienced the benefits for myself. At the time, I was a medical resident at the Brigham and Women's Hospital in Boston. Most of my waking (and non-waking) hours were spent at the hospital, learning to manage a constant stream of life-threatening emergencies from motor vehicle accident injuries to "code blues," when patients would go into cardiopulmonary arrest. Experiencing the exigency of the final moments of life, and the incredible gratification of changing that outcome, along with all the emotions and vulnerabilities in between, was an incredible privilege. But it came at a cost: working seven days a week with grinding thirty-six-hour shifts of often relentless stress was exhausting and kept me on alert.

My apartment at the time was in an old brownstone in Beacon Hill, the oldest district of Boston, which boasts charming antique shops, narrow cobblestone streets, historic hand-carved doorways, and the antiquated plumbing and heating systems that go along with all that old-world charm. One morning, in my rush to get to the hospital, I didn't have time to wait for the water to warm up, so I jumped into a freezing cold shower. It knocked the breath out of me, and two minutes later I came out shivering.

Later that morning, though, I noticed feeling peculiarly energized and focused. I repeated my morning experiment, and not only did the cold showers become more tolerable, but I also felt uplifted, inspired, and calmer, although nothing else in my life had changed. As much as I dreaded the cold, morning showers became a ritual that helped me get through those tough training years.

Once I moved and a hot shower became readily available to me, I stopped my daily cold shower habit, despite knowing how good it made me feel. We are comfort-seeking creatures, after all. Exposing ourselves to extremes of cold or heat isn't something most of us would do voluntarily. For starters, it can feel miserable. In the extreme, it can also be dangerous. Spending extended time in frigid temperatures without proper attire can cause frostbite, or, worse yet, hypothermia, and enduring a heat wave without taking precautions can cause a heat stroke. But while chronic or extreme exposure to heat and cold can overwhelm and damage our bodies, brief, intermittent, and tolerable exposures to thermal stress can make us healthier, happier, and more resilient.

Of course, deliberate cold exposure, also called cold therapy or cryotherapy, and deliberate heat exposure, also called heat therapy or thermotherapy, aren't new. They have a long and rich history as ancient healing practices. The renowned Greek physician, Hippocrates, believed cold water therapy relieved fatigue. And in Nordic countries like Finland, sauna bathing has been a cultural tradition for centuries. But interest in these time-honored practices has been renewed in recent decades because of a growing number of studies showing their extensive physiological and psychological benefits.

The connection between cold exposure, mental performance, and resilience relates to how deliberate cold exposure works as a stress stimulus. When sensory nerves in your skin detect extreme cold, they quickly send a message to your brain, triggering a stress response. Because the skin is densely packed with cold sensors, the nerve impulse to your brain is like a jolt that spikes the blood level of the stress hormone noradrenaline up to five times the normal level. The immediate effect is that it makes you feel energized, alert, and focused—exactly how I felt from my morning showers. The effects don't stop there. Cold immersion rapidly increases dopamine levels by 250 percent, which can increase your sense of reward, pleasure, and motivation. If you stay in the cold and take deep breaths or try to do a mental task while your brain and body are flooded with stress hormones, you essentially train your mind to stay calm and perform well under stress in other situations. It's no coincidence that cold water diving is used as a technique to train elite military forces.

Brief, deliberate cold stress activates your neurochemicals differently than the classic fight-or-flight response. During the fight-or-flight reaction, your brain perceives a threat and releases adrenaline and noradrenaline throughout your body. The alarm system stays activated through the release of the stress hormone cortisol. During cold stress, which is mainly triggered by cold receptors on the skin, the neurochemical profile is different. Cold exposure does spike noradrenaline, but the other key stress hormones that increase during the fight-or-flight response, such as adrenaline and cortisol, don't change. In fact, brief exposures a few times a week can actually lead to *lower* baseline cortisol levels in as little as four weeks, which explains the calm I felt during those intensely stressful years. Not all stress responses are the same. Good stressors create a different biochemical profile in our body that benefits rather than harms us.

Of course, I knew none of this when I stumbled on cold showers. In fact, none of these studies existed. Every one I am mentioning here has come out since 2000, most of them in the past decade. I just knew I felt better, and that is ultimately the true purpose of any healthy habit. Judging by the growing number of studies explaining how cold exposure improves mental states like anxiety, depression, focus, and resilience, other people feel this too, and that speaks to our natural inclination toward good stress. However, thermal stress does so much more—it heals the body. And that opens the door to an entirely new way of thinking about how temperature affects our health and longevity.

Are You Ready for a Feel-Good Story, Literally?

Deliberate heat also increases mental resilience, and one of the coolest ways both heat and cold exposure boost your mood is by increasing the production of beta-endorphins. These are often referred to as "feel-good" hormones because beta-endorphins are natural painkillers and can give you a sense of euphoria, similar to the sensation known as a "runner's high." However, with heat exposure, there is an added twist. Along with endorphins, heat triggers the release of a different natural opioid called dynorphin. Unlike endorphins, dynorphin can temporarily cause a feeling of discomfort. While this might seem like a downside, it actually leads to a benefit. The short feeling of discomfort you experience from deliberate heat exposure enhances your body's sensitivity to the pleasurable effects of beta-endorphins. Essentially, the presence of dynorphin makes the resulting euphoria from beta-endorphins more pronounced. By regularly using a sauna, you are training your body to become more responsive to these feel-good hormones.

THERMAL STRESS AT THE GENESIS OF DISEASE

Like other good stressors, episodic, intentional cold and heat exposure hormetically trigger protective mechanisms. When exposed to discomforting temperatures, our core body temperature changes to the point where we are either mildly hypothermic (cold exposure) or mildly hyperthermic (heat exposure). The thermal threat is sensed by the hypothalamus, the part of the brain that acts like an internal thermostat. It kicks on the "wisdom of the body" through a process called thermogenesis, whereby signals get communicated throughout your body to restore your core temperature. This ripples down to your cells, which have their own complex and interconnected coping mechanisms that increase antioxidant defenses, reduce inflammation, repair damage, and increase expression of genes involved in stress resistance. Although the exposure is brief, the benefits are longer-lasting. With repeat exposure, the body acclimates to the cold and heat, and in the process, builds adaptations that reduce the risk of chronic disease, improve mental health, and slow aging.

While they work differently, both cold and heat exposure cause your body to burn extra calories to restore body temperature. The process increases metabolism, which makes it particularly helpful for people with conditions in which metabolic health is compromised, such as insulin resistance, type 2 diabetes, metabolic syndrome, and cardiovascular disease. Like exercise stress, cold and heat exposure break down fat stores and increase glucose uptake, which helps manage these conditions and prevent their development.

Our bodies thrive so much from thermal stress that the mismatch created by *not* being exposed to it—by living in thermoneutral air-conditioned and heated indoor spaces which are so different from the outdoor exposure our ancestors experienced—is an overlooked risk factor for our modern chronic disease and mental health epidemics.

NOT ALL FAT IS CREATED EQUAL: THE BRILLIANCE OF BROWN FAT

Have you ever wondered how kids can run around in the dead of winter in nothing more than a T-shirt, insisting they're not cold? It's not just because they're stubborn; it's because they have a lot of something called "brown fat," which protects them from cold temperatures by essentially working as the body's space heater. For a long time, scientists believed that brown fat was only the province of children and that it disappeared as we age. However, about a decade after my own experiment with cold therapy, researchers at Harvard Medical School made a fascinating discovery. Using a technology called positron emission tomography (PET scans), they found that adults have brown fat, too. Unlike white fat, which deposits in unwelcome places and contributes to obesity, brown fat is found only around the neck, collarbone, and upper chest—areas strategically close to vital organs such as the heart, lungs, and nervous system. While white fat is designed to store energy (calories), brown fat is designed to use it: brown fat rapidly burns energy to keep these crucial areas warm under cold conditions. The discovery that adults have brown fat was hugely exciting because it opened the possibility of activating it to burn stored energy and speed metabolism. It meant that we could leverage our body's innate thermogenesis to reduce accumulating excess white fat and the risk of developing insulin resistance and other health-related consequences.

Research shows that the more brown fat you have and the more you activate it, the healthier you're likely to be. More brown fat is associated with lower body mass index, and vice versa, suggesting that activating brown fat or increasing its volume—or both—could potentially combat obesity and its metabolic and cardiovascular consequences. Brown fat is also associated with reduced visceral fat, the dangerous belly fat that releases hormones and pro-inflammatory chemicals that increase the risk of diabetes, metabolic syndrome, and heart disease.

We are just at the cusp of understanding this special type of fat, but it is clear that activating brown fat, and getting more of it, can improve metabolic and cardiovascular health by regulating blood sugar and insulin levels and lowering cholesterol. Glucose is your body's main fuel source for generating heat. So when brown fat is fired up by cold exposure, it helps lower the risk of diabetes by burning more glucose and increasing insulin sensitivity to uptake glucose out of the circulation faster. As it replenishes its fuel supply, brown fat also clears triglycerides and cholesterol from your bloodstream, reducing the risk of cholesterol plaques forming in the arteries.

If you don't use brown fat, you lose it, and as you get older or develop conditions like obesity and diabetes, you have less of it. However, brown fat has incredible plasticity and adapts quickly. You can grow and activate brown fat regardless of your current health. By doing so, you can utilize your body's ability to do all the amazing things I just described: increase metabolism, reduce body fat, lower your cholesterol, improve your insulin sensitivity, and reduce the risk of diabetes and heart disease. To activate brown fat, all you need to do is expose yourself to cold temperatures. You don't even have to take a freezing shower. Simply lowering your indoor thermostat can be effective. In one study, people who spent six hours a day in a 60°F (15°C to 16°C) room while wearing shorts and a T-shirt saw a 37 percent increase in their brown fat volume after just ten days!

This is how cold exposure activates brown fat. When you're cold, your body produces heat through two types of thermogenesis: shivering and non-shivering. With shivering thermogenesis, as the name suggests, you shiver as your muscles rapidly contract to generate heat. But as your muscles tire, shivering slows down, and your brown fat takes over. It quietly burns calories to produce heat through non-shivering thermogenesis. Brown fat is effective at non-shivering thermogenesis because it has lots of mitochondria. In fact, it's the iron in the mitochondria that gives it its brownish appearance. Cells with more mitochondria can burn more energy and generate more heat. Animal studies suggest that we can even "hack" our bodies to use white belly fat as a fuel source for heat-generating brown fat, as some white fat cells can transform into a type of fat that's more like brown fat called "beige fat," or "brown in white fat," by increasing their mitochondria. Just like exercise improves metabolism by increasing mitochondrial density in muscle cells, cold stress improves metabolic health by increasing mitochondrial density in fat cells. Isn't that fascinating?

At a molecular level, the process of heat generation works through hormesis, too. The sensory nerves in your skin trigger a stress response; however, in this instance, instead of preparing you to escape danger, the fivefold-higher circulating noradrenaline attaches to receptors on your brown fat cells, activating a proccess that turns on heat production. This process is driven by a switch called uncoupling protein 1 (UCP1), a unique protein in brown fat cells that converts mitochondria from using fat to make ATP to using the energy from fat to generate heat instead. You can think of UPC1 as a match that ignites a fire in the mitochondria of brown fat cells. The fat stored in brown fat is like firewood for this metabolic fire. The neat part is that if you need more firewood, you will break down white fat to supply your brown fat, reducing your white fat stores.

Like all hormetic stressors, cold stress triggers multiple protective pathways. In addition to creating new mitochondria and increasing glucose and lipid metabolism, cold exposure activates antioxidant and anti-inflammatory pathways that build immunity and reduce inflammation—including the low-grade, invisible kind that is a common factor contributing to long-term diseases and aging. By depleting the body's energy reserves, cold exposure stimulates AMPK and SIRT1, the energy sensors that are also activated by exercise and plant toxins such as resveratrol. As a result, repeatedly exposing yourself to cold temperatures builds stress resistance, increases your natural disease defenses, and slows aging.

HEAT UP FOR HEART HEALTH AND HEAT SHOCK PROTEINS

Heat exposure also boosts metabolism, improves cardiometabolic health, and even helps you live longer—but it does so by getting rid of heat to cool off, rather than generating it to warm up. Sitting in a sauna, for instance, triggers a response that is remarkably similar to what happens during moderate or high-intensity exercise! Sauna can actually raise your body's core temperature to the range of a low-grade fever. To cool down, your body produces sweat. Just as brown fat is your body's space heater, sweating is your built-in air conditioner.

When you sweat, your body is pumping as much blood as possible to your skin, where the heat evaporates to cool you down. During this process, your heart rate may nearly double, up to 120 to 150 beats per minute, and your heart may pump out around 70 percent more blood. So while you are relaxing in a sauna, the deliberate heat exposure can act like a workout without requiring you to move. I am not recommending that you replace exercise with heat exposure, but it can be considered an alternative for those who can't exercise. In fact, some of the long-term benefits of heat exposure are remarkably similar.

For starters, all this blood flow happens to be very good for your heart and blood vessels. It improves the health of the lining of your blood vessels, called the endothelium. Picture your blood vessels as highways connecting every organ in your body. There are approximately sixty thousand miles of delicate endothelium between the blood vessel walls and the circulating blood. When this lining doesn't function properly—due to oxidative stress and low-grade inflammation often caused by factors such as a poor diet, lack of exercise, or smoking—it can lead to cardiovascular disease. Poorly functioning endothelium, known as endothelial dysfunction, is one of the earliest changes leading to atherosclerosis, heart attacks, and strokes. Heat therapy can improve endothelial function by activating the body's natural defense against oxidative stress and inflammation. Another way the blood pumping to the skin from heat exposure helps the heart is that the shearing forces of the blood on the endothelium cause it to release a magical molecule called nitric oxide (NO). Nitric oxide helps blood vessels relax and dilate, which lowers blood pressure. It also makes blood vessels less susceptible to inflammation and clotting. In fact, the discovery of its role in cardiovascular health was so groundbreaking that it earned three scientists a Nobel Prize in 1998.

Heat has a healing effect on your heart in ways you can't see or feel because precursors to cardiovascular disease happen long before we get a heart attack or stroke. The health of the lining of your blood vessels is one of these early markers. It's so critical that the direction of medical research is toward finding earlier and earlier markers of chronic diseases so we can address them when they are reversible. By focusing on early indicators, such as mitochondrial health and endothelial dysfunction, we can treat the root causes of heart-related diseases before they escalate to life-threatening problems. It's a way of being proactive about your health.

Heat stress also activates heat shock proteins, which protect the shape of proteins and their ability to carry out most of the functions in our cells. (Cold exposure, exercise, and fasting all activate this same healing process, but heat is one of the most powerful!) Any change in the shape, assembly, or action of proteins can be detrimental to our health and is another root cause of many chronic diseases and aging. A higher core body temperature can harm and damage proteins, but our body has a natural defense that activates heat shock proteins to counter this. These proteins act as a cleanup crew that rescue misfolded proteins and maintain their function. Within just thirty minutes of experiencing heat stress, the levels of heat shock proteins can increase by almost 50 percent. If you recall from Chapter 2, heat shock proteins are part of our natural cellular stress response defense system and they kickstart other repair and regenerative mechanisms within our cells. The increase in heat shock proteins and other protective defenses helps improve our cardiovascular and metabolic health. They allow our body to handle future stress better and help us live a longer, healthier life.

Heat therapy activates other responses that slow down aging and disease processes, too. Since conditions like heart disease, stroke, and diabetes result from multiple processes that progress over decades, you can see why heat therapy can be so beneficial for our health. For example, heat stress reduces low-grade chronic inflammation. Heat shock proteins play a role in this anti-inflammatory response. These proteins also improve metabolic health by enhancing insulin sensitivity and lowering blood sugar levels. Additionally, heat stress activates certain genes that help combat cellular aging by activating a gene regulator called FOXO3, one of the same regulators triggered by beneficial plant toxins like resveratrol and curcumin. These genes regulate stem cells and promote tissue repair and regeneration, among other functions that support healthy aging and longevity.

HOW TO USE TEMPERATURE FOR HORMESIS

Rather than plunging straight into an ice bath or overheating in a sauna, it is important to gradually build up your tolerance. Remember, you are deliberately choosing to challenge yourself with cold and heat exposure. This is what distinguishes good stress from bad stress. You have control over the kind, dose, and duration of exposure, and you should tailor these variables to make yourself feel invigorated and stronger.

Choosing the Right Kind

Studies on cold exposure typically use immersion in cold water up to the neck, whether it be in a cold bathtub, a chilly lake, or an ice bath. While this method is the most effective, cold showers are more readily available and are the next best option. The temperature from the tap in a cold shower is comparable to the cold temperatures used in cold water immersion studies. After that, exposure to cold air or sleeping in a cold room have also been proven to increase brown fat activation and volume. If you have access to whole-body cryotherapy, protocols using cold air in cryotherapy chambers for a few minutes are also very effective.

Sauna is a popular form of heat exposure that has been widely studied in clinical trials. The most common type used in studies is the dry sauna, which is low in humidity (10 to 20 percent), typically made of wood, and heated by an electrical heater. Dry sauna is preferable to a wet sauna, which has higher humidity (50 percent or more) to reduce sweat evaporation and is harder on your body. Infrared saunas are also available, which use thermal radiation to directly warm the body and surrounding air. While safe, they haven't been as well studied. However, the simplest and most affordable way to get started is using a hot tub. Studies have shown that hot tubs can significantly reduce blood sugar, enhance cognitive function, improve mood and reduce depressive symptoms, increase heat shock proteins, and lower cortisol levels.

Dosing Thermal Stress

When considering the dose—or how cold or hot the temperature needs to be—the most important thing you need to know is that there isn't a specific temperature or duration you have to use. Although you can use the parameters from clinical trials as a guide, I recommend you adjust them to your individual needs. Every person's tolerance to cold and heat is different. The key is to listen to your body. The benefits depend more on how your body reacts to the exposure than the temperature itself. Begin with a temperature that feels challenging but bearable—for example, just at the point before you start to shiver—and gradually increase the intensity over time as your body adapts to the exposure.

The temperatures in cold water immersion protocols are typically between 50°F and 59°F (10°C to 15°C). The cold water tap in a city water supply generally falls in that range, often between 45°F and 65°F (7°C to 18°C), depending on the region and season. The duration of exposure also varies and is usually between twenty seconds to three minutes. In comparison, whole body cryotherapy chambers use much colder temperatures, ranging from –166°F to –256°F (–110°C to –160°C), for one to three minutes. Cryotherapy chambers use lower temperatures than water immersion protocols because the heat transfer rate of water is approximately thirty times greater than in air. This means that we lose heat much faster in water than when exposed to the same air temperature. Cold air exposure protocols typically use temperatures between 59°F and 64°F (15°C to 18°C).

Studies that incorporate dry saunas have used temperatures ranging from 158°F to 203°F (70°C to 95°C). Sessions are usually between five and twenty minutes. As a general recommendation, you can increase the duration of sessions by five minutes every two to three days. Infrared saunas use lower temperatures, ranging from 113°F to 140°F (45°C to 60°C). Hot baths are effective at temperatures around 102°F to 104°F (39°C to 40°C).

Keep It Episodic

Brief, intermittent episodes of thermal stress, followed by recovery, provide a healthy amount of stress to our body. However, when stress becomes excessive or lasts for a long time, it can overwhelm your nervous system and cellular coping mechanisms and become detrimental chronic stress. The milder the temperature, the longer you can expose yourself and stay in the hormetic, or optimal, zone for benefits. On the other hand, the more uncomfortable the temperature, the shorter the duration of exposure you need. For example, studies using cold air exposure use protocols up to six hours; a water immersion study at 57°F (14°C) used a one-hour exposure; and a protocol using gasping cold water temperatures at 32°F to 36°F (0°C to 2°C) kept the exposure to twenty seconds—and all were effective! My advice is to acclimate by increasing the number of sessions per week before increasing the duration of each session. You benefit more from repeated, brief episodes of thermal stress rather than fewer, longer sessions. The goal isn't to build tolerance to lengthy sessions.

If you want to maximize the benefits of thermal stress, you can practice contrast therapy, which involves alternating between brief cold dips and hot sauna sessions, as commonly practiced in Scandinavian culture. A noteworthy 2021 study by Dr. Susanna Søberg and her colleagues at University of Copenhagen found that a minimum threshold of eleven minutes of cold exposure and fifty-seven minutes of heat exposure per week, divided over two to three days with several sessions per day, was the "sweet spot" for health benefits. It's more beneficial to end hot and cold cycles with cold and allow for a recovery period of about a half hour for body temperature to normalize.

◆

The ancient practices of cold and heat therapy are natural good-stress therapies for our most common health challenges. They are a perfect example of how molecular technology is enabling us to decipher the aspects of ancestral life that we need to reintroduce to correct the mismatch between our genes and our comfort-seeking lifestyle. The technology is also allowing us to go a step further and fine-tune thermal stress protocols to optimize our mental and physical health and longevity.

CHAPTER 7

Cycles of Fasting, Eating, and Our Circadian Biology

For much of our existence, the primary threat faced by our species, *Homo sapiens*, was starvation. Over many generations, our ancestors developed various internal safeguards to increase their chances of survival during times when food was scarce, with layers of cellular pathways that helped their bodies detect and efficiently respond to a lack of nutrients. As a result, food scarcity triggers one of our most robust "good" stress responses. We have inherited three interconnected nutrient and energy sensors that work together to signal our cells to grow and multiply when food is available and to halt growth and conserve energy when food is scarce. In times of low nutrient and energy availability, our three-alarm-fire response not only mobilizes a chain of processes that make our cells more efficient, but it also protects, heals, and regenerates them.

Fasting has become a popular health trend promoted for benefits ranging from weight loss to balancing hormones and lifespan extension. I'm less interested in it as a "biohack" and more as a hormetic stress: when done at the right intensity, for the right duration, and followed by recovery, fasting creates just enough stress to activate our conserved stress responses, which restore our body's balance. In the process, fasting turns on our natural disease defenses and regenerative pathways, improving health from the cellular level.

Our ancestors experienced natural cycles of fasting and eating. They often went long intervals without food, as the hunter-gatherer way of life involved spending much of their day searching for food. This led them to adapt to being alert, agile, and physically capable in the fasted state. Today, our eating patterns are starkly different. The average person now eats for fifteen hours or longer a day, starting with juice or coffee shortly after waking and ending with a glass of wine or snack before bed. This constant eating, especially combined with the stress of consuming high-fat, high-sugar processed foods, is a significant departure from the dietary pattern to which we are adapted.

The problem with this is that it disrupts the natural balance between building up and breaking down—or you might say between stress and recovery—that our bodies developed over many generations. When you eat, you supply your body with energy. When you fast, you use up stored energy. The key behind this back-and-forth between eating and fasting is a metabolic switch from burning glucose for energy when it's available from food to burning stored fat for energy when you fast.

Insulin is the primary hormone orchestrating this switch. When you eat a bagel, for example, your blood sugar level rises, which signals your pancreas to secrete insulin. If your body needs the energy right away, insulin distributes it to the cells that need it. If you're not active and don't need the energy immediately, insulin stores the extra energy—first, a small amount as glycogen, a short-term energy reserve form of glucose, and then the rest as fat for long-term use.

When you don't eat for a while, these processes reverse. Insulin levels drop, telling your body to break down its stored energy instead of building it up. After about twelve to twenty-four hours of fasting, your body runs out of its short-term energy glycogen store and switches to burning fat instead. This fat is converted into ketones in the liver, which your body uses as an alternate energy source. You can either be in one phase or the other, buildup or breakdown.

Both phases are important—we need buildup to create reserves as a buffer, and we need breakdown to avoid excess energy storage. When we don't take long enough breaks from eating, our bodies create excess fat buildup, throwing us out of metabolic balance. Excess fat can spread from adipose tissues to organs like the liver, muscles, and pancreas, leading to insulin resistance, meaning these organs resist insulin's signal to store more fat. To cope, the pancreas secretes even more insulin, making the resistance worse. This creates a harmful cycle: insulin stores excess energy as fat, excess fat causes insulin resistance, and insulin resistance leads to even higher insulin levels, which drives more fat storage. A 2022 study estimates that 93 percent of Americans are caught on this roller coaster of poor metabolic health.

Many people think insulin resistance is linked only to obesity and type 2 diabetes, but it actually underlies many chronic diseases such as high blood pressure, abnormal cholesterol, fatty liver, heart disease, stroke, cancer, and neurodegenerative diseases. Insulin resistance can even increase the risk of death, regardless of diabetes or obesity. Remember that improving metabolic health—and reversing metabolic dysfunction—is pivotal for health and longevity. That's why it's so important to balance buildup with breakdown.

Eating throughout all our waking hours is a form of bad stress that tips the balance toward too much buildup and growth. Just as working around the clock would wear us down and make us inefficient, nonstop eating does the same to our cells. By intentionally alternating eating with fasting, we allow our cells the necessary downtime for maintenance and repair—similar to how we need time for self-care and recharging. Fasting regularly is the most effective way to lower insulin levels and restore insulin sensitivity. And by improving how your body responds to insulin, you can reverse the root cause of a whole chain of diseases. However, unlike our ancestors, for whom this eating pattern was natural and instinctive, we must now make a deliberate choice to maintain this balance.

Fasting is simpler than traditional diets because it doesn't require tediously counting calories. Nor does it involve counting nutrients, which can be incredibly confusing with all the debates and opinions about the best diet. With fasting, you simply count time. The timing of your meals alone profoundly impacts your health and longevity. Your body has an innate intelligence to adapt to the stress of fasting and, in the process, improve your mood and energy; build your defenses against a wide range of chronic diseases such as obesity, diabetes, cardiovascular disease, cancer, and neurodegenerative disease; and ultimately, help you live longer.

Chris's Story

Chris was surprised to see his blood sugar test come back in the prediabetic range. He'd never had health problems in the past and was worried I'd suggest he needed to take blood sugar medication for the rest of his life.

While most diabetes medications are effective at lowering blood sugar, what I really wanted for him was to reverse the underlying cause, which was insulin resistance. Besides, even if we were to control his blood sugar with medication, that wouldn't prevent insulin resistance from progressing and causing micro-level damage to his blood vessels, which over time, would increase his risk of erectile dysfunction, heart attacks, stroke, and cancer. I wanted to help him get to the bottom of this.

As we talked about his lifestyle, I learned that Chris's routine already included one good stress—he lifted weights several days a week. But I noticed he had a habit of starting his day with coffee and a quick breakfast first thing before heading to work and eating a late-night dinner with his family followed by a glass of wine before bed. It became clear to me that the most powerful change we could make to improve his insulin resistance was adding good fasting stress by altering the timing of his meals.

We started with shifting his breakfast to at least an hour after waking. He could still have his coffee first thing but without cream. Evenings were more difficult because dinner with his family was among the few times they were all together. I encouraged him to start by making his dinner a lighter meal and instead eat a bigger lunch. If he wanted to have wine, he could have it earlier. We gradually worked toward his last calorie being consumed two to three hours before bed, giving enough time for his body to switch from buildup to breaking down his energy stores and restoring insulin sensitivity.

At his six-month follow-up appointment, Chris was thrilled that his blood sugar was back to normal. His blood pressure and cholesterol had also improved, and he had lost an inch from his waistline. The best part was that Chris's diagnosis had a positive impact on his family as they began having dinner earlier, too!

BEYOND BALANCING CALORIES

The benefits of fasting go beyond balancing energy by matching calories in with calories out. They even go beyond continuously cutting back on calories without periods of fasting. That's because fasting triggers adaptations at the molecular and cellular level, which prevent disease even further upstream than correcting the mismatch between buildup and breakdown at the whole body level.

At the cellular level, when you eat, cells use the energy to grow and build new cellular components from proteins and fats. When you fast, your cells halt growth and shift to survival mode to conserve energy. In this mode, cells ramp up their stress defenses and do internal cleanup. They fix damaged parts, remove what they can't repair, and recycle usable parts. After you start eating again, the rejuvenated cells grow, proliferate, and reconfigure their connections so they are better prepared to handle future stress. That's plasticity at work. And this ongoing switching between creating new parts and growing, and degrading worn parts and recycling them, is critical for better health and longevity.

Think of growth and repair as the cellular equivalent to the buildup and breakdown that happens in our body systems. Fasting corrects the imbalance of too much growth (creating new cells and proteins) and not enough repair (breaking down and recycling old and damaged cells). While constant growth might sound good, too much of it can damage cells and accelerate aging.

Studies show that fasting reduces inflammation and oxidative stress, cleans up waste, improves energy metabolism, and helps repair DNA. It works through three nutrient-sensing pathways—mTOR (mammalian target of rapamycin), AMPK, and SIRT1—that surveil energy and nutrient levels. They read long-range signals from insulin and insulin-like growth factor, as well as more direct ones from nutrients, mainly glucose and amino acids. These nutrient-sensing pathways have been conserved in our genome for ages. They help us adapt and thrive, just as they did for our ancestors.

Among these nutrient-sensing pathways, mTOR is the master controller, determining whether cells grow and multiply, or repair and recycle. The other two sensors, AMP-activated protein kinase (AMPK) and the sirtuins (SIRTs), are separate pathways that gauge cells' energy status and initiate different protective cellular functions. They communicate energy-related information to mTOR and influence its activity. Think of mTOR as the central hub, like Grand Central Station. The other pathways are like train routes that operate independently but intersect and exchange information at the central hub, which then coordinates cellular activity.

As a growth regulator, when mTOR senses that energy and nutrients are available, it commits to making new cells. However, overstimulating the mTOR pathway can lead to problems like diabetes, cancer, and aging. When there is a drop in energy and nutrients, mTOR activity is inhibited, which shuts down growth and initiates the remarkable process of autophagy. As I mentioned previously, autophagy eliminates damaged or dysfunctional cellular parts to make cells more efficient and disease resistant. If we don't periodically restrict our nutrient intake, we limit autophagy. Just as too much growth can lead to chronic diseases and aging, impaired autophagy can, too. The buildup of cellular junk and damage is linked to diseases like Alzheimer's, Parkinson's, heart disease, diabetes, and cancer, as well as aging.

Inhibiting mTOR is one way to stimulate autophagy. Autophagy can also be turned on by activating the AMPK and SIRT1 pathways, which communicate and work together with mTOR. Remember from Chapter 5, AMPK is the energy sensor that detects when we run low on fuel, like during exercise, and boosts metabolism by triggering mitohormesis. Just as with exercise, depleting energy by fasting initiates the formation of new mitochondria and removes old and damaged ones. During fasting, AMPK also promotes the breakdown of glycogen and fat stores for energy, which is precisely what we want to be metabolically healthy. Additionally, when we run low on nutrients, particularly when glucose levels drop, sirtuin 1 (SIRT1) gets activated, which also stimulates autophagy, along with the other ways it helps cells survive that I mentioned in Chapter 2. The key point is that our natural ability for autophagy decreases with age, but by inhibiting mTOR and activating AMPK and SIRT1, we can keep this self-renewing process going longer.

Our nutrient-sensing pathways show that *when* we eat greatly affects our health and longevity. We don't access these natural disease defenses when we stick to the belief that we must eat three meals a day, with snacks in between!

Can You Get the Benefits of Cycling
Fasting from a Ketogenic Diet?

If you've heard of "keto," or ketogenic, diets, you may have heard that they work by a similar kind of "switching"—switching your body from burning glucose for energy to burning fat. But do they work the same way?

Ketogenic diets typically include about 10 percent carbs, 70 percent fat, and 20 percent protein, which means eating mostly meat, fish, eggs, cheese, butter, full-fat dairy, avocado, and nuts, and keeping carbs very low (20 to 50 grams per day). Proteins are kept moderate because excess protein can be converted to glucose. While keto diets do make your body burn fat and produce ketones for fuel just like fasting, they're not quite the same.

With intermittent fasting, you are continually switching between burning fat (ketosis) and burning glucose, which improves your metabolic flexibility and cycles you between growth and repair. With a ketogenic diet, you are constantly in ketosis. You don't get the benefit that comes from switching between fuel sources. Another key difference is the level of autophagy. That's because the mTOR pathway, which controls autophagy, adjusts its activity based on the types of nutrients and overall calories that are available. It's not just an on-off switch; it's more like a dimmer switch that fine-tunes the body's response. Limiting carbohydrates and proteins but consuming energy doesn't fully turn on autophagy. However, fasting sends a strong, combined signal through all three nutrient-sensing pathways that maximizes our cellular defense.

Another downside of a ketogenic diet is that it severely restricts carbohydrates—and since all plant foods have carbohydrates, it limits the intake of super-important phytochemicals. Keto might be useful in the short term for extending a fast, but intermittent fasting is a healthier, more sustainable option in the long run.

ENHANCING FASTING STRESS BY SYNCING
WITH YOUR CIRCADIAN RHYTHM

There are many ways to fast, and all involve extending the time we naturally don't eat while sleeping. The protocols studied include daily time-restricted eating (TRE), which is consuming all your calories during a specified time window and fasting the remainder of the day; eating fewer calories twice a week (5:2 fasting); fasting every other day (alternate day fasting); or occasionally doing a longer fast with a special diet that mimics fasting (fasting-mimicking diet). Each has proven hormetic benefits, and no studies have compared them to determine whether one is superior to another.

I prefer to practice time-restricted eating because of the way the repeated switching back and forth from fasting to eating, or from stress to recovery, leverages the most hormetic benefit for our cells. This rhythm allows us to benefit from fasting in another way: by syncing the eating window with our circadian rhythm. Just as the pattern of fasting and feasting, or stress and recovery, honors our biology, so does aligning that back-and-forth with the natural biorhythm of our circadian rhythm, or the roughly twenty-four-hour body clock.

The first study to show how profoundly important TRE is for our biology was conducted in 2012 by a team of researchers led by Dr. Satchin Panda. They fed mice a high-fat diet, similar to the Western diet, and divided them into two groups. One group could eat around the clock, while the other could eat only within an eight-hour window. Both groups ate the same amount of calories, but the mice with all-day access to food gained weight and developed metabolic diseases. The ones with restricted eating times were protected from obesity, high insulin levels, and fatty liver and maintained better circadian rhythms. This seminal study led to subsequent studies in humans on how restricting eating to a limited time window on a daily basis benefits our health and risk of common chronic diseases.

The importance of circadian biology owes to the discovery a couple of decades ago that we don't have just one internal clock—the master clock in the brain's hypothalamus that controls our sleep-wake cycle. Almost every organ in the body has its own clock governing its daily activities. These are called peripheral clocks. While light and darkness influence our sleep-wake cycle and main circadian clock, our peripheral clocks can be adjusted by food availability. The timing of our first and last meal sets these clocks. Our circadian rhythm is very adaptable, and when our mealtimes don't align with our sleep-wake circadian biology, it can make our central and peripheral clocks fall out of sync. It's like having different parts of our body operating in different time zones, with one part ready for sleep and another part gearing up for a late dinner.

Eating out of sync with our sleep-wake cycle, by having a big meal late at night when our body is winding down for the day, can interfere with the repair and maintenance processes that happen during sleep. Worse yet, eating irregularly at different times each day and snacking late at night can disrupt our circadian rhythm, which is often overlooked and underestimated as a reason why people struggle with metabolism and develop conditions like insulin resistance and metabolic syndrome. By combining fasting with eating in alignment with our sleep-wake cycle, meaning eating most of our calories earlier in the day when our body is primed for digesting and processing food, we can get the most metabolic and restorative benefits from our fasting cycles.

Eating most of our calories earlier in the day matters because our daily rhythm includes a rise in melatonin level at night to prepare us for sleep. Melatonin also makes the pancreas release less insulin. As a result, eating the same food late at night, like a bagel, will cause a bigger blood sugar spike than if eaten earlier in the day. Fat burning also changes during the day—the genes regulating fat burning are expressed 38 to 82 percent lower before dinner than before breakfast. A study of over eight thousand adults followed for nearly four years found that men who ate dinner before bed and snacked after dinner were twice as likely to be obese compared to those who didn't eat late at night. For women, the risk of obesity was three times higher. These studies highlight the detrimental impact of circadian disruption on our physiology. Consuming your bigger meals earlier in the day leads to better blood sugar control, more calorie burning, and more efficient digestion.

The activities in our cells also occur in a cyclical manner, with thousands of genes turning on and off at roughly the same time every day. This cycle is partly controlled by our nutrient- and energy-sensing systems, which have their own daily rhythm, regulating when cells are hungry or full. Cells also have their own schedule for maintenance: they are programmed to repair themselves at night during sleep and grow during the day. TRE helps reinforce these cycles for us. A study showed that eating within a restricted time period early in the day increases the expression of genes related to cellular stress responses (autophagy and SIRT1) while fasting, and later increases expression of genes related to growth (mTOR and brain-derived neurotrophic factor [BDNF]) after eating. Daily eating and fasting within a time frame that matches our body's natural rhythms reinforces our nutrient-sensing pathways and the cellular stress responses they activate to improve the efficiency of our cells. It strengthens us from this fundamental unit up.

Is Breakfast the Most Important Meal of the Day?

A large study with nearly eight hundred thousand adults found that most Americans who follow time-restricted eating often choose eating windows in the afternoon or evening, likely to share meals with family and friends. I understand this, and not being much of an early-morning eater, I did the same when I started time-restricted eating. However, research shows that the timing of the eating window can significantly affect the health benefits you get from time-restricted eating.

For example, a rigorous controlled trial with prediabetic men showed that eating within a six-hour window early in the day improved blood sugar after meals, insulin sensitivity, blood pressure, and oxidative stress levels. Studies with midday eating windows show similar results, with lower body weight, body fat, fasting glucose, insulin level, insulin resistance, cholesterol, and inflammation. However, trials with late afternoon or evening eating windows have not shown the same health benefits and, in some cases, even made post-meal blood sugar, blood pressure, and cholesterol levels worse.

From these studies, we can say that you don't need to skip dinner or start every morning with an early breakfast. In fact, the notion that we need to start the morning with breakfast didn't originate from scientific studies but rather during the Industrial Revolution, when workers moved to cities and started eating before going off to a full day's work. (And breakfast later became known as "the most important meal of the day" as part of a breakfast cereal ad campaign!) However, to get the most benefit from time-restricted eating, it's better to eat most of your calories earlier in the day and have a lighter dinner, aligning with your natural biorhythm.

USING FASTING AS GOOD STRESS

Switching between different cellular fuel sources is how we activate our natural self-healing and regenerative capabilities. If the thought of restricting your eating feels intimidating, remember that your body was made for this—what it *wasn't* designed to handle is our current cultural eating patterns. Your genome thrives on cyclically switching back and forth between metabolic states, from buildup to breakdown, and from growth to repair. You can start wherever you are and slowly expand your fasting window so that you give your cells enough time to adapt.

Choosing the Right Kind

Time-restricted eating supports combining the good stress of fasting with optimizing your natural circadian biology. A lot of people who fast don't realize how important it is to sync their eating times with their sleep-wake cycle. By doing this, you get the advantages of fasting stress plus those of eating in line with your body's natural biorhythm during recovery.

TRE is also the easiest and most sustainable method. Many people can stick to a plan for a short time, but the real test is whether it is feasible long term. Most intermittent fasting studies are short term, from weeks to a few months, but a 2023 study published in the *Annals of Internal Medicine* showed impressive long-term results: participants kept an eight-hour daily eating window for a whole year with an 87 percent success rate. This is significant because it means people can consistently follow this method without the struggle they face counting calories like in traditional diets. In comparison, another group in the study reduced their daily calories by 25 percent and had a lower success rate of 61 percent over the year. Those who followed time-restricted eating lost about 5 percent of their body weight, reduced their body fat and waist circumference, and improved insulin sensitivity. Plus, the study confirmed it's a safe method.

While you have the flexibility to choose whichever fasting protocol speaks to you, you'll find detailed instructions for practicing time-restricted eating in Chapter 13.

Dosing Fasting Stress

Those following time-restricted fasting often have questions about the duration: How long should the fast be, or how short should the eating window be?

I think about dosing fasting the way I do when dosing medication (after all, good stress can be as effective and, at times, even more effective than drugs!). We first want to start with the "minimal effective dose," which is the smallest amount that has a noticeable effect. Then, we want to gradually increase it to find the optimal dose, where you get the most benefits with the fewest side effects—this is the peak of the hormesis inverted U curve. And we want to avoid overdosing fasting, where it becomes harmful rather than beneficial.

The minimum effective fasting dose is more than twelve hours (or restricting eating to less than twelve hours). This is based on how long it takes your body to metabolically switch from burning glucose to burning fat. Ketones, which form when using fat for energy, appear in the blood after about eight to twelve hours of fasting. An intense workout that burns glucose stores more rapidly will hasten that transition. A large, heavy meal before fasting will delay it. While ketones start to increase after eight to twelve hours of fasting, they go up even more with longer fasts. So, fasting for longer can give you more benefits, but starting with an over twelve-hour fast is a good beginning. A study showed that when overweight, healthy adults narrowed their eating window from over fourteen hours to ten to eleven hours (fasting for thirteen to fourteen hours) for sixteen weeks using feedback from an app for guidance, they lost weight, had more energy, and slept better. The benefits persisted for a year.

Most people assume that the optimal TRE protocol is the 16:8 diet, where you fast for sixteen hours and eat for eight hours. However, the idea of 16:8 comes from early studies in rodents. In humans, the ideal duration can depend on the benefits you want to get from fasting, your overall health, and your current eating habits.

If you are fasting for cardiometabolic improvements, like in your weight, body composition, blood sugar, insulin sensitivity, cholesterol, and blood pressure, the sweet spot from most human studies is a ten-hour eating window. A ten-hour window has significant benefits compared to a twelve-hour eating window and offers similar benefits to shorter six-to-eight-hour windows. Narrowing the window to eight hours might offer additional benefits but is harder to follow. Once you restrict to an eating window of six hours or shorter, you may run into mild side effects like headaches.

If you are aiming for autophagy, you'll need to fast for a longer time. This process starts when cells are deeper into their stress survival response. Initially, when your body senses it's not getting food, it makes cells more efficient at using their energy reserves. This leads to metabolic benefits like burning fat and better glucose uptake through increased insulin sensitivity. As fasting continues, your body looks for other sources of energy. This is when cells start breaking down and recycling their own components. Shorter fasting periods, like those in time-restricted eating, lead to a modest amount of autophagy. But fasting more than sixteen hours, and up to forty-eight hours or more, can lead to more significant cellular renewal. Although much of this information comes from animal studies, we know that a special targeted kind of autophagy, known as chaperone-mediated autophagy, starts around three days of fasting.

In the Stress Paradox Protocol, we will aim for a 14:10 circadian fast, fasting for fourteen hours and eating in a ten-hour window, in phase with our natural daily rhythm. This method combines the "sweet spot" metabolic advantages of fasting stress with those of developing a more robust circadian rhythm.

The optimal fasting duration, or "dose," also depends on your health. You may be surprised that people with obesity or diabetes may benefit more from longer fasts than healthy people. That's because the more fat, or energy, a person has stored, the more reserves they have to burn during an extended fast. A yearlong study using an app found that people of normal weight or underweight didn't lose much weight, while obese individuals lost significant weight over time, with more weight loss observed in those who fasted more per day. Think of your body's fat stores as a well-stocked pantry. The more supplies you have, the more you'll use up if you go longer without grocery shopping or, in this case, eating.

Another factor influencing your optimal fasting duration is your current eating pattern. Time-restricted eating works as a good stress when it's a change compared to your eating window. Most studies haven't looked at what people's eating schedules were like before they started fasting. We don't know yet if the benefit depends on how much you change from your baseline eating window. I believe it does, and that you will need to continue adjusting your eating window as your body adapts.

It's also important to consider fasting in relation to your overall health. For instance, when rodents fast for fewer than eight hours, they also end up eating fewer calories. While that may seem beneficial in the short term, it can be detrimental in the long term. When I started time-restricted eating, I followed the common 16:8 method. However, I wasn't eating enough protein, which is essential for preventing muscle loss and the effects of aging on muscles, called sarcopenia. Losing muscle can slow metabolism, increase the risk of falls with aging, and is linked with higher death rates. In one study, most weight lost during an eight-hour time-restricted window was lean muscle mass, which the authors speculated was likely due to less overall protein intake. Balancing the benefits of fasting with nutritional needs, I have found that a ten-hour eating window works better for me.

Our bodies are made to adapt to prolonged durations of fasting, but you need to find the duration that is optimal for you. The key is that you want a little discomfort and the benefit of repeated cycles of fasting and recovery.

Keep It Episodic

Regular cycling between fasting and eating is key to the hormetic benefits of fasting because we not only have distinct adaptations to fasting but unique signaling pathways that are engaged during recovery. Switching from glucose to ketones bolsters our cellular stress resistance and sets the stage for the subsequent plasticity and growth that occur when we switch from ketone to glucose utilization. In addition to autophagy and repair pathways, fasting induces expression of specific genes involved in plasticity and making new mitochondria. It is during recovery that the proteins encoded by those genes enable remodeling and strengthening our body's efficiency and resilience. It's like Batman and Robin, Tom and Jerry, peanut butter and jelly. Fasting and recovery work together to improve our metabolic flexibility, insulin sensitivity, lipid metabolism, gut bacterial balance, inflammation, thinking, and mood. It's the repeated cycles of switching between fasting and eating, or between stress and recovery, that lead to the long-term changes that build resilience to disease and aging.

Do you have to do time-restricted eating every day? There aren't studies on doing it a limited number of days a week. However, we know that in trials where people are assigned to a group that is supposed to be fasting daily, they stick to it about 70 to 93 percent of the time. (Because we are humans! We're imperfect.) So, all those benefits reported from time-restricted eating trials come from studies where people aren't fasting perfectly every day. This means you're still going to get benefits even if you do it about 80 percent of the time. Of course, the more consistent, the better. But don't let perfect be the enemy of good. And avoid anything that feels too restrictive or impossible to stick to. What works in your favor is that we are more likely to maintain habits that make us feel better and healthier.

Repeat Cycles of Fasting and Recovery Can Help Your Thinking and Mood

Our body's ability to get stronger from good stress is a gift. It makes all our cells, including brain cells, more resilient. As a result, challenges like fasting help not just our physical health but also our mental and emotional well-being. When we regularly fast and recover, our brain is able to form new brain cells and connections. These changes in our brain structure translate to improvements in how our brain functions: they make us more creative, solve problems better, and handle emotions more flexibly.

The plasticity of our brain and entire nervous system depends on a growth factor called brain-derived neurotrophic factor (BDNF), which is ramped up by ketones formed during fasting. BDNF is crucial for the growth, repair, and upkeep of brain cells. Low levels of BDNF are linked to brain diseases like Alzheimer's and Parkinson's. BDNF also helps develop new mitochondria in brain cells, enhancing their energy. Additionally, fasting promotes autophagy in brain cells, which helps them remove damaged components and repair themselves. In other words, fasting activates different protective responses in the brain, which, in turn, lowers the risk of neurological disorders and helps our brain cope with aging.

Fasting can also make you feel more mentally alert and calm, and improve your mood. It does this by increasing the activity of the parasympathetic "rest and digest" part of your nervous system. This is reflected in increases in heart rate variability (HRV)—a sign of well-being—just like what happens with thermal stress and exercise. A key factor here again is likely BDNF, which, interestingly, plays a role in how the widely prescribed antidepressant class of drugs called selective serotonin and noradrenaline reuptake inhibitors (SSRI and SNRI) reduce anxiety and depression. This suggests that intermittent fasting and other good stressors might be new ways to improve mood and decrease anxiety similar to how antidepressant medications work.

◆

Our bodies have an incredible capacity for self-healing and regeneration. Regular fasting followed by eating aligned with our natural biorhythm balances our need for buildup with breakdown and cellular growth with repair. It builds cellular stress resistance and helps with weight loss, mainly losing fat instead of muscle, lowering insulin levels, reducing blood pressure, and lowering LDL cholesterol and triglycerides, which makes it an effective way of forestalling the most common health conditions we face today.

CHAPTER 8

Finding the Golden Mean
in Emotional and Mental Stress

So far, we've been looking at how good physiological stresses activate our cellular response pathways to make us healthier and more mentally and emotionally resilient—a "bottom-up" approach; now we're going to see how psychological stress can also work at the cellular level to strengthen us and make us more resistant to chronic stress, disease, and aging—a "top-down" approach.

It's easier to see how physical stress can help us grow and adapt, partly because we have a cultural reference for the way weightlifting builds muscle by first breaking it down. But the truth is that our brains respond similarly to good psychological stress: they reshape and grow stronger afterward. We're more familiar with the idea of harmful stress, like a hectic day at work, and the need to unwind from it by unplugging, scheduling downtime, or getting a massage. Yet, by bringing good psychological stresses into our daily lives with activities that positively change our brain chemistry and reconfigure our nervous system, we can increase our capacity to deal with harmful stress and be better prepared the next time we encounter it.

Modern-day stressors like financial hardship, caregiver stress, social adversity, childhood trauma, and contentious relationships are forms of chronic stress. For sure, these stressors can harm. But we're stuck in a mindset that believes psychological stress is inherently harmful. In the effort to manage or reduce stress from our lives, we risk inadvertently eliminating the "good" stress that we need for happiness, health, and, ironically, for building resilience to the very stress that we are trying to avoid.

The notion that all psychological stress is harmful goes back a long time. The concept comes from Hungarian endocrinologist Hans Selye. In the

1930s, Selye, who is known as the father of stress research, did a series of experiments on rats. He exposed them to harsh conditions like extreme cold, spinal shock, sublethal doses of toxic agents like formaldehyde and morphine, and even surgical injury. No matter how he stressed them, the poor creatures had a similar response. They developed what he called "general adaptation syndrome": their immune systems failed, they developed bleeding gastro-intestinal ulcers, their adrenal glands enlarged, and, after getting sick, they eventually died. He published his findings in a seminal paper in the journal *Nature* in 1936, and that is how stress, as a medical concept, originated.

In the eighty years since Selye's general adaptation syndrome theory, our methods for measuring stress hormones and our understanding of stress have greatly improved. Now, we know that while life-threatening stress triggers a standard fight-or-flight response, similar to what Selye's rats went through, everyday stressors cause different kinds of stress responses, depending on their type, intensity, and duration. In other words, we don't respond in the same patterned way to every stressor. Different ones activate a range of dif-ferent chemicals and hormones. Some of the ones involved in our response to good stress include dopamine, which increases reward and motivation; endocannabinoids, which help regulate our physical, mental, and emotional response to stress; and oxytocin, which is involved in nurturing and seeking support when stressed. They control behaviors that help us cope and respond in a sophisticated way to a variety of stressors. Our stress responses are in-tended to help us, not to cause harm.

Despite decades of progress in stress research, Selye's theories have per-sisted and are still widely used today. Maybe that's because Selye was very persuasive and spent a good part of his career traveling to spread his ideas and teach medical professionals and the public about his concept of stress. A Google search for "general adaptation syndrome" still brings up 460,000 re-sults that describe stress in the three phases Selye identified: alarm, resistance, and exhaustion. And even though Selye's third stage, exhaustion—where he believed the adrenals tire out and fail to make enough cortisol in the face of intense or prolonged stress—has been replaced by the understanding that cortisol is actually made in excess amounts during chronic stress (an impor-tant concept we will come back to), the disproved theory of "adrenal fatigue" is still used today to explain various symptoms like exhaustion, trouble sleeping, and difficulty concentrating.

The biggest legacy we have from Selye is our fear of psychological stress. From his rat experiments, Selye assumed all stress—*"anything, pleasant or unpleasant"*—would trigger the same triad of ulcers, immune deterioration, and enlarged adrenal glands as the life-threatening stress he inflicted on rats. Furthermore, he extrapolated that we, as humans, respond the same way to stress. However, just as with other hormetic challenges, research on psychological stress shows an inherent paradox: while excessive or chronic amounts can be detrimental, the right amount, in the right duration, with adequate recovery, can be good. It's time to let go of a century-old theory that's been disproved many times. Even Selye acknowledged eustress (good stress) late in his career. Good psychological stress is a valuable internal resource that can contribute to a long, healthy, and purposeful life.

STRESS 2.0: RETHINKING PSYCHOLOGICAL STRESS AND RESILIENCE

The first hint that low to moderate levels of psychological stress might be beneficial to our mental health actually preceded Selye's studies on the harmful impact of extreme stress in rats. In 1908, Robert M. Yerkes and John Dillingham Dodson did a classic experiment to see whether stress could help mice learn a new habit. They found that too little or too much stress slowed habit formation, but moderate stress helped mice learn the fastest. Known as the Yerkes-Dodson law, this finding is often illustrated as a curve shaped like an upside-down U, where performance improves as stress increases to a certain point, after which more stress makes performance worse. This is like finding a "golden mean" in psychological stress. It's similar to Schulz's findings in yeast, which led to the concept of hormesis in biology.

The inverted U-shaped curve is now considered the single most important concept in psychological stress research. Unlike early experiments on rodents, present-day stress experiments, like the Human Connectome Project, use groundbreaking MRI technology to analyze human brain structure, function, and connectivity in unprecedented detail. About a decade ago, Assaf Oshri, PhD, and his team at the University of Georgia used data from this consortium to put hormesis to the test with psychological stress, just as it had been proven with physiological stress. They analyzed data from over twelve hundred young adults that rated their stress levels, tested many aspects of their cognitive function, and assessed their feelings and behaviors. They hypothesized the traditional stress model, which presumes that the harms of stress are linearly proportional to the amount of stress, might not capture the complete picture of how psychological stress affects our cognitive functions. They worked around this blind spot by looking for a Goldilocks amount of stress where stress may paradoxically be beneficial. In 2022, they published a study showing that low to moderate stress helps young adults' cognitive abilities and resilience under stress—a finding that would have been missed without applying the inverted U-shaped hormesis curve to psychological stress.

Dr. Oshri's study showed that everyday stress can make us stronger and more resilient. Think of the process like this: When stress levels increase from low to moderate, our brain undergoes changes that strengthen our cognitive abilities. Our thinking improves, which makes us better at handling challenges. The improvements in our thinking protect us from the negative effects of higher stress levels, so that we not only manage stress better but also build a defense against mental health problems. Far different from Selye's view that all stress is harmful, studies like Oshri's show that stress can have varied effects, with some types increasing our tolerance and safeguarding us against future stress.

The idea of healthy psychological stress may seem contradictory, just like the concept of healthy aging did as recently as the 1980s. Back then, it was considered an oxymoron because most of the literature up to that time had been on the debility and decline that occur with aging. A massive MacArthur Foundation study on successful aging changed that, leading to a surge of studies exploring what helps people age well—a rethinking that led to aging 2.0. In the same way, most stress research has focused on how stress increases vulnerability to mental and physical health problems. Today, we are learning more about what makes stress good—and we are just beginning to understand how measured psychological stress, like physiological stress, works its way down to our cells to make us mentally and physically stronger.

My Surprising Road to Good Psychological Stress

A decade ago, my patient John came to me concerned that stress from his job was damaging his health. John was an engaging and charismatic executive whose work involved intense negotiations and high-stakes, multimillion-dollar decisions. He was particularly concerned about his risk of a heart attack and dying young.

At the time, my first thought was he needed to slow down for his own good. However, as I listened, I could sense the satisfaction and excitement he got from closing deals and bringing new products to consumers. He also used his position to mentor and create opportunities for people who might not have the chance otherwise, which he found very fulfilling. For him, his work was invigorating and meaningful. Was he stressed? Absolutely. He rated his stress level an eight out of ten. Did he believe he handled the stress well? Yes. He rated himself an eight out of ten in dealing with it. He said he seldom felt overwhelmed.

I felt uneasy about simply suggesting that he reduce his stress level. I remembered reading about psychological stress being different when it had to do with altruism, which intrigued me. I wondered if that was true for John. So, I decided to put on my researcher hat and investigate.

Eventually, this led me to design clinical trials measuring stress and resilience through biomarkers and questionnaires and evaluating their association with health and longevity. What I discovered was that stress indeed affects people differently at a biochemical level depending on their stress and resilience hormone levels. We also found that the risk of heart disease associated with stress was greatly influenced by a person's resilience. This meant that even though John had a high level of stress, it wasn't necessarily causing harm. Furthermore, we observed that stress can work hormetically on aging, in some cases beneficially impacting longevity. This suggested that stress wasn't only not harmful in some instances but that certain types and amounts could even be beneficial.

Before understanding stress in this new way, I was a poster child for Selye's message that stress harms and has far-reaching effects on every

part of our body. I even collaborated with the TED team to create a popular video titled "How Stress Can Make You Sick"! However, I learned something from John that I could measure in the research: there are many types
of stress, and they affect each person differently. John didn't feel drained
from stress. He continued to work out regularly and enjoy trips with his family. His tests indicated that he had no signs of early heart disease, and the
level of systemic inflammation in his body was exceptionally low. The "good"
psychological stress from his work may have even helped him develop resilience. There is still much to learn about stress, but we definitely need to
move beyond a one-size-fits-all understanding of its role in our lives.

THE NEUROBIOLOGY OF
GOOD PSYCHOLOGICAL STRESS

The Yerkes-Dodson law and Dr. Oshri's research show us, from a psychological perspective, that good stress improves mental health. The groundbreaking work of Bruce McEwen, who was a world-renowned neuroscientist at
Rockefeller University, explains this psychological principle from a biological
standpoint. His research links stress hormones involved in our sympathetic
nervous system and hypothalamus-pituitary-adrenal (HPA) axis response to
the inverted U concept. McEwen found that stress-related chemicals like
adrenaline and cortisol, which we commonly think of as harmful in high
amounts, can have both protective and detrimental effects, depending on
their dose. This finding perfectly aligns with the inverted U curve that describes our psychological response to stress. Essentially, the same stress
chemicals that contribute to wear and tear during severe or prolonged stress
can help us adapt during moderate, short-term stress. A healthy stress response system is designed in such a way that both too little or too much
cortisol can increase susceptibility to stress, while a moderate amount can
strengthen resistance to it.

Dr. McEwen's research changed how we think about our physiological
response to psychological stress. He saw it as more than an emergency

fight-or-flight reflex. Instead, he redefined it as a system that helps us adapt, similar to our cellular stress response. It's a built-in tool for dealing with challenges and being strengthened by them. When we face real or imagined threats, our conserved nervous system stress response kicks in to restore balance in our body. Through this process, it recalibrates our psychological stress set point, either making us more resilient or, if there is too much cortisol, more vulnerable to stress.

The brain is the epicenter of stress in our body. It decides what is stressful and manages our response to it. Until the 1960s, it was believed that the brain stopped changing after it developed. But in 1968, Dr. McEwen and his colleagues discovered that the brain has receptors for hormones like cortisol, which are known as glucocorticoids. This indicated that stress affects the brain in the same way it affects the body. When stress hormones are at a mild to moderate level, they help brain cells communicate more effectively and increase the brain's adaptability, which helps us learn new things. But if these hormone levels are very high, for example from long-term stress, they have a negative effect. They can reduce resilience and the brain's adaptability by making the communication between brain cells less efficient, and even damage brain cells.

Just as good stress molds our body through bioplasticity, it can also mold our brain through neuroplasticity. This suggests that when you experience stress, your brain doesn't just return to how it was before; instead, it sets a "new normal." Your brain's current state reflects all the stress you've experienced in your life. You can actively reshape your future brain to be more resilient by deliberately exposing yourself to certain types of stress.

The same hormone, cortisol, can have opposite effects on our ability to grow from stress depending on its dose because of the different downstream effects of attaching to distinct glucocorticoid receptors, reflecting the inverted U-shaped pattern of hormesis. The hot spot in the brain where glucocorticoids act is the hippocampus, our learning and memory center. The cells in the hippocampus have two distinct receptors for cortisol. When they are occupied, these receptors act as switches controlling gene expression and other cellular activities, including how mitochondria function. The presence of different receptors allows varying "doses" of stress hormones to have different effects on brain growth. With a mild to moderate amount of stress, cortisol primarily binds mineralocorticoid receptors, which have a high affinity for cortisol. These receptors enhance plasticity at synapses, the connections between neurons that allow them to communicate with each other. Enhancing plasticity is like speaking louder in a conversation, allowing our brain to adapt to new information and learn from the experience. The second class of receptors, glucocorticoid receptors, have lower affinity for cortisol and are not substantially occupied until there is a major surge in glucocorticoids. When they are switched on, they decrease plasticity, turning down the volume of the conversation.

The glucocorticoid and mineralocorticoid receptors also play a key role in rapidly activating and then efficiently turning off our response to psychological stress. Mineralocorticoid receptors are the on switch, helping us remember, assess risks, and select a response strategy. They help us pick the best way to deal with things while conserving our energy. If we perceive danger, more stress hormones are released, and both receptors work together. After stress, glucocorticoid receptors act as the off switch, ending the stress reaction to prevent it from going too far. They help us regulate our reactions and emotions and store the memory of the stress experience, so we can do better next time. This system first works rapidly, triggering cellular responses within minutes, and then through a slower process that controls how a cell's genes are expressed. The latter process takes at least thirty minutes to begin and can last for days or even a lifetime. This on-off mechanism is built into our stress response to keep it short-lived and beneficial. Subsequently, stress can be "memorized" by cells through epigenetic changes, which are alterations to your DNA that don't change the underlying DNA sequence but affect how it's read. These epigenetic changes record your stress history. They are an important way we adapt to progressively higher doses of stress, and how intermittent bursts of stress mold our body to build resilience.

Besides being important for glucocorticoid activity, the hypothalamus is one of only two brain areas where new neurons can grow, a process called neurogenesis. While chronic stress can reduce neurogenesis and impair memory, intermittent, brief stress may help the growth of new neurons. In a fascinating experiment, Daniela Kaufer, an associate professor at the University of California, Berkeley, and then postdoctoral fellow Elizabeth Kirby found that briefly stressing rats by immobilizing them for a few hours stimulated a growth factor that caused new neurons to mature from stem cells two weeks later. When the stressed rats were then given a memory test, they performed better, which they traced to the new nerve cells. Kaufer believes the same happens in humans— that short bursts of stress can improve memory by promoting stem cell growth and differentiation. Our highly conserved psychological stress response, like our cellular stress response, is designed to help us deal with and learn from stress—in a natural biorhythm that likely developed in response to the types of intermittent psychological stress that our ancestors faced.

The discovery that the hippocampus has receptors for stress hormones led scientists to find similar receptors in other brain areas related to thinking and emotions, such as the prefrontal cortex and amygdala. Stress makes the brain reorganize by changing the neuron's branches (dendrites) that receive information. In some brain areas sensitive to stress, these branches retract, while in others, they expand. This ability of the brain to change helps it adapt to and process stress, shaping how we become resilient to stress effects.

In the world of psychology, resilience means being able to handle tough situations well and to adapt and bounce back from stress, even when there's a lot of it. From a biological standpoint, resilience is an active process of re-wiring our brain circuitry. This leads to differences in how we feel, remember things, and make decisions. It lays the groundwork for managing our emotions and actions better and more flexibly when we face stress in the future. It's a process we're just beginning to understand by studying stress at a molecular and cellular level.

Good Psychological Stress Makes
Our Cells Healthier

A hormetic amount of psychological stress can do more than help us cope better with future stress; it can make our cells healthier. In one study, Elissa Epel and her colleagues found that acute low to moderate psychological stress reduced oxidative damage in postmenopausal women who were not chronically stressed at baseline. Early research also indicates that good psychological stress, like exercise, phytochemicals, and intermittent fasting, might improve our mitochondrial health, making us more resilient to chronic diseases and helping us live longer. Interestingly, mitochondria are the parts of our cells that produce stress hormones like cortisol. Therefore, the healthier our mitochondria from physiological stressors, the better we might handle psychological stress. It's all part of the cross-stressor resilience we form when we deliberately expose ourselves to good stress.

USING PSYCHOLOGICAL STRESS AS GOOD STRESS

Each person's brain reacts differently to stress. While some aspects of the response are universal, others depend on your genes and your own history with stress. The stressors you have experienced have contributed to shaping your passive resilience through epigenetics. You cannot change the biological impact of your past experiences, but you can influence your future by seeking new experiences that enhance your ability to handle stress. Your brain's adaptability and plasticity give you the chance to actively build your resilience over your lifetime.

Choosing the Right Kind

Science gives us a very clear picture of "bad" psychological stress: stress that is either unpredictable, like getting a sudden call about your child being injured, or stress that feels uncontrollable, such as a cancer diagnosis. Stress tends to harm us when it's from uncertainty or when we think we can't do anything about it.

Good psychological stress, in contrast, is a choice. By its very nature, it is predictable and controllable. It's stimulating but not overwhelming. It's a challenge that comes with a motivating amount of doubt, where there is potential for reward, but it's not guaranteed. This kind of stress arises from situations that lead to personal growth, inspiration, and a feeling of accomplishment. Good stress sharpens our focus and attention, boosts our confidence, and makes us feel excited. When we anticipate "good" stress, it releases bursts of dopamine in brain areas associated with reward and motivation that interact with our classic fight-or-flight stress response. Examples of good stress include starting a new job, tackling a challenging project, participating in sports, or going on a thrilling adventure.

Another key feature of good psychological stress is that it aligns with our sense of purpose and contributes to the greater good. Steve Cole, a professor of medicine and psychiatry at the University of California, Los Angeles, has spearheaded a field called social genomics, studying how our life experiences affect our cells on a molecular level. He discovered that stress we perceive as threatening, like a cancer diagnosis, activates a specific set of genes in our immune cells. This gene profile, known as the conserved transcriptional response to adversity (CTRA), is linked with inflammation, which can lead to conditions like anxiety, depression, and chronic illness. Cole then went on to show that eudemonic happiness, which comes from feeling purposeful and being part of something bigger, has a healthier impact on our gene expression compared to hedonic happiness, which comes from purely pleasurable activities like enjoying a gourmet meal. Eudemonic happiness showed less expression of the CTRA genes, suggesting that meaningful and socially beneficial pursuits positively affect our biology.

In research our team, led by Dr. Jennifer Mascaro, did with Cole, we found something similar in healthcare workers. Those who were flourishing, meaning they felt a sense of well-being that enabled them to work effectively and make valuable contributions, showed downregulated CTRA pro-inflammatory gene expression. These studies collectively indicate that engaging in meaningful and generative endeavors beneficially affects us at a molecular level. So the right kind of psychological stress involves choice, control, and predictability; stimulates and excites with a degree of uncertainty but not to the point of overwhelm; and aligns with our sense of purpose and social good.

Dosing Psychological Stress

The neurochemistry of good psychological stress shows that stress doesn't need to come close to killing you to make you stronger. In fact, rather than extreme adversity, moderate everyday psychological stress may be optimal for building resilience.

Karen Parker, a scientist at Stanford University, conducted a series of experiments on baby squirrel monkeys that illustrates this theory. She exposed them to short bursts of early life stress by separating them from their mom for an hour each week for ten weeks when they were four months old. Although this wasn't as severe as some forms of trauma, she thought the separated monkeys might become emotionally unstable. She and her team followed these monkeys as they grew up. When they were nine months old, the ones that were separated for short intervals clung less to their moms and explored more when they were placed in a new environment with different food and toys than the monkeys that weren't separated. They showed signs of being less anxious, and levels of stress hormones in their bodies were lower. Their early life stress made them more resistant to subsequent stress. In preadolescence, they had more self-control, and as they got older, they remained more curious and explored new things more than the ones that hadn't been separated.

When scientists looked at their brains, the monkeys exposed to early, intermittent stress had developed resilience through neuroplasticity. Their prefrontal cortex, the part of the brain responsible for decision-making and controlling behavior, was larger in areas that reduce impulsiveness, retain the learning of overcoming fear, and manage and control the response to stressful situations. In other words, their brains adapted to stress by building areas that made them better at handling it.

Experiments like these show that stressful experiences that are challenging but not overwhelming can create a form of stress protection referred to as "stress inoculation"—good stress acts as a vaccine and builds tolerance against more challenging future stress in childhood and beyond. Based on this framework, the dose we are aiming for is moderate. Keep in mind that we each react differently to the *same* psychological stress—the sweet spot of psychological stress for you won't look the same as it will for others. The optimal dose of psychological stress should stretch your comfort zone but not feel overwhelming.

To assess whether you are at a healthy dose of stress, ask yourself: Did the experience increase my belief in my ability to handle stress? Did it leave me feeling alert and energized? Did it encourage creativity and big-picture thinking? Or: Did I feel overwhelmed? Did the situation make me want to fight or flee?

The right dose of good stress should leave you with positive emotions. Much as negative emotions like fear benefit us in threatening situations, positive emotions from good stress provide a survival advantage. They allow problem-solving and psychological flexibility. Our ancestors used the benefits of good psychological stress to navigate new terrain, build new tools, outsmart prey, and conquer their environment. The goal today remains the same—to dose good stress to enhance your mental, emotional, and physical flexibility. Ultimately, the aim is to shift your personal inverted U stress curve toward greater resilience.

How Can You Measure Your Stress Level?

People often believe checking cortisol levels through a blood or saliva test will reveal if they are stressed. However, a single cortisol measurement can provide only limited insight because cortisol levels can fluctuate within minutes and naturally rise in the morning and fall at night. In our studies, we have measured cortisol from hair to get a better estimate of chronic stress levels, as each centimeter of hair from the scalp represents one month of cortisol. Another shortcoming is that cortisol is just one aspect of our stress response.

A practical way to check your stress level is to monitor your heart rate variability (HRV), which can be done with specialized wearable devices or smartphone apps. HRV measures the variation in time between successive heartbeats. It is affected by the balance between your sympathetic nervous system (which activates the fight-or-flight response) and parasympathetic nervous system (which controls "rest and digest"). A higher HRV generally indicates better stress resilience and overall health, whereas a lower HRV may indicate increased stress and a reduced ability to respond flexibly during stress.

Keep It Episodic

A key pillar of what makes stress good is being able to turn off our stress response after a challenge. Just as fasting activates a metabolic switch from glucose to fat metabolism to enable repair and regeneration—and the switching back to glucose metabolism during feeding enables growth—a similar turning on and off of our stress response is critical for resilience. I call this "psychological switching"; it's our body's natural rhythm of switching on and off our response to stress. If the brain gets stuck in the on position and doesn't have the cognitive flexibility to cope with stress, the natural mechanism for resilience is disrupted. Stress becomes chronic, the balance between the receptors gets thrown off, and that makes us more vulnerable to stress.

At the core of our body's response to a challenge, then, whether running from a burning building, public speaking, or courageously expressing ourselves in service of our values, is not just our ability to turn on a stress response to initiate adaptation but also our ability to efficiently turn off this response after the threat is past to avoid overwhelming our system.

Recovery after experiencing good psychological stress is essential to prevent the harms of prolonged stress. Allowing stress hormones like cortisol to return to their baseline levels, instead of remaining continuously elevated, reduces vulnerability to the potential adverse health effects of stress. Recovery is in fact the time that we learn and grow from stress.

The stress response doesn't end immediately after a challenging event. Even after your heart stops racing, stress-recovery hormones continue to be released for a few hours so that you can learn from the experience. The brain releases growth factors, such as brain-derived neurotrophic growth factor, which reinforce neural pathways, and make you more prepared to tackle similar stressors in the future. During this period, purposeful rumination—examining what went well, understanding its significance and outcomes, and contemplating alternative approaches—is part of constructive recovery. This is distinct from repetitive rumination, which is when we worry or brood excessively and can't let go of a real or perceived threat.

◆

We've come a long way from Selye's relentless and largely successful campaign to convince us that all stress is damaging; in fact, we can now see that our physiology requires good psychological challenges in order to grow, heal, and buffer harmful stress. When activated chronically, our elegant fight-or-flight response can indeed harm us, but when we take control and engage it with moderate, manageable psychological stressors followed by recovery, we're actually training our brain like a muscle to be stronger and more flexible so we become better able to handle whatever life throws our way. Good psychological stress expands our capacity to ride the waves of life without going under.

PART III

LIVING LONGER, HEALTHIER, AND HAPPIER

Using Good Stress to Age Better, Fight Illness, and Live Fully

CHAPTER 9

The Hallmarks of Aging

When Good Cells Go Bad

Much as with the study of stress, most research on aging historically focused on the negative aspects of aging, such as debility and decline. That is, until the mid-1980s, when a perfect storm of the most comprehensive aging studies changed our perspective. The MacArthur Foundation study I mentioned last chapter introduced the term "successful aging" for the first time, focusing on factors that enable better functioning as we age; and the Baltimore Longitudinal Study on Aging revealed that we all age at different rates, depending on our genetics, lifestyle, and environment—which, at the time, was groundbreaking. Living proof of this subsequently came from the Blue Zones project, led by Dan Buettner, which found that in the five regions of the world where people live exceptionally long, healthy lives, the inhabitants have remarkably similar lifestyle patterns.

Since then, scientists have discovered specific molecular and cellular changes that occur as we age, providing an even more detailed understanding of aging. In 2013, Carlos López-Otín and his colleagues took on the monumental task of compiling these processes into nine "hallmarks of aging." Each hallmark plays a role in the aging process and, when altered, can speed up or slow down aging. These hallmarks are conserved across different species and represent a significant shift from just observing aging to understanding the actual mechanisms behind it—the accumulation of cellular damage that underlies everything from wrinkles to frailty.

The hallmarks of aging provide us a blueprint for guiding what we need to do to slow down the aging process and its related decline. They offer a way to evaluate how health habits, supplements, or new drugs affect the rate at which we age. These hallmarks are interconnected, so influencing one can change our overall aging trajectory; influencing several could significantly alter how fast we age. The implication is that aging is adaptable, and we can identify ways to control our biological age, which is different from our chronological age. Since aging is the biggest risk factor for common chronic diseases, understanding and altering these hallmarks forms the foundation for extending our healthspan and lifespan.

One of the biggest insights from this longevity research is the connection between our aging biology and our stress biology—which intersect through hormesis. The cellular survival circuits that are activated by stress counter many of the same hallmark processes that lead to aging. In other words, exposing ourselves to good stressors is one of the most effective strategies we have for slowing down the aging process.

A landmark study on Danish twins in the 1990s found that genetics only contributes 25 percent to longevity. Most of how we age is influenced by our lifestyle, environment, and health habits. This means that an overwhelming 75 percent of the aging process is under your control. Although we have known this since the 1990s, what's new is how you can use good stress to remodel the 75 percent that's in your control.

Lifespan Versus Healthspan

Most researchers believe our *maximal* lifespan, which is the number of years a human can live, is around 120 years, with only one person, Frenchwoman Jeanne Calment, exceeding that by living to the age of 122. While some longevity experts predict that we will push this boundary beyond 120 years in our lifetime, the aging process is complex and driven by many interconnected pathways. It's uncertain whether we can find a "master switch" to stop it.

However, longevity scientists agree on the cellular and molecular processes that cause aging, which means that you can slow these processes down to increase your lifespan—or life expectancy—which is the number of years a person is expected to live. The average life expectancy in the

United States in 2021 was 79.1 for women and 73.2 years for men, which is the lowest it has been since 1996. By bridging the gap between your life expectancy and the maximal lifespan, you can gain many more years of life. That is what we are aiming for, and it's a very real and achievable possibility.

Living a long life isn't the only goal. By itself, it may not even be desirable. It's also important to ensure that those extra years are fulfilling and healthy—in other words, to extend healthspan as well as lifespan. If you have ever watched someone close to you suffer a slow and painful decline, you understand the importance of this. The concept of "compression of morbidity" was introduced by Dr. James Fries in 1980, which proposes that we can shorten the period of time that a person spends suffering from illness or disability; in other words, we can live long and then die fast. This goal is the cornerstone of healthy aging, and extending both lifespan and healthspan is where the science of good stress plays a crucial role. You can make sixty the new forty in your cells.

Mark's Story

Mark was a sixty-year-old successful entrepreneur who was at a stage in life where what mattered most to him was living longer and with enough vigor to continue traveling and enjoying his grandchildren. He was in good health, which boded well. However, the absence of disease is different from maximizing health and longevity. His goal was the latter.

We began by testing his cardiorespiratory fitness with a VO_2 max test because, interestingly, research shows this is a stronger predictor of longevity than whether a person has an underlying chronic disease like heart disease or diabetes. He had high expectations for himself and was disappointed to learn that he was in the fiftieth percentile. This meant that he was on a trend of age-related decline that would make it difficult for him to climb stairs in another two decades and may compromise his ability to live independently by his nineties. Fortunately, his muscle mass and strength, also strong predictors of longevity, were in the seventy-fifth percentile. Still, the rate of muscle strength decline per decade with aging wasn't meeting his goal. Additionally, his blood sugar, lipids, insulin, and inflammation levels were normal but not optimal. (These measures and recommended ranges are listed in Chapter 12.) He didn't like the news but was very motivated to improve them. I assured him they were all in his control.

The most powerful way I could help him reach his goals was by incorporating hormetins. One by one, we did that. Over months, he challenged himself to reach the "sweet spot" hormetic zone of maximizing his capacity for cellular regeneration and resisting, repairing, recycling, and recharging his body. When we tested these measures six months later, they had all improved. He was on track toward his goal of optimizing his healthspan and lifespan.

THE PROFOUND CONNECTION BETWEEN GOOD STRESS AND THE HALLMARKS OF AGING

You can view aging as a process of "remodeling" that is shaped by the stress we experience throughout our lives. When we experience good stress, our bodies adapt and remodel at the cellular level; a similar plasticity occurs with our biological age. Good stress helps activate mechanisms that counteract the hallmarks of aging, allowing us to repair DNA, reverse negative epigenetic changes, activate protein chaperones, improve the elimination of damaged proteins and other cellular components, remove aged cells, trigger mitohormesis, activate our nutrient-sensing pathways, rejuvenate stem cells, and reduce inflammation.

Hormesis is a holistic process that doesn't just target one aspect of aging; it combats multiple aging processes. The overlap between aging hallmarks and stress-activated pathways suggests a deep relationship between the stress we experience and how we age. By exploiting the tremendous potential inherent in hormesis, we can age better using our most effective natural antiaging strategies, which align with our evolutionary history.

Take a look at the nine hallmarks of aging and see if some familiar concepts from the science of good stress stand out:

1. **Genomic Instability:** Accumulation of DNA damage over time.
2. **Telomere Attrition:** The protective tips on our chromosomes, called telomeres, wear down, affecting the stability and replication of chromosomes.
3. **Epigenetic Alterations:** Changes to genes that impact their expression.
4. **Loss of Proteostasis:** Loss of ability to eliminate damaged proteins and replace them with healthy ones.
5. **Deregulated Nutrient Sensing:** Impairment in our body's ability to sense and respond to nutrients through insulin, mTOR, AMPK, and sirtuin pathways.
6. **Mitochondrial Dysfunction:** Our mitochondria become less effective at producing energy (ATP) and more prone to releasing harmful reactive oxygen species that cause cell damage. Since mitochondria control cell metabolism and energy, this hallmark plays a disproportionately large role in longevity.
7. **Cellular Senescence:** The buildup of old or damaged cells that can no longer divide but release harmful chemicals that inflame surrounding cells. Factors like shortened telomeres, oxidative damage, and DNA damage can trigger senescence.
8. **Stem Cell Exhaustion:** A decline in our body's ability to regenerate from stem cells due to factors like DNA damage, telomere attrition, and other forms of cellular damage.
9. **Altered Cell Communication:** Changes in how cells communicate, for example, through hormones and nerves. Altered communication can lead to "inflammaging," a persistent low-level inflammation associated with aging. As we age, our gut health can change. The loss of balance in gut microbes contributes to inflammation, which affects stem cell function and other aging hallmarks, and accelerates the aging process. While related to cellular communication, gut dysbiosis and inflammation were added as new hallmarks of aging in 2022.

Sounding familiar? Let's take a look at how each good stress slows these hallmarks.

Phytochemicals

Of the nine molecular and cellular hallmarks, phytochemicals have been found to delay seven: genomic instability, epigenetic alterations, loss of proteostasis, deregulated nutrient sensing, mitochondrial dysfunction, cellular senescence, and altered intercellular communication.

Scientists are zeroing in on the phytochemicals in our top ten list in Chapter 4. For example, a 2019 study analyzed data from 22,811 individuals who were followed for a median of 8.2 years and found that regular chili pepper consumers (at least four times a week) had a 23 percent lower overall mortality risk and over a 50 percent reduced risk of cerebrovascular-related deaths. Similarly, a United States study involving 16,000 participants followed for a median of 18.9 years found that those who consumed hot red chili peppers had a 12 percent lower mortality rate. These are observational studies, and so we can't conclude that chili peppers caused a reduction in mortality, but they support that spicing up your life with the toxin capsaicin may help you live longer.

The toxins quercetin, curcumin, luteolin, and fisetin combat the buildup of senescent cells, which emit harmful pro-inflammatory substances that damage neighboring healthy cells. These compounds act as senolytics, triggering the self-destruction (apoptosis) of senescent cells, thus promoting health and longevity. Pomegranate contains another promising phytochemical, ellagitannins, which our gut converts to urolithin A. This compound rejuvenates cells by activating mitophagy, which clears out damaged mitochondria, countering another aging hallmark. In a study with inactive older adults, urolithin A enhanced mitochondrial health, indicating its potential to promote cellular health in later years.

Exercise

Exercise is the most potent hormetin in our longevity toolkit because a substantial part of our genetic makeup relies on exercise to be expressed optimally.

When we exercise, we activate genes that enhance metabolic efficiency and energy production. Since a significant portion of our genes govern metabolism, regulating how effectively we store and use energy to ensure our cells function optimally, metabolic efficiency plays an outsize role in our health and longevity.

The primary reason exercise is so effective at slowing aging is because it decelerates, at least in part, *all* of the hallmarks of aging. For example, a 2017 study found a stark correlation between exercise and telomere length: people who exercised frequently had telomeres that were nine years biologically younger than those who were more sedentary. Exercise also protects against the age-related decline in regulating the primary nutrient-sensing pathways. By rapidly depleting nutrients and energy, exercise inhibits the mTOR pathway to increase autophagy and removal of damaged proteins, and activates the AMPK and SIRT1 pathways to combat mitochondrial dysfunction and increase stress resistance. Additionally, exercise induces production of reactive oxygen species (ROS) that activate the transcription factor nuclear factor erythroid 2-related factor 2 (Nrf2), which turns on over five hundred genes of our vitagene system. As a result, exercise stimulates our natural ability to produce antioxidant enzymes that reduce cellular damage. Exercise also counters another hallmark, altered intercellular communication and "inflammaging," by stimulating secretion of drug-like molecules called myokines that reduce systemic low-level inflammation.

The list of cellular antiaging effects from exercise on aging hallmarks is long, but perhaps most remarkable is the effect of exercise on our natural, stem cell-based, regenerative capacity. Exercise acts as a potent trigger for the growth and movement of different adult stem cell groups from their original tissue (like bone marrow) to the damaged tissues, where they help in repair and regeneration. For example, regular exercise helps counter the age-related decline in the repair capability of certain cells that help rejuvenate the lining of blood vessels. Exercise also stimulates mesenchymal stem cells, which are versatile origin cells with a range of therapeutic uses (like being carriers for anticancer genes), and encourages the growth of neural stem cells, aiding in brain regeneration and better cognitive functioning.

Heat and Cold Therapy

Heat exposure has been found to slow down the loss of protein homeostasis that occurs as a hallmark of aging. Heat creates low-grade protein damage, just enough to activate the heat shock protein response above baseline levels, leading to the repair of damaged proteins and reducing clumping and disordered proteins. Additionally, heat exposure triggers the process of mitochondrial biogenesis, which slows age-related mitochondrial dysfunction. It also increases endogenous antioxidant enzymes and lowers systemic inflammation, which helps counter additional hallmarks.

Similarly, cold exposure promotes longevity by activating cold shock proteins, which play a key role in maintaining protein balance in response to cold. These proteins activate the proteasome, a cellular complex that disposes of unneeded or damaged proteins and helps maintain proteostasis (protein homeostasis). Like exercise, cold exposure also increases cellular energy demand, leading to the creation of new mitochondria, which counters the age-driven decline in mitochondrial function. Cold exposure also boosts the body's natural antioxidant defenses and reduces overall inflammation, creating a more favorable internal environment for longevity.

The most compelling data on the longevity benefit of heat exposure is from a large study in Finland, a country with more than three million saunas. (That's a Guinness World Record for the most per citizen and enough for every single Finn to be in a sauna at the same time!) The study followed more than twenty-three hundred men for over two decades and found that men who used the sauna two to three times per week had a 24 percent reduced risk of dying from all causes of premature death than people who used the sauna once a week. The risk reduction was even greater for those who used the sauna four to seven times per week. They had a 40 percent reduced risk of all-cause mortality. The duration of sauna sessions also played a role in reducing all-cause mortality. Participants who spent eleven to nineteen minutes per session had a 9 percent reduced all-cause mortality, while those who spent more than nineteen minutes per session had a 17 percent lower risk than participants whose sauna bathing sessions were less than eleven minutes. These results took into account various potential confounding factors, including age, body mass index, systolic blood pressure, serum low-density lipoprotein cholesterol, smoking, alcohol consumption, previous myocardial infarction, type 2 diabetes mellitus, cardiorespiratory fitness and resting heart rate, physical activity, and socioeconomic status.

The Origin of Fasting for Longevity: Calorie Restriction

In the 1930s, nutrition researcher Clive McCay discovered that rats on an approximately 30 percent calorie-restricted diet lived longer and had fewer age-related diseases than those who ate freely. This was among the earliest evidence that limiting food intake was linked to lifespan. Over the next eighty years, this finding was replicated in other animals, such as yeast, worms, flies, fish, rodents, and rhesus monkeys. Studies consistently showed that starving animals without malnutrition increased their lifespan by 30 to 50 percent. However, these animals also became more susceptible to infections and frailty. So, if these organisms were in their natural environment outside a lab, their mortality from calorie restriction may have differed from that observed by these studies. For beings as complex as we humans are, there isn't evidence that calorie restriction has the same longevity effect: we don't live in a lab; we may succumb to frailty and infection from it; and calorie restriction is nearly impossible to sustain for a lifetime for us to study its long-term effects.

While severe calorie restriction isn't feasible for extending our lifespan, the value of these studies is that they led to discovering conserved mechanisms that underly longevity—the primary nutrient and growth signaling pathways of insulin signaling, mTOR, AMPK, and sirtuins. Certain genetic modifications in these pathways were observed to significantly enhance lifespan in model organisms, mirroring the effects of calorie restriction. Since calorie restriction isn't viable long-term, researchers sought alternatives like calorie restriction–mimicking drugs or dietary interventions that could emulate the effects of calorie restriction. Intermittent fasting, which activates these longevity pathways, emerged as a more practical and sustainable approach with potential for similar lifespan benefits.

Intermittent Fasting

Intermittent fasting regulates numerous genes involved in defending against the hallmarks of aging. Cells respond to intermittent fasting by increasing their expression of antioxidant protection, DNA repair, protein quality control, mitochondrial biogenesis, autophagy, and downregulation of inflammation. Studies in humans have shown that intermittent fasting improves healthspan by improving obesity, insulin resistance, dyslipidemia, hypertension, and inflammation. Interestingly, this improvement is greater than what can be attributed just to reducing calorie intake. Although these studies have been short term, conducted over several months, I expect we will see similar findings in longer-term studies. Based on these positive effects on healthspan, intermittent fasting is very likely to extend average lifespan by mitigating common causes of mortality.

Research on calorie restriction has mostly focused on the effects of continuously restricting calories. However, a pattern of restricting calories for a short period followed by unrestricted eating presents a unique benefit. It triggers regenerative processes that are not activated during continuous calorie restriction. Cycles of inhibiting and then reactivating nutrient-sensing pathways powerfully promote a self-renewing rejuvenation process in cells, tissues, and organs. They activate cell death and autophagy, followed by stimulation of stem cells. The refeeding period plays a crucial role in this regeneration process. It facilitates the replacement of senescent or damaged cells with new ones.

These studies on calorie restriction and intermittent fasting suggest that how much and when we eat plays a significant role in our longevity. Certain pharmacological agents that can mimic the effects of calorie restriction are also being investigated for their potential longevity benefits, with the lead ones being metformin (activating AMPK), NAD (activating sirtuins), and rapamycin (inhibiting mTOR). Although they have shown some promise and may have a role in adding healthy years to life, I doubt that their safety and effectiveness will match the benefits of naturally triggering our body's innate longevity pathways in the rhythmic pattern practiced by our ancestors.

Good Psychological Stress

We don't have nearly as much research on the effects of good psychologi-cal stress on longevity as we do of bad psychological stress, but one of the key hallmarks connecting psychological stress and aging is mitochondrial dysfunction. Our bodies react to both good and bad stressful experiences by affecting the health of our mitochondria. The kind, dose, and duration of psychological stress may impact our mitochondria in the inverted U pattern characteristic of hormesis: too little or too much stress may harm our mito-chondria and accelerate aging, while moderate hormetic psychological stress can optimize our mitochondrial health and slow down the aging process.

Much of the research in this area is from studying caregiving and stress. A study on the influence of caregiving stress and daily mood on mitochondrial function found that high stress levels negatively affect mitochondrial health, and that this is likely a key way stress influences cellular aging. Mitochondrial health was measured by a mitochondrial health index, which was a measure of mitochondrial content per cell or mitochondrial functional capacity. The study found that mothers who had an autistic child and experienced higher levels of stress had a lower mitochondrial health index compared to mothers with neurotypical children.

Another key hallmark linking stress and cellular aging is telomere length. A groundbreaking study found that women who were caregivers of a chron-ically ill child and had the highest level of perceived stress had shorter telo-meres, on average by the equivalent of at least one decade of additional aging, compared to women with low perceived stress. Telomeres and mitochondrial dysfunction work together in a reinforcing pattern. Critically short telomeres damage mitochondria, and they can cause cells to enter a state of senescence, where they can no longer replicate or regenerate. Senescent cells can release harmful inflammation and contribute to inflammaging, which can further damage telomeres and mitochondria.

You can see how important it is for caregivers to get breaks—and to bring in good stress challenges to support health and longevity when dealing with chronic stress. In a study I conducted on a group of executives that included CEOs and senior vice presidents of Fortune 500 companies, we found that perceived stress is hormetically associated with biological aging. We asked the executives to rate their stress level over the past month using a standardized questionnaire and similarly measured their resilience as a stress coping ability. Through a single blood sample, we profiled more than eight hundred thousand methylation sites across their genome to calculate their biological age. We found experiencing stress levels comparable to national norms was paradoxically associated with a *younger* biological age than lower amounts of stress among executives with low resilience. This association held even after controlling for other lifestyle factors such as sleep and exercise, which also impact biological age.

◆

Longevity science is uncovering the aging process at a molecular level, revealing the progressive accumulation of cellular damage and dysfunction that occurs as we age; hormesis shows us how good stress works at a cellular level to heal and reverse this damage by directly countering the hallmarks of aging. Hormesis is a giant step forward in our quest for longevity. While much longevity research focuses on pills or supplements to extend life, we often overlook our body's built-in, side effect–free solution: our genetic ability to regenerate from good stress.

CHAPTER 10

Turning Bad Cells to Good

New Ways to Combat the Most Common Killers

When Jen first walked into my office, she appeared frustrated and over-whelmed. She told me she had been healthy most of her life, only struggling with her weight on and off for years. That had changed several months ago, when she was diagnosed with prediabetes, high cholesterol, and high blood pressure. "The thought that keeps running through my head is watching my mother suffer with progressively worse stages of dementia," she said. She was terrified that the same would happen to her. "I haven't been as good at taking care of myself as I should have been." Jen explained that work and taking care of her family had been her priority. She knew she needed to make some changes. She tried cutting out sugar and fast food but kept craving them, espe-cially when she felt stressed. She was trying to take more standing breaks and move more throughout the day. Her frustration was mounting. "I am tired all the time, I don't sleep well, and I am getting sicker," she said. She didn't just want another blood test, a referral to a specialist, or more medication. She wanted to feel good and become healthier.

Every day in my office, I work with patients like Jen who are struggling, along with millions of Americans, with chronic health issues. And if you are among them, I want you to know you don't have to just watch them pro-gress and respond reactively to lessen their complications. You can change their course and possibly even reverse them. And if your goal is prevention, you are very likely to succeed because 80 percent of chronic disease is pre-ventable.

This is where our approach of building cellular resilience shines. It's what drew me to the science of good stress. Using hormetic stress activates your cells' ability to counter the disease processes that are shared by many chronic illnesses. We'll go through the four most common killers— metabolic disease, cardiovascular disease, cancer, and dementia. We'll see how they develop, and I will explain how good stressors work effectively to manage and prevent them, in many ways that are unique to the resilience we build from stress. Once you connect the forms of cellular damage that lead to these diseases, you will see how deeply powerful good stress is not only at tackling them upstream but also at giving you a unified strategy for building your chronic disease defenses.

GOOD STRESS AS MEDICINE FOR
METABOLIC DISEASE

Abdominal obesity, insulin resistance, metabolic dysfunction-associated steatotic liver disease (MASLD), prediabetes, and type 2 diabetes may seem like distinct conditions, but they are progressive stages of metabolic disease and share a common underlying cause: energy intake in excess of expenditure.

At the root of all metabolic disease is insulin resistance, a condition where your cells are less sensitive to insulin. There are many causes of insulin resistance, but, by far, the most common is overloading your body's fat storage capacity. This is not the same as obesity: obesity doesn't necessarily indicate insulin resistance, and you can have insulin resistance if you are not obese. In fact, a large study found that nearly half of young adults with insulin resistance are not obese. The primary problem is that you've exceeded your body's unique storage capacity for fat. We each have a different genetic capacity to store fat where it's meant to be stored, which is in the layer of fat, or adipose, cells that sits just beneath our skin. Even without being obese, you can exceed the genetic capacity of your adipose cells to expand and accommodate more fat.

As the subcutaneous fat cells get stuffed beyond their capacity, they begin to die or function abnormally. They, along with the immune cells within adipose tissue, release inflammatory molecules, resulting in chronic low-grade inflammation that disrupts insulin signaling. Additionally, the subcutaneous fat cells spill triglycerides into the bloodstream, and fat begins to store in places not designed for fat storage, such as the liver, muscles, pancreas, and heart. This leads to a state known as lipotoxicity, where toxic by-products are generated that interfere with insulin signaling, which further contributes to insulin resistance. Fat accumulation in these organs also strains the mitochondria in their cells, compromising their ability to utilize and produce energy efficiently.

Even though insulin resistance is commonly thought of as a disease, it's really more a protective mechanism of your body's organs, especially muscle and liver, to "resist" insulin's signal to build up by storing fat. The body is trying to protect itself from the excessive energy influx that it can no longer safely accommodate. The good news is this process is reversible and good stressors are some of the most powerful ways of restoring insulin sensitivity and reclaiming metabolic health.

Fasting Stress

When you fast, your body switches from using glucose to fat as its primary fuel source. Breaking down excess fat stored in subcutaneous adipose cells is the first step toward reducing inflammation and restoring proper insulin signaling. Less fat in the liver, muscles, and pancreas also decreases lipotoxicity, restoring insulin responsiveness in these critical metabolic organs. Fasting also depletes glycogen (glucose) reserves. This stresses liver and muscle cells, and they activate pathways that make them more sensitive to insulin so they can uptake glucose more efficiently the next time it is available. In other words, the stress primes the cells to be more insulin sensitive so they are better prepared for a drop in glycogen reserves in the future. Last, the stress from fasting triggers adaptations in hormones, and a decrease in leptin and increase in adiponectin further decrease inflammation and insulin resistance. So, how does all this measure up in terms of metabolic health? In one twelve-month study, participants on an intermittent fasting regimen decreased their fasting insulin levels by 52 percent and insulin resistance by 53 percent.

Exercise Stress

When you exercise, muscles use glucose for energy. After exercising, muscles want to restock this energy, so they become more sensitive to insulin. In one small study, just one forty-five-minute session of moderate exercise improved insulin sensitivity, resulting in a greater than threefold increase in the muscles' ability to make glycogen after a carbohydrate-rich meal. Exercise also activates an alternate pathway for glucose uptake into muscle cells that doesn't involve insulin. That makes it a powerful way to lower blood sugar, particularly in people with insulin resistance or diabetes.

Exercise is also the most potent way to increase mitochondrial content and restore their function. This becomes critically important when metabolic health is declining. Poor metabolic health often leads to poor mitochondrial health as fat that spills into muscle and other organs strains the mitochondria in their cells. When mitochondria don't function efficiently, they can't manage glucose or burn fats effectively, which further worsens metabolic health. It's a downward spiral of metabolic and mitochondrial dysfunction that you don't want to get caught in. Exercise disrupts this harmful loop. When you exercise, your muscle cells respond by producing more mitochondria, preparing them to use oxygen and burn fat more efficiently the next time they face exercise stress. The improvement in your mitochondrial health translates to better metabolic health.

Thermal Stress

Cold exposure makes your body produce heat by burning more energy. Brown fat and muscles generate this heat using glucose and fats. As your cells use up energy stores, blood glucose and insulin levels go down. In response, cells increase their sensitivity to insulin to replenish their fuel. A small study showed that living in a mildly cold environment improved response to insulin by 50 percent in healthy young men within a month. Are you noticing a theme? Stress—whether from fasting, exercise, or temperature—is a potent stimulus for reversing insulin resistance and improving metabolic health.

Similarly, heat therapy can help manage metabolic diseases by reducing inflammation, improving insulin sensitivity, and lowering blood sugar levels.

Phytochemical Stress

You can think of phytochemicals as *nutraceuticals*—natural remedies powerful enough to use like pharmaceuticals. Plant phytochemicals improve metabolic health in many ways, including:

- Slowing down the rate the intestines break down and absorb sugars from food.
- Stimulating the pancreas to produce insulin.
- Adjusting how the liver manages sugar.
- Making body tissues more responsive to insulin.
- Reducing oxidative stress and inflammation, both of which contribute to metabolic dysfunction.

Psychological Stress

There's no doubt that elevated cortisol levels from chronic stress can cause abdominal obesity, metabolic disease, and eventually, cardiovascular disease. However, the metabolic effects of psychological stress are different when it's intermittent and followed by recovery. Intermittent psychological stress stimulates the release of catecholamines like epinephrine and norepinephrine, which help break down fat, mobilize energy, and increase heat production in brown fat.

GOOD STRESS AS MEDICINE
FOR CARDIOVASCULAR DISEASE

The primary cause of most cardiovascular diseases is atherosclerosis, a process in which fatty deposits (plaques) accumulate in the walls of arteries, leading them to narrow and lose elasticity. A crucial factor as to whether atherosclerosis develops or causes complications is the integrity of the innermost lining of blood vessels, called the endothelium.

Damage to the endothelial lining, called endothelial dysfunction, is one of the earliest detectable vascular changes in developing atherosclerosis. The endothelium forms a special barrier between the circulating blood and the vessel wall. More than a passive layer of cells, the endothelium is an organ that produces many factors to help blood vessels dilate, reduce inflammation, and prevent clotting and cholesterol plaque buildup. When this lining is damaged, it allows low-density lipoprotein (LDL) to enter the arterial wall, where it can become oxidized and highly inflammatory. Oxidized LDL can then get transformed into "foam cells," which form early fatty streaks. If left unchecked, the process snowballs into more oxidative stress and chronic low-grade inflammation. Over time, the fatty streaks grow into progressively larger cholesterol plaques that reduce blood flow and can eventually rupture, precipitating a heart attack or stroke.

(Can you measure chronic low-grade inflammation and your vascular health? Yes! Check out Chapter 12: Getting Out of Your Comfort Zone.)

Fasting Stress

Intermittent fasting can help reduce the risk factors for cardiovascular disease by improving blood sugar and insulin resistance, reducing abdominal obesity, and decreasing cholesterol and blood pressure levels. What's interesting is that the reduction in blood pressure may be from activation of the parasympathetic system by brain-derived neurotrophic factor (BDNF), which doesn't depend on weight loss.

Beyond reducing risk factors, intermittent fasting can improve the health of endothelial cells. It can increase their production of nitric oxide, a molecule made by the endothelium that is crucial for dilating blood vessels, reducing inflammation and oxidative damage, and preventing blood clots. A study showed that in men with heart disease, intermittent fasting significantly increased the production of nitric oxide, which is important because when the endothelium is damaged, it produces less of this magic molecule, leading to atherosclerosis and an increased risk of heart attacks and strokes. Additionally, intermittent fasting reduces inflammation, reflected in lower levels of inflammatory markers like homocysteine and C-reactive protein, and reduces oxidative stress, both of which help slow the progressive buildup of cholesterol in arteries. Intermittent fasting also has an impact on the balance of hormones produced by fat cells, which further reduces damage from immune cells. Moreover, intermittent fasting helps prevent macrophages from turning into foam cells, limits the buildup of harmful substances in blood vessels, and reduces the movement of endothelial cells into the inner layer of arteries, all of which are crucial steps in developing atherosclerosis.

Exercise Stress

The way the heart and blood vessels adapt to cycles of exercise stress and recovery is remarkable. During exercise, the heart has to work harder due to increased blood flow and blood pressure. To handle this extra work, it adapts by making its cells bigger, which remodels the heart to grow larger, and it becomes stronger to pump more blood into the circulation. During this growth, muscle cells in the heart create new mitochondria, which makes the heart muscle more efficient at producing energy to meet the increased demands of exercise.

Blood vessels also get stronger and healthier from the intermittent stress caused by exercise. The increase in blood flow puts a special kind of stress, called shear stress, on the walls of the blood vessels. This stimulates the endothelium to adapt by producing more nitric oxide, which results in more widening and anti-inflammatory, antioxidant, and anti-clotting protection. The stress also triggers an increase in endothelial progenitor cells, a type of stem cell that's like a repair worker. These cells fix and renew the endothelium, especially when it's damaged by aging, high blood pressure, diabetes, or atherosclerosis. That means that when you exercise, you activate your ability to repair and regenerate your endothelium.

Phytochemical Stress

Phytochemicals that activate cellular stress responses can help prevent and treat cardiovascular disease:

- Flavonoids, including quercetin, EGCG, luteolin, and genistein, are particularly effective at preventing endothelial dysfunction. These phytochemicals can be found in foods such as cocoa, apples, tea, citrus fruits, and berries. Consuming these foods can improve the production of nitric oxide in your blood vessels and reduce your overall cardiovascular risk, whether you are healthy or at risk. They can even improve endothelial dysfunction in the face of bad stress from a high-fat or high-sugar meal.
- Sulforaphane is a compound found in cruciferous vegetables like broccoli, cabbage, cauliflower, and kale. It activates a defense mechanism against oxidative stress and can treat cardiovascular disease by scavenging free radicals and reducing inflammation.
- Allicin, found in garlic, onions, and leeks, lowers cholesterol.
- Curcumin, found in turmeric, reduces blood pressure and prevents platelets from clumping, which could lead to a blood clot and cause a heart attack or stroke.

Thermal Stress

The most convincing study to date on the cardiovascular health benefits of sauna bathing is the Kuopio Ischemic Heart Disease Risk Factor (KIHD) Study, which followed more than twenty-three hundred Finnish men for over two decades. The risk of fatal cardiovascular disease was 50 percent lower in men who used a sauna four to seven times per week compared to those who used it only once per week. Regular sauna use can decrease blood pressure and improve endothelial function within two to twelve weeks. At a molecular level, heat stress can positively influence pathways that increase nitric oxide production, reduce oxidative stress, and decrease vascular inflammation. Heat shock proteins (HSPs) are believed to play a role in these improvements, and their activation might be the main reason behind the hormetic benefits of heat therapy on cardiovascular function.

Psychological Stress

Stress that is chronic, such as work stress or private life stress, is underappreciated as a risk factor for cardiovascular disease. However, in studying the role of resilience, I've found that resilience is a strong protector against heart disease, and our results suggest that building resilience is a way to mitigate chronic stress-related heart disease. Other researchers have similarly found that positive psychological well-being is consistently protective against cardiovascular disease, independent of traditional risk factors.

When you participate in activities that you find stressful but fulfilling and rewarding or give you a sense of purpose—whether it's a personal passion, a professional achievement, or a creative endeavor—your stress response triggers the release of endogenous opioids, including endorphins, in the brain. These natural opioids help improve endothelial function and reduce the negative effects of cortisol and pro-inflammatory cytokines. Additionally, performing acts of kindness or helping others also releases endogenous opioids in the brain, commonly referred to as the "helper's high." There is a beautiful interconnectedness in our biology—being kind not only benefits others but also has a positive impact on your own heart health.

GOOD STRESS AS MEDICINE FOR CANCER

While we have made significant strides in early detection and treatment, cancer continues to be the second leading cause of death in the United States and globally. Nearly two million cases of new cancers are diagnosed each year in the United States, and around six hundred thousand people will die from the disease. The encouraging news is that our lifestyle choices impact our cancer risk more than our genetic makeup. We have the power to be proactive about lowering our chances of developing cancer. Good stressors can help combat cancer at every stage, from preventing it and slowing its spread, to improving treatment responses and reducing its recurrence.

Cancer cells behave differently from normal cells in many ways. They can metabolize nutrients differently, avoid detection by the immune system, and escape the usual process of cell death. Under normal conditions, these characteristics enable them to grow uncontrollably. However, good stressors can challenge these advantages, potentially weakening cancer cells.

Fasting Stress

Cancer is traditionally viewed as a disease arising from genetic mutations. However, the way cancer cells process energy—their metabolism—is also crucial in how they grow and survive. From our perspective, this matters because we can use good stress to have some control over this aspect of cancer.

When people fast, there's less glucose available in their bodies. Normal cells can adapt to this because they can switch to using other energy sources. Cancer cells, on the other hand, reprogram their metabolism to use a unique energy system that depends on glucose for rapid replication. This makes cancer cells less metabolically flexible, and unlike healthy cells, many cannot readily use ketones for energy. As a result, fasting can weaken cancer cells and make them more susceptible to chemotherapy. Note, however, that the response varies depending on the type of cancer. Moreover, when energy supplies are low during fasting, normal cells halt their growth and shift to repair and housekeeping functions, while cancer cells continue to grow and proliferate. This difference is another way fasting can protect healthy cells during chemotherapy treatment while cancer cells remain vulnerable. In addition to potentially improving efficacy and reducing toxicity of treatments, fasting may reduce recurrence in some cancers. For example, a 2016 study found that women who fasted less than thirteen hours per night were 36 percent more likely to experience a breast cancer recurrence than those who fasted more than thirteen hours.

Meal timing is also more important than we may realize. Disrupting our natural body clock, or circadian rhythm, has been classified by the World Health Organization as a probable carcinogen in humans. Our built-in repair systems, such as DNA repair and autophagy, are scheduled to work most efficiently at specific times within our circadian rhythm. Optimizing our circadian rhythm may give cells more time to repair damage properly.

Exercise Stress

Exercise helps fight cancer in multiple ways, but I think the most impactful are how it affects metabolism, making it harder for cancer cells to grow and survive; and the body's immune system, by sending specific immune cells on a search-and-destroy mission.

When we exercise, we use a lot of glucose for energy. Cancer cells also need glucose to grow and survive. So during exercise, they have to compete with the rest of the body for this precious energy source. This competition may divert energy away from high-energy-utilizing tumors to other active tissues, leaving tumors energy deprived.

Exercise can also activate immune system cells that are specialized to be natural attackers, such as cytotoxic T cells (also known as CD8+ T cells) and natural killer (NK) cells. We all have these immune cells working for us, and they can recognize and destroy cancer cells. However, cancer cells have clever ways they can put the "brakes" on these immune cells. Exercising can increase the presence of these immune cells in the bloodstream and potentially help them reach cancer sites. A 2023 study on newly diagnosed breast cancer patients found that even a single ten-minute exercise session increased CD8+ T cell count by 34 percent and NK cells by 130 percent. The more intense the exercise, the more immune cells were mobilized. Additionally, exercise and fasting can change the tumor microenvironment. The unique glucose-using metabolism of tumor cells creates an acidic environment around tumors that can evade immune cells. Exercise can reduce this immune suppression by competing for glucose and reducing acidity, making cancer cells more "visible" to the immune system.

Phytochemical Stress

The National Cancer Institute has found more than one thousand phytochemicals with the potential to prevent cancer, based on laboratory studies. Cancer develops in multiple stages, and phytochemicals can intervene at each stage to reduce the chance of it developing and progressing from an early phase to malignancy. They can detoxify and remove carcinogens from the body; block the DNA damage they might cause; lower inflammation, which is linked to cancer development; induce the death of potentially cancerous cells; block abnormal cells from multiplying; inhibit cancer cells from invading other tissues and spreading; and stimulate the body's immune system to defend against cancer. While they might not completely prevent cancer, phytochemicals can significantly lower its risk, much like other good stressors. More than 250 population-based studies show that people who consume about five servings of fruit and vegetables a day have about a 50 percent lower cancer risk, especially cancers related to digestive and respiratory systems, compared to those who consume less than two servings.

Psychological Stress

Improving your ability to cope with psychological stress can have a positive impact on how stress hormones influence tumor initiation and growth and the immune system's ability to fight cancer. In other words, stress resilience could lead to better cancer outcomes. Adopting good stress strategies to improve psychological stress resilience can also improve the response to cancer therapies. If your resilience is low, especially in the face of cancer, remember that good stressors work collaboratively. You can consume a diet rich in phytochemicals, such as the Mediterranean diet, which, unlike consuming a Western diet, is linked to increased psychological resilience.

Thermal Stress

In 2022, a study published in the journal *Nature* showed for the first time that cold exposure could markedly hinder the growth of tumors. Mice kept at 39°F

(4°C) had an 80 percent reduction in tumor growth twenty days after being inoculated with a tumor compared to mice in an 86°F (30°C) environment. The effect is attributed to cancer cells' dependence on glucose. Cold exposure triggers heat production in brown fat, which draws glucose from the blood to fuel brown fat, and consequently slows down cancer growth. An initial human trial in a cancer patient showed that mild exposure to cold significantly activated brown adipose tissue (BAT) activity and reduced glucose uptake by tumor cells.

Heat can be another incredibly simple and effective way to enhance the effects of chemotherapy and radiation therapy. Hyperthermia treatments can increase the sensitivity of cancer stem cells to radiation, disrupt tumor cells' ability to repair radiation damage, enhance the delivery of chemotherapy, and strengthen the immune system's ability to attack cancer cells. While there is not enough evidence to say that sauna use offers the same benefits as medical hyperthermia treatments, sauna can help with pain relief, stress reduction, and overall well-being during cancer treatments.

GOOD STRESS AS MEDICINE AGAINST NEURODEGENERATIVE DISEASE

Neurodegenerative diseases, of which Alzheimer's dementia is the most common, are a group of disorders that lead to progressive deterioration of brain cells and their connections, which ultimately changes the structure and functionality of the nervous system. The human brain has eighty-six billion brain cells, or neurons, that connect to each other through thousands of connections, called synapses. Conditions like insulin resistance, metabolic syndrome, and vascular disease can increase the risk for developing Alzheimer's disease by contributing to loss of synaptic connections and neuronal death, particularly in brain regions crucial for memory and cognitive functions, such as the hippocampus and cerebral cortex. Intermittent good stress followed by recovery helps counter the risk from these conditions by increasing brain growth factors that stimulate neuroplasticity, creating new and stronger connections between brain cells, and neurogenesis, which involves growing new brain cells.

Good stressors offer another unique advantage: they make neurons more resistant to cellular injury, which helps them better withstand changes associated with Alzheimer's disease. The cellular processes involved in Alzheimer's include neuroinflammation and mitochondrial dysfunction, oxidative stress, and impaired clearance of damaged proteins in neurons. Good stressors activate cellular stress responses that reduce neuroinflammation and oxidative damage, repair and recycle damaged molecules and proteins, and improve mitochondrial energy efficiency. As a result, they not only safeguard against disease but also improve cognitive functions like thinking, memory, and mood. In other words, lack of good stress is an overlooked risk factor for cognitive impairment and dementia. I strongly believe that we need good stressors to keep our brain health optimal throughout life.

Psychological and Mental Stress

One of the most fascinating findings is that up to a third of people who have a high amount of plaques and tangles in their brain at autopsy, which are hallmark findings associated with devastating cognitive impairment, do not exhibit clinical symptoms of dementia during their lifetime. Part of the reason may be that the more we engage in intellectually challenging real-life experiences, such as professional work or recreational activities, the more we develop what is known as "cognitive reserve."

By continuously exposing our brains to cognitive challenges, we can "exercise" circuits in our brains and push them to adapt to mental stress. Such activities help build a buffer for the brain, enabling it to better cope with and compensate for any damage it might suffer. Enriching activities help by increasing synaptic activity, which stimulates the brain to produce growth factors, such as brain-derived neurotrophic factor (BDNF). They also promote mitochondrial biogenesis, DNA repair, and the creation of protein chaperones that aid in the proper functioning of other proteins within brain cells. A study that analyzed data from over twenty-nine thousand people across twenty-two papers found that cognitive reserve reduced the risk of developing dementia by 46 percent. This effect was proportional to the "dose," and the benefits were consistent throughout all stages of life. Our research on late middle-aged adults found that whether a person had a purpose in life, which often involves intellectual challenges, was an even better predictor of cognitive decline than having a family history of dementia, underscoring the importance of good stress.

Fasting Stress

The ability to learn, reason, and remember depends on processing signals across synapses, forming and pruning them, and creating new neurons. This brain remodeling requires an enormous amount of energy. While the energy our neurons use gives us, as humans, distinctively advanced cognitive abilities, it also makes the brain vulnerable to disruptions in its energy supply.

The brain's primary fuel is glucose. Glucose is delivered to the brain via transporters in the blood-brain barrier, which selectively allows nutrients in and toxins out. However, an inadequate amount of glucose can get delivered to the brain from lowered glucose uptake through these transporters, which can happen with central insulin resistance or from age-related changes that reduce blood flow to the brain. This causes an "energy crisis" in neurons, leading to a cascade of events, including oxidative stress, neuroinflammation, and mitochondrial dysfunction, which can damage and destroy neurons.

Fasting helps protect against this energy crisis. When glucose supply is limited, the brain can use ketones as an alternate energy source. Besides serving as an energy source, ketones, especially beta-hydroxybutyrate, can directly inhibit oxidative stress, neuroinflammation, and mitochondrial dysfunction. Fasting also upregulates brain growth factors such as brain-derived neurotrophic factor (BDNF) and clears abnormal proteins through autophagy, which further helps reduce neurodegeneration.

Phytochemical Stress

In a 2018 study, Martha Clare Morris and her colleagues found that individuals who consumed one to two servings of green leafy vegetables per day had a rate of cognitive decline that was the equivalent of being eleven years younger compared to those who rarely or never consumed them. Green leafy vegetables, such as spinach, kale, collard greens, and lettuce, are a rich source of lutein, folate, vitamin E, beta-carotene, and flavonoids, which may work together to slow some of the processes implicated in Alzheimer's dementia, such as tau phosphorylation, oxidative damage, mitochondrial dysfunction, and neuroinflammation.

Berries, particularly blueberries, also offer strong protection for the brain. They are uniquely high in flavonoids, which include quercetin, luteolin, genistein, and EGCG. Flavonoids can cross from the blood to the brain to influence proteins critical for brain cell activity. Other phytochemicals, such as sulforaphane in broccoli, cauliflower, and cabbage and resveratrol in dark chocolate, grapes, and peanuts, also work in various ways to reduce beta-amyloid and phosphorylated tau proteins, in addition to activating antioxidant, anti-inflammatory, and other stress responses that make neurons more resistant to injury.

· Exercise Stress

During prolonged exercise, the brain's production of brain-derived neurotrophic factor (BDNF) increases two- to threefold, promoting the formation of new brain cells and connections, particularly in the hippocampus and cerebral cortex, which are areas that Alzheimer's disease most commonly affects. While aerobic workouts, particularly with high-intensity exercise stress, have the strongest evidence for brain health, resistance training and other forms of exercise have also been linked with improved cognitive function. An analysis including nearly 164,000 people showed that those with the highest level of exercise had as much as a 45 percent reduced risk of developing Alzheimer's disease. Although exercise has the greatest benefit for prevention, numerous studies have found aerobic exercise can also improve cognitive function in older adults with mild cognitive impairment and Alzheimer's dementia.

Thermal Stress

The data linking sauna use to heart health is just as compelling for brain health. Using a dry sauna four to seven sessions per week, for at least twenty minutes, can lower the risk of Alzheimer's disease by 65 percent. Thermal stress may help prevent dementia by increasing the production of heat shock proteins. A common problem in diseases like dementia is the buildup of damaged and improperly folded proteins in the brain. Heat shock proteins act like helpers, preventing the accumulation of these harmful proteins and maintaining the balance needed for the brain to function properly. Heat therapy also increases blood flow to the brain, reduces chronic low-grade inflammation, and improves metabolic health. It may be a particularly good option for risk reduction in people who cannot be physically active.

THE FUTURE OF MEDICINE

As we learn more about good stress and develop ways to measure cellular health, such as monitoring the efficiency of mitochondria and levels of autophagy, we can better individualize good stress prescriptions with the optimal kind, dose, and frequency. Modern technologies are empowering us to move from a "one-size-fits-all" approach in medicine toward personalizing care, where you and your physician can adjust the dose of good stressors with greater precision. They are also showing the importance of reintroducing the natural good stressors that are missing in our modern lives. The advantage of good stressors is that using them to improve any of these common chronic conditions will also improve the course of the others. They are accessible and affordable ways to reduce human suffering, decrease mortality rates, increase lifespan, and ease the social and financial strain caused by chronic disease, which will continue to be a major challenge in most societies in the future.

CHAPTER 11

Living in Balance

The Cellular Connection to a Better Life

We've been wrong about what our job is in medicine.
We think our job is to ensure health and survival, but really,
it is larger than that. It is to enable well-being, and
well-being is about the reasons one wishes to be alive.
—Atul Gawande, *Being Mortal: Medicine and What Matters in the End*

Our aim is not just to prevent disease and make life longer, but also to make each day better by improving the quality. By that I mean our mood, pain level, quality of sleep, energy level, digestive symptoms, motivation, and happiness. However, because medicine often struggles to effectively address these components (as they typically respond better to changes in behavior rather than medication), many people suffer from these symptoms for years.

Beyond health and longevity, good stressors can rapidly improve well-being, often within days or weeks. In addition to activating our cellular stress responses, good stressors influence two vital ancient cellular networks intimately tied to our well-being: the endocannabinoid system and the gut microbiome. These systems coevolved with our adaptive responses to good stress and have far-reaching effects throughout our body. Their main function is to maintain our body's balance, or homeostasis. When our body is balanced, we are not only healthier but also feel better. By calibrating these critical internal systems, good stressors amplify their effect on our life quality.

Sally's Story

When Sally came to see me, she was having pain in her hips and knees. She was doing exercises her physical therapist had given her but was needing nonsteroidal anti-inflammatory medications daily for pain. She didn't like the idea, but she was trying to put off surgery, which her orthopedic doctor said she would need eventually. The pain was getting her down and limiting her ability to do things she loved, like going on hikes and gardening.

I suggested a different approach to help with joint pain and mood by focusing on systemic inflammation and neurotransmitter imbalance. Instead of directly treating her joints, we decided to support her endocannabinoid system and improve balance in her gut bacteria. To this end, we introduced potent phytochemicals in turmeric and green tea to help with gut dysbiosis. I shared my favorite smoothie and latte recipes. I explained how endocannabinoids influence pain perception and feeling good, and suggested that if she was willing, she could increase her levels through cold immersion. She was apprehensive but said that her neighbor had recently purchased an ice plunge and swore by it, making her curious. We also discussed doing daily acts of kindness to reduce her cortisol level and help her endocannabinoid system and gut function more efficiently.

The next time I saw her, Sally told me she couldn't believe it when she woke up one morning without pain and stiffness. She also felt her stress level was lower, and in retrospect, she realized that the chronic family stress she had been dealing with had been escalating her pain and inflammation. She was glad to be in a much better place.

THE GOOD STRESS–ENDOCANNABINOID CONNECTION

Although not widely known, the endocannabinoid system is one of the most crucial systems in our body. Discoveries since the 1990s suggest this vast network is the master regulator of homeostasis, affecting how we feel hunger, learn information, regulate body temperature, manage pain, balance mood and energy, digest food, and sleep. The endocannabinoid system consists of three parts: endocannabinoids, which are chemical compounds we make; enzymes that make and break down these compounds; and cannabinoid receptors that activate certain signals when endocannabinoids attach to them.

Endocannabinoids, as their name suggests, are similar to the cannabinoids found in cannabis. The prefix "endo" means our bodies naturally make these cannabis-like molecules. The first endocannabinoid discovered was anandamide, named after the Sanskrit word "ananda," meaning joy or bliss. A handful of others have since been found.

Cannabinoid receptors are on cells throughout our brain and body. Cannabinoid type 1 (CB1) receptors are most densely packed in the brain. They act like air traffic controllers, directing and adjusting the levels of most neurotransmitters so that when a body system is out of balance, they help correct the problem. Once balance is restored, enzymes break down the endocannabinoids to prevent overcorrection. A second type of cannabinoid receptor, called CB2 receptors, are mainly in immune cells. They can regulate inflammation and other immune functions to lessen the effects of autoimmune conditions and adjust intestinal inflammation, motility, and pain.

The endocannabinoid system has likely evolved over five hundred million years. However, we are still learning many of its potential roles. For example, chronic pain conditions like fibromyalgia, irritable bowel syndrome, and migraines, which can be hard to treat, may be due to a lack of endocannabinoids. By supporting our endocannabinoid system, good stressors can impact many ways we feel and function.

The Science Behind the Wim Hof Method
and Adapting to Cold Stress

You may have heard of Wim Hof, the "Iceman," known for his ability to withstand extreme cold temperatures for long durations. He is the perfect case for studying how the body adapts to cold challenges. Using a functional MRI brain imaging technique, researchers found that his Wim Hof Method—a combination of forced breathing, cold exposure, and meditation—masterfully activates hormesis. The stress response happens when changes in his oxygen level and cold exposure activate a part of the brain called the periaqueductal gray. This area is a primary control center for how we perceive pain. It releases endocannabinoids, leading to a stress-induced analgesic response. The endocannabinoids not only act as natural painkillers but also play a role in the good feeling and reduced anxiety we get from cold exposure. Other studies have similarly shown that cold exposure increases endocannabinoid levels and the density of CB1 receptors in the brain. The endocannabinoid system plays a central role in helping us adapt to repeat cold challenges and reap its benefits. The communication between good stress and the endocannabinoid system makes cold therapy a useful method for managing pain and inflammation, especially after exercise and in arthritis and rheumatologic conditions.

"Cannabimimetic" Plants

If the *Cannabis sativa* plant (i.e., cannabis) can hijack our endocannabinoid system, can other edible plants work similarly?

The cannabis plant contains compounds called phytocannabinoids, with THC (tetrahydrocannabinol) and CBD (cannabidiol) being the most well known. These phytocannabinoids are a type of phytochemical, which the cannabis plant makes as part of its defense against parasites and herbivores. (They haven't deterred humans!) Other plants make phytochemicals that mimic the actions of cannabinoids found in the cannabis plant, called cannabimimetics. They either stimulate or inhibit cannabinoid receptors, or prevent the breakdown of endocannabinoids. Although the discovery of cannabimemetics is relatively new, plants likely make cannabimimetic phytochemicals for their own defense. When we consume these compounds, they benefit us by acting on our endocannabinoid system, suggesting cannabimimetics may work through xenohormesis. Apples, blueberries, kale, broccoli, grapes, red onions, and tomatoes are some of the fruits and vegetables that contain cannabimimetic phytochemicals.

For instance,

- Curcumin, resveratrol, EGCG, and quercetin may either attach to cannabinoid receptors or increase their activity.
- Genistein inhibits the enzyme that breaks down anandamide, prolonging its pleasant effects in our system.
- And, if you crave the feel-good effect of chocolate, an intriguing theory is because dark chocolate and cocoa powder contain small amounts of anandamide and compounds like N-oleoylethanolamine and N-linoleoylethanolamine that may mimic the effects of anandamide and slow its breakdown, allowing it to circulate longer in the body.

Although cannabimimetics are a fascinating discovery, there's not enough research to tell whether the amounts in these foods are sufficient to make a difference in our health or how much we would need to consume to get a healing or pleasurable effect.

Runner's High

I have been a runner since my middle school years and run avidly because it makes me happy, relaxed, and almost euphoric—commonly known as the runner's high.

Exercise stress produces endocannabinoids in your body. The sweet spot, based on studies, is running for thirty to forty-five minutes at a pace that is 70 to 85 percent of your maximum heart rate, where you can talk in short phrases or breathy sentences. During exercise, the endocannabinoid system sends signals to stimulate the parasympathetic nervous system, which helps restore balance with the sympathetic nervous system. These endocannabinoids act as short-term "circuit breakers" in response to stress and help to reduce pain and create a feeling of a high, which might have helped our ancestors endure running long distances. This is an additional way exercise acts as a good stress, using the endocannabinoid system to lessen pain, alleviate anxiety, and improve well-being.

For a long time, scientists thought that endorphins, our body's natural painkillers, were responsible for the happy feeling we get from exercise. Endorphins are naturally produced opiates that work much like morphine to reduce pain, but they are large molecules that cannot cross the blood-brain barrier to reach the brain, where the "high" feeling happens. We now know that endocannabinoids, which are smaller, can get to the brain and create this exercise stress–induced high.

Feeling Good by Doing Good

Keeping psychological stress in a hormetic range helps your endocannabinoid system work more efficiently. Short-term good stress activates signals between CB1 receptors and endocannabinoids, which can reduce the potential harm from stress. In contrast, chronic stress with high cortisol levels can have the opposite effect, reducing CB1 receptors and their ability to bind to endocannabinoids. This weakens the signals from the endocannabinoid system and contributes to the negative effects of chronic stress. The relationship between stress and the endocannabinoid system works both ways. Different kinds of stress fine-tune the endocannabinoid system, and maintaining a well-functioning endocannabinoid system provides resilience against stress. As a regulator of homeostasis, the endocannabinoid system, when functioning at its best, prevents the unnecessary activation of stress responses and helps return the body to baseline after a threat has passed. This reduces the wear and tear caused by stress. In other words, the stress-endocannabinoid connection is crucial to nurture because the endocannabinoid system plays a role in nearly every aspect of our biology, with its regulation of our stress responses being one of the most significant.

My favorite way of keeping stress in a hormetic range to optimize the endocannabinoid system is doing small acts of kindness on a daily basis. The upside of this type of good stress is that it raises oxytocin (the "cuddle hormone" involved in social bonding and trust), dopamine (the "reward hormone" related to pleasure and motivation), and serotonin (the "calming hormone" that regulates mood, anxiety, and happiness)—the trifecta for buffering our cortisol levels. Helping others gave our ancestors a survival advantage because it gained trust and social cohesion. Our brains are wired to motivate us to do good, and this, in turn, improves our well-being.

Fasting and Endocannabinoids

The hormetic cycle between fasting and feeding changes the levels of endocannabinoids in the brain. These endocannabinoids help control our hunger, desire to eat, and our metabolism. Most of our understanding of how fasting affects the endocannabinoid system comes from animal studies. We also know that what you eat during recovery is important. Endocannabinoids are made from polyunsaturated fatty acids. So, eating plant foods rich in omega-3s, like flaxseed, walnuts, chia seeds, and avocados, not only activates hormesis but also supports your endocannabinoid system.

THE GOOD STRESS–GUT AXIS

Our stress responses developed alongside another ancient system: our gut microbial ecosystem. Our gut is home to about a hundred trillion microorganisms, mainly bacteria but also viruses, fungi, and other single-celled organisms such as archaea and protozoa. Together, they form our gut microbiota, which influences our immune system, neurotransmitters, metabolism, hormones, and even our gene expression. The gut microbiome, the collective genome of these microorganisms, is estimated to be a hundred times larger than our human genome.

Stress—good and bad—influences our gut microbial composition. A poor diet, sedentary lifestyle, or chronic psychological stress can lead to dysbiosis, an imbalance from too much harmful bacteria or loss of good bacteria. This can cause a leaky gut and inflammation throughout the body, leading to symptoms like bloating, cramping, fatigue, mood imbalance, constipation, diarrhea, food sensitivity, anxiety, and depression.

Good stressors, on the other hand, support gut health by promoting balance and diversity in our microbiota. This creates a healthier gut ecosystem, which amplifies the benefits of good stress. A balanced gut keeps the body in homeostasis and protects against symptoms that can compromise quality of life.

Phytochemicals for a Balanced Gut

The composition of bacteria in your gut is greatly influenced by the amount of good edible stressors, or phytochemicals, in your diet. Phytochemicals are key players in gut health, just like fiber. Since they don't get absorbed quickly, they remain in the gut for a longer time. This is actually a good thing because it gives them time to improve our gut microbial community. Phytochemicals promote the growth of beneficial bacteria and suppress harmful ones. Luteolin, EGCG, quercetin, genistein, curcumin, ferulic acid, resveratrol, and allicin are some of the phytochemicals that help balance our gut ecosystem. The more of these you consume, the better it can be for your gut.

Interestingly, the health benefits of most phytochemicals (especially the largest family of phytochemicals called polyphenols) come from the by-products created when gut bacteria interact with the unabsorbed phytochemicals rather than from the phytochemicals in the form present in food. This process is another way phytochemicals work with our gut bacteria to improve our health and well-being.

Making Gut Bacteria Fitter with Exercise Stress

Exercising at the right intensity and duration, followed by adequate recovery, benefits physical and mental well-being, and part of the reason may be through its beneficial effects on gut bacteria. Exercising for thirty to sixty minutes three times a week for six weeks can change gut microbial composition, even in people who were previously inactive. A 2018 study found this amount of exercise also increases the production of butyrate, an important short-chain fatty acid (SCFA) produced when gut bacteria ferment fiber. Butyrate is a key energy source for gut cells, improves the gut wall barrier, has anti-inflammatory and antioxidant properties, and can protect intestinal stem cells, which help repair and regenerate the gut wall. However, if you stop exercising, the improvements in gut health can disappear, so you need to exercise regularly to maintain these benefits.

Athletes have more beneficial bacteria like *Faecalibacterium prausnitzii* and *Akkermansia muciniphila* and higher levels of SCFAs like butyrate compared to non-exercisers. Higher fitness levels, measured by high VO_2 max, are associated with a more diverse mix of gut bacteria. Although diet matters for gut health, the impact of physical fitness is often underestimated. Cardiorespiratory fitness (VO_2 max) can account for about 22 percent of the differences in an individual's gut bacteria. However, it's important to balance exercise intensity hormetically; excessive or prolonged high-intensity exercise can harm gut health by possibly increasing gut wall permeability.

Fasting, Eating, and Your Gut

Given that our gut bacteria have their own circadian rhythm, it's not surprising that the natural rhythm of stress and recovery from daily cycling between fasting and eating is good for our gut bugs. Among the ways fasting builds our defenses is that it increases the levels of specific beneficial bacteria and the overall diversity of our gut microbiota, along with the genes they encode, which constitute our microbiome. In one study, healthy men who followed a sixteen-hour fasting, eight-hour eating pattern had enhanced gut microbial richness, with an increase of *Prevotellaceae* and *Bacteroidaceae*, beneficial bacteria linked to better metabolic health. Other studies link intermittent fasting to an increase in other beneficial bacteria, such as butyric acid–producing *Lachnospiraceae*. Furthermore, by improving the gut microbial ecosystem, fasting can protect the intestinal barrier wall and block systemic inflammation. Here again, our gut bacteria are a common pathway by which good stress can have far-reaching effects on our well-being.

Another housekeeping function that happens in our gut when we are not eating is a series of cyclical, recurring stomach and small bowel contractions that occur about every 130 minutes, called the migrating motor complex.

These contractions sweep the gut's contents down to the lower gastrointestinal tract between meals, moving gut microbes to the colon to minimize bacteria in our small intestine and support a healthy balance. Eating stops the contractions immediately—another reason our constant grazing pattern is hurting our health and quality of life. Caloric drinks, such as those containing sugar and fat, also interfere with the migrating motor complex because they need to be digested. However, noncaloric beverages like water, tea, or black coffee generally do not disrupt the migrating motor complex and allow it to continue its cycle.

The Psychological Stress–Gut Connection

The brain and gut are connected, and gut bacteria play a big role in this brain-gut communication. Psychological stress can change the composition of your gut bacteria, and your unique gut microbiome controls many aspects of your mental health and psychological resilience. The vagus nerve is an important part of this communication, sending messages about your psychological state to your gut and feeding back information from your intestines to your brain. Your immune system, of which a large part resides in the gut, can also impact gut bacterial composition and function via stress-induced immune changes, as can neurotransmitters involved in mood, motivation, and reward that are made both by the brain and the gut. Managing psychological stress in a hormetic range can keep your gut bacteria balanced and improve your physical and mental well-being.

Cold and Heat Microbiota

Studies on animals show that gut bacteria play an important role in thermogenesis. When exposed to cold, gut bacterial composition changes to increase insulin sensitivity and browning of white fat. Both heat and cold stress can change the gut's mix of bacteria, protective barrier, antioxidant ability, and inflammatory markers. However, we are still learning about how temperature stress affects gut health as a means of improving our well-being.

◆

The connection between good stress, our endocannabinoid system, and gut bacteria is another way we access our body's natural wisdom when we follow the rhythm of stress and recovery. The evidence is pointing us toward a life-style with good stress as how we were meant to live for optimal aging, health, and well-being.

PART IV

STRESS, RECOVER, REPEAT

Putting the Power of Hormesis to Work

CHAPTER 12

Getting Out of Your Comfort Zone

> You've always had the power my dear, you
> just had to learn it for yourself.
> —Glinda, the Good Witch of the North, *The Wizard of Oz*

Now you know the power of good stress in unlocking the potential of your genes and the right stressors to activate your regenerative stress responses. You've seen how powerful they are for slowing your biological age, preventing disease, and improving your well-being. Now it's time to put good stress into action.

I created the Stress Paradox Protocol to guide you through the process of challenging yourself with stress and recovery. My intent is to give you a practical and sustainable way of living that will make you feel strong and energized, restore your health, and ultimately live a longer, happier life. I am so excited to be a part of this journey with you. Before we get into the good stress protocol, let's set you up for success.

GET INTO A GOOD STRESS MINDSET

Deliberately choosing stress and overcoming the inclination toward comfort may seem challenging, but I know you can do this. I've done it and I've helped thousands of patients transform their lives through good stress. The key is arming yourself with the right mindset.

You've already begun just by reading this book and letting this little idea about the benefits of good stress take root in your mind. This alone can transform your health. It might seem hard to believe, but brief, simple, one-time "wise interventions" that aim to alter a specific way in which you think, particularly about stress, can change your health for years. This is why I want you to take a moment and get in the right mindset for your good stress journey. If you're going to believe in your power to embrace challenges and come out stronger on the other side, you need to take ownership of your life and your potential.

Mindset Shift #1:
Shift Your Perspective on Your Locus of Control

The way you interpret your life and your health may seem unchangeable, but in fact it's determined by your "locus of control." If you believe that your actions significantly impact the outcome, you have an internal locus of control. People who do are more proactive about their health, set higher goals, and actively work toward achieving them. In contrast, people with an external locus of control believe that external factors such as fate, luck, or others are responsible for their well-being.

Your locus of control can influence your health-related behaviors and, therefore, your overall health. In studies, people with an internal locus of control are happier, more satisfied with life, and enjoy greater well-being. They are more likely to adopt healthier habits, such as eating a balanced diet and exercising regularly. In other words, if you believe you have control over your health, you will. In contrast, people with an external locus of control don't cope as well with life's challenges and are more likely to experience anxiety and depression. So, the first step to taking control of your health is to be aware of your locus of control and cultivate an internal one, which will lead you to a more empowered and proactive approach to life.

Not sure how? Start by setting small, achievable goals. Meeting these goals can reinforce the idea that your actions have a direct impact on outcomes. Another good practice is, in any situation, identify what aspects you have control over and focus your energy there rather than on external factors beyond your control.

Mindset Shift #2:
Be the Hero of Your Story

You can tell a lot about yourself by how you tell your story—the character that you play and the arc of your journey. Your personal narrative is how you make sense of the world.

Dan McAdams, a psychologist at Northwestern University, has spent over thirty years studying how people create their "narrative identity" —an internal and evolving life story made up of significant memories. These personal stories don't just leave a lasting impression on the people to whom we tell them. Our stories and the way we tell them have a profound impact on *ourselves*—our mindset, health, and well-being.

When you tell your story, the role you assign to yourself matters. Are you a hero, a caregiver, or a victim? The way my patients describe their experiences shows me their readiness to face challenges and improve their health. A key factor here is self-agency—feeling in control of your own actions and decisions. This sense of empowerment is crucial for shaping your life path, growing during mental health recovery, and believing in your success. The great thing about storytelling is that you can change parts of your story to become more active and in control of your life.

Research shows that even small edits in how we tell our stories can greatly improve our health and well-being. For instance, one study had forty-seven adults write their life stories and undergo mental health assessments over twelve therapy sessions. The results showed that as their stories evolved to reflect more control, their mental health improved. They lived their way into the story versions of themselves.

I want you to perceive yourself as the hero of your story. The hero is the one who is prepared to go through a journey of challenges and become transformed. The iconic hero during my formative years was the fictional character Rocky Balboa, the protagonist of the *Rocky* film series. He is a down-on-his-luck boxer who has a chance to fight the world heavyweight champion. To earn his self-respect, he has to go through grueling training and overcome numerous challenges, guided by his trainer and significant others, that build his resilience and prepare him for the biggest fight of his life. The inspiration from Rocky's journey is that there is a hero in all of us. Once we perceive self-agency, we shift internally to feeling in control over our actions and decisions.

Shelly's Story

Shelly's days were busy getting her three children ready for school, planning meals, running errands, and shuttling her kids to their activities. Her mother had recently fallen, so Shelly was also caring for her mom, including driving her to all her doctors' appointments. As she was telling me this during her annual visit, I could sense her exhaustion. I have known Shelly for over a decade. She is a kind, compassionate, and selfless mother, daughter, and wife whose nature is to be a caregiver. She is the first person her family would ask for help. And she is always there for them. Year after year she tells me the events that have unfolded and her hope that in the coming year, things would slow down and she would have more time for herself. She was completely depleted.

"If you had time, what would you do?" I asked. After a long pause, she confessed, "I would get back to painting." She had a love for art and majored in art history in college. She had a longing to one day return to it. However, it seemed unrealistic to her. "Life may never simplify on its own," I replied. With good stress on my mind, I boldly suggested to Shelly that she add art to her weekly schedule. Her jaw dropped and she asked me if I was crazy. "I'm already stretched so thin, how could I possibly add one more thing, especially something just for me?"

I explained to Shelly that adding something positive for yourself, even if it would add stress, would lead to a different physiological state. "I know this seems implausible," I said. I encouraged her to take deliberate action anyway.

Shelly took my advice and enrolled in a community art class. During the small islands of time when she was painting, she felt fully immersed, losing track of time, creative, and joyful. She emerged calmer and with inner happiness. With time, something shifted in her. She envisioned more possibilities for herself and her family. She was brighter and more confident, and that carried over to everyone around her.

DO SOME OBJECTIVE ASSESSMENTS WITH
HEALTH AND LONGEVITY BIOMARKERS

Tracking and measuring progress is an important part of improving health and vitality, but so often we get blood test results we don't really understand (or just partially understand) or we get confused by the options for mail-in tests that proliferate on the internet. As someone who works at the forefront of developing ways to analyze your health and aging using real-time, preventive data, I want to give you my recommendation for ten biomarkers that best predict your long-term health and longevity. My criteria for selecting these is that they are easy to obtain, inexpensive, and very modifiable through a lifestyle based on the science of good stress. This means you have significant control over these markers, and by managing them, you can actively improve your health and longevity. I also want you to have insight into understanding what these markers mean and how to assess your progress in shifting them.

You often can't see or feel the early stages of declining health, but biomarkers help you gauge whether you're on track. The most important thing to remember is that it's not about where you start, but how much you improve. These assessments are for awareness, not judgment. Don't be hard on yourself—lower scores just show where you have the most room to grow. Measurements are tools, not something to dread or fear.

Since no single test gives the full picture of your risks and aging trajectory, I recommend getting as many of these ten tests as you can before starting the Stress Paradox Protocol and retesting every six to twelve months to track your progress.

My Top Ten Biomarkers for Assessing Health and Longevity

1. Body composition

Unlike fat that is stored safely under your skin, abdominal fat, or visceral fat, is where metabolic problems begin, and it is a significant predictor of your risk of diseases such as diabetes, heart disease, stroke, cancer, and premature mortality. While body mass index (BMI) is commonly used to estimate overall body fat, it does not always accurately reflect abdominal obesity, especially in muscular people. A simple way to estimate your abdominal fat can be done at home: with a tape measure, measure your waist circumference midway between the top of your hip bone and the bottom of your ribs. For men, a waist measurement of over 94 cm (37 inches), and for women, over 80 cm (31.5 inches), indicates higher health risks. Your waist-to-height ratio, which is your waist circumference divided by your height, is an even more reliable predictor of early health risks because it takes into account height differences. To minimize the risk of health problems, your waist should be less than half your height.

If you have access to a dual-energy X-ray absorptiometry (DEXA) scan, you can measure the amount and distribution of your body fat more accurately. Bioelectrical impedance analysis (BIA) is an alternative method, but its accuracy can vary from medical grade to less-precise home scales. These machines not only allow you to measure your abdominal fat but also your muscle mass, which is another component of body composition that is strongly correlated with longevity. According to a large national study of over thirty-six hundred people fifty-five years or older, those with muscle mass index in the top 25 percent (fourth quartile) had a 20 percent lower risk of dying compared to those in the bottom 25 percent (first quartile) of muscle mass index. Muscle mass index measures muscle amount in kilograms divided by height in meters squared. For women, the twenty-fifth, fiftieth, and seventy-fifth percentiles of muscle mass index were 6.2, 6.9, and 7.6 kg/m² and for men, it was 9.2, 10.0, and 10.8 kg/m². To be in the top range in skeletal muscle mass percentage for your age, women should aim for about 31 percent muscle mass if they're between thirty-six and fifty-five years old, and 30 percent if they're between fifty-six and seventy-five years old. Men should aim for 40 percent if they're between thirty-six to fifty-five years old, and 35 percent if they're between fifty-six and seventy-five years old.

2. Muscle strength

Grip strength, the force exerted by your grip, is not just a measure of hand and forearm muscle strength but a reliable indicator of overall muscle strength and a valuable biomarker for healthy aging. A large 2018 meta-analysis of approximately two million men and women found that individuals with higher grip strength had a significantly lower risk (31 percent) of mortality from all causes compared to those with lower grip strength. A handgrip dynamometer is a simple, portable, and reliable device for measuring your grip strength.

3. Cardiorespiratory fitness

Cardiorespiratory fitness is a powerful indicator of your overall health and longevity. It is most commonly measured by a VO_2 max test, which determines the maximum amount of oxygen that you can consume during exercise. While there is no simple and readily available test to directly measure mitochondrial function, you can use your cardiorespiratory fitness as an indirect estimate. A higher VO_2 max indicates better mitochondrial efficiency and cardiorespiratory fitness.

The gold standard for measuring VO_2 max involves running on a treadmill while wearing a mask that measures your volume of oxygen consumed per minute (VO_2) and volume of carbon dioxide produced per minute (VCO_2) as well as your heart rate. Although many smartwatches provide an estimate of your VO_2 max, they calculate it using your heart rate only. I recommend using the Rockport Walk Test or the Cooper 12-Minute Run Test, which are more accurate. They are both simple, scientifically validated ways to estimate your VO_2 max on your own.

The Rockport Walk Test is ideal if you are new to exercise, older, or have joint issues that make running difficult. To perform this test, plan a one-mile course on level ground and have a stopwatch on hand. Start walking as fast as you can without running along the one-mile course and time how long it takes you with the stopwatch. As soon as you finish, count your pulse for fifteen seconds and multiply by four to get your heart rate. Then use this formula to calculate your VO_2 max in milliliters of oxygen used per kilogram of body weight per minute (ml/kg/min):

VO_2 max = 132.853 - (0.0769 × your weight in pounds) - (0.3877 × your age) + (6.315 if you are male or 0 if you are female) - (3.2649 × your walking time in minutes) - (0.1565 × your heart rate at the end of the test)

The Cooper 12-Minute Run Test, developed by Kenneth Cooper, MD, in 1968, is better suited for people with a higher fitness level. To perform this test, you warm up with a light jog, then run on a level surface, ideally a track, for twelve minutes, and cool down. Count the laps or distance you covered. You can also use a treadmill set at a 1 percent incline. You can calculate your estimated VO$_2$ max result (in ml/kg/min) using either of these formulas:

$$\text{Kilometers: VO}_2 \text{ max} = (22.351 \times \text{kilometers}) - 11.288$$
$$\text{Miles: VO}_2 \text{ max} = (35.97 \times \text{miles}) - 11.29$$

You can determine your cardiorespiratory fitness by comparing your VO$_2$ max results with charts that have norms based on age and gender. If you are starting in the least fit quartile, the good news is you stand to gain the most significant benefits by improving your VO$_2$ max. Even modestly improving your VO$_2$ max can substantially reduce cardiovascular disease risk and mortality by half, which I think is remarkable. There simply isn't a pill I could prescribe that comes close to that.

4. Insulin resistance

It might be surprising, but there isn't a widely accepted clinical test specifically for insulin resistance. Usually, it's diagnosed through the presence of metabolic syndrome, which means having at least three of these conditions: a large waist size (over 35 inches for women or 40 inches for men), high blood sugar, high blood pressure (130/85 or higher), low HDL cholesterol (below 50 mg/dL for women or 40 mg/dL for men), and high triglycerides (150 mg/dL or higher). However, insulin resistance can start much earlier than the onset of metabolic syndrome. To diagnose insulin resistance earlier, a combination of several simple blood tests can be useful.

A reliable way to check for insulin resistance is to calculate your insulin resistance score using a mathematical model called the homeostatic model assessment of insulin resistance (HOMA-IR). Ask your doctor for your fasting insulin and glucose levels. Then, use this formula to calculate your insulin resistance (HOMA-IR) score: multiply your fasting insulin level (in mIU/L) by your fasting glucose level (in mg/dL) and divide the total by 405. This method correlates well with the research gold standard for measuring insulin resistance, called the euglycemic insulin clamp technique. Note that just measuring your fasting insulin level isn't always reliable for checking for insulin resistance. This is because your body releases insulin at varying levels throughout the day, and in later stages of metabolic diseases, your insulin levels might not be high if your pancreas is worn out.

Calculating your triglyceride-to-HDL ratio is another simple way to test for insulin resistance. You can easily calculate your ratio by asking your doctor for a standard lipid panel, and then dividing your blood triglyceride value by your HDL cholesterol level and checking your ratio against the chart on page 178. This ratio strongly correlates with the euglycemic insulin clamp method and is a strong predictor of cardiovascular disease, which is significantly increased by insulin resistance.

You can get more detailed information about how your body handles insulin with a Kraft test, which shows you your glucose and insulin levels after you drink a glucose solution. However, this test is more costly and takes a few hours to complete.

5. Blood glucose

Fasting blood glucose, which is your blood sugar level when you haven't eaten in more than six hours, depends on how much glucose your liver produces. Insulin signals your liver to stop making glucose when there's enough in your blood. In insulin resistance, the liver doesn't respond well to insulin. So, it keeps making glucose even when there is enough in the blood, leading to higher fasting blood sugar levels. High fasting blood glucose typically indicates your body's ability to manage glucose is already quite compromised, meaning insulin resistance is more advanced.

Hemoglobin A1c (HbA1c) is a blood test that measures your average blood sugar over the past two to three months, including your fasting and post-meal blood levels. When there is too much sugar in your blood, it attaches to hemoglobin in your red blood cells, creating glycated hemoglobin. Since red blood cells live for around 120 days, HbA1c reflects average blood sugar during this time. It's a better indicator of your blood sugar control than a single fasting blood sugar. Both fasting glucose and HbA1c are common blood tests, and you can check your number against the chart on page 178 to find your range.

6. Lipid profile

A standard lipid blood test will give you your low-density lipoprotein (LDL) cholesterol, high-density lipoprotein (HDL) cholesterol, and triglycerides information. Together, they can help you assess your risk of heart disease.

Low-density lipoprotein (LDL) cholesterol is often called "bad" cholesterol because it can cause plaque buildup in your arteries, leading to atherosclerosis. However, it measures the concentration of cholesterol in your LDL particles rather than your actual number of LDL particles. This means the test isn't a perfect estimate of your risk for heart disease since you could have many small particles or fewer large ones with the same LDL cholesterol level. To get a clearer picture of your heart disease risk, an ApoB blood test is helpful, which is next on the list.

High-density lipoprotein (HDL) is often referred to as "good" cholesterol because it is associated with a lower risk of heart disease. HDL protects against cholesterol plaque formation by carrying cholesterol from other parts of the body to the liver for elimination, lowering inflammation, protecting LDL particles from oxidation, and promoting vasodilation.

Triglycerides are fats in your blood, different from cholesterol. Unlike cholesterol, which is used to build cells and certain hormones, triglycerides store calories your body doesn't immediately use. High levels can indicate health issues like type 2 diabetes, prediabetes, or metabolic syndrome. Triglycerides account for most of the fat in a diet. The liver also turns processed carbohydrates, such as pastries and white bread, into triglycerides. Elevated triglycerides, especially with high LDL or low HDL cholesterol, raise the risk of heart disease.

7. Apolipoprotein B (ApoB)

ApoB is a structural protein that carries lipoproteins in your blood that can cause plaque buildup, particularly LDL, VLDL (very-low-density lipoprotein), and IDL (intermediate-density lipoprotein). Each of these lipoproteins contains one ApoB molecule. Measuring ApoB directly counts the number of these atherogenic particles. ApoB is a more accurate marker for cardiovascular risk than the LDL-C obtained from a lipid panel because the number and size of these particles are more closely linked to cardiovascular risk than the concentration of cholesterol in these particles. ApoB is especially useful for people with diabetes or metabolic syndrome, who often have high ApoB despite normal LDL cholesterol levels, due to smaller, denser LDL particles. ApoB is a blood test you can add when getting a routine lipid profile.

8. Inflammation

High-sensitivity C-reactive protein (hs-CRP) is a blood test commonly used to measure inflammation, with higher levels indicating increased risk of heart disease, stroke, diabetes, certain cancers, anxiety, depression, and other conditions. This marker is particularly useful for identifying people who are at higher risk of cardiovascular disease because persistent low-grade inflammation can cause plaque formation, instability, and rupture, leading to heart attacks or strokes. The liver produces hs-CRP in response to inflammation, and it is "high-sensitivity" because it detects even low levels. However, hs-CRP is a general marker of systemic inflammation and doesn't tell you what's causing the inflammation or whether it's acute or chronic. You can get this test done by your doctor or at a commercial lab. Keep your eye out for more specific inflammation tests that are being developed.

9. Blood pressure

This simple and common test directly affects your risk of heart disease, stroke, kidney disease, dementia, and many other conditions. Getting your number down, ideally as close to 115/75 as possible, has many benefits. Between the ages of forty to sixty-nine, for every 20 mm Hg increase in systolic blood pressure (SBP) or 10 mm Hg increase in diastolic blood pressure (DBP) from this ideal number, there's more than a doubling in the rates of stroke and heart disease deaths. You can get your blood pressure checked at your doctor's office with a blood pressure cuff, called a sphygmomanometer. Many pharmacies and supermarkets also have machines that check it for free. Alternatively, you can buy an automated blood pressure monitor to use at home.

10. Psychological resilience

Just as we should be proactive in measuring disease markers, we need to recognize potential emotional health problems early on. However, identifying emotional health problems can be difficult because they aren't always as evident as changes in body composition or fitness. Emotional health problems differ from mental illness and can be easily overlooked since they aren't categorized under diagnoses like depression or schizophrenia, and medication is not used as a treatment. Developing psychological resilience is a key aspect of emotional health and requires continuous effort, just like other health measures.

There is no gold standard for measuring psychological resilience, but there are scientifically validated questionnaires available that you can use for self-assessment. A good option is the Brief Resilient Coping Scale, created by Vaughn Sinclair and Kenneth Wallston. One of the advantages of this scale is that it's very short, consisting of only four questions. Scores on this scale can range from 4 (indicating low resilience) to 20 (indicating high resilience). You can find this questionnaire online and take it with zero cost at https://emdrfoundation.org/toolkit/brcs.pdf.

Big Data, Wearables, and Health Technology Are Changing How We Practice Medicine

Imagine being able to get your genes, epigenetics, proteins, metabolites, and even the microbes in your gut analyzed at a low cost and having machine learning tools and algorithms analyze all that big data to predict your disease risk before it becomes clinically apparent. Or picture a simple blood test, a liquid biopsy, that can detect signs of cancer far earlier than traditional methods by analyzing DNA fragments from a tumor in your bloodstream. These aren't futuristic ideas; they are technologies my colleagues and I currently use in our clinical studies.

In the near future, I foresee combining these large datasets with medical assessments, lab results, and health metrics from wearables like Apple Watch, Samsung Galaxy Watch, WHOOP, and Oura Ring to personalize medicine with unparalleled precision. Wearables are already providing reliable data on metrics like activity, heart rate variability, sleep quality, and our recovery needs. Artificial intelligence can also enable us to access real-time and customized health advice to support healthier habits and live longer, healthier lives.

◆

Check your test results against the chart on the next page to identify areas that need improvement. The chart shows different ranges because health is a continuum and can't be defined as "normal" or "abnormal." Diseases can start developing before reaching the at-risk stage. Also, reference ranges for normal results are based on average values from a healthy population. However, with declining health in the general population, being in the normal range doesn't mean you're in optimal health. Even lower-end normal results could point to potential health issues. Aim for the optimal range, ideally through healthy lifestyle habits that include good stress rather than with medication.

YOUR GOOD STRESS JOURNEY

The right mindset and knowledge about your health set you up for success. Nonetheless, encountering setbacks is expected in any journey. Be kind and compassionate to yourself, as you would with a close friend. Remember that you don't have to do things perfectly. Any challenge is progress compared to the good stress mismatch that exists for most people. And know that you are not alone in this. We're going to work together, and you will have easy-to-follow tools to live your healthiest and most vibrant life. You can also tap into the strength of a community by joining me online, partnering with a friend, or working with your physician.

Health and Longevity Markers and Their Recommended Ranges

Marker	At risk	Room to improve	Optimal	Peak
Body composition				
Waist circumference (male)	≥102 cm (40 in)	94 to 101 cm (37 to 39.8 in)	86 to 93 cm (34 to 36.6 in)	<86 cm (<34 in)
(female)	≥88 cm (35 in)	80 to 87 cm (31.5 to 34 in)	69 to 79 cm (27 to 31.1 in)	<69 cm (27 in)
Waist to height ratio	≥0.5		<0.5	
Muscle strength				
Grip strength*	Below average (50% or less)	Above average (51 to 75%)	High (76 to 94%)	Elite (Top 5%)
Cardiorespiratory fitness				
VO$_2$ max*	Below average (50 % or less)	Above average (51 to 75%)	High (>75%)	Elite (Top 2.3%)
Insulin resistance				
Fasting insulin level	≥15 mIU/L	7 to 14 mIU/L	3 to 6 mIU/L	<3 mIU/L
HOMA-IR	2.0 or higher	1.5 to 1.9	1 to 1.4	<1.0
Triglyceride/ HDL ratio	>2	1.5 to 2	1 to 1.4	<1.0
Blood sugar				
Fasting blood sugar	>100 mg/dL	91 to 100 mg/dL	85 to 90 mg/dL	<85 mg/dL
HbA1c	>5.6%	5.3 to 5.6%	5.0 to 5.2%	<5.0%

Inflammation				
hs-CRP	>2.0 mg/L	1.1 to 2.0 mg/L	0.5 to 1.0 mg/L	<0.5 mg/L
Blood pressure				
	>130 mmHg/ >80 mmHg	121 to 130/ >80 mmHg	115 to 120/ 75 to 80 mmHg	<115/ <75 mmHg
Lipid profile				
LDL-C	≥100 mg/dL	85 to 99 mg/dL	70 to 84 mg/dL	<70 mg/dL
HDL-C (male)	<40 mg/dL	40 to 49 mg/dL	50 to 59 mg/dL	≥60 mg/dL
(female)	<50 mg/dL	50 to 59 mg/dL	60 to 69 mg/dL	≥70 mg/dL
Triglycerides	≥150 mg/dL	100 to 149 mg/dL	50 to 99 mg/dL	<50 mg/dL
Cardiovascular risk				
ApoB**	>90 mg/dL	81 to 90 mg/dL	71 to 80 mg/dL	≤70 mg/dL
Psychological resilience				
Brief Resilient Coping Scale (BRCS) score	Low-resilient copers 4 to 13	Medium-resilient copers 14 to 16	High-resilient copers 17 to 20	

* Percentile ranking vary by age and gender
** ApoB and lipid goals can vary based on cardiovascular risk

CHAPTER 13

The Stress Paradox Protocol

I often cringe when I come across "detox" regimens because the word is frequently misused. However, this is literally a detox program. A genuine one. It will activate your body's natural detoxification enzymes and help you remove damaged proteins and senescent cells. Stimulating your cells with good stress will rejuvenate you at a cellular and molecular level. In just a few weeks, you will feel stronger, more confident, and more mentally, emotionally, and physically flexible as you build your resilience.

When I'm teaching doctors and students about how important resilience is for health and longevity, I use the analogy of thinking about your body like a bustling city. Just as a city needs essential roadways, utilities, and government to prosper, our bodies need a solid foundation. This foundation must be strong enough to withstand unforeseen natural disasters or catastrophes. To prepare, we can fortify our infrastructure with durable bridges, concrete-enforced walls, emergency response teams, and a reliable food and water supply. That way, when something goes wrong, we have the best chance of overcoming it and recovering quickly. Instead of brainstorming and planning for every possible emergency—a hurricane, flood, wildfire, or pandemic—it's more effective and efficient to build our overall defenses. That is exactly what we are doing when we increase our biological resilience through good stress.

You need—and deserve—a protocol for life. This isn't a fourteen- or thirty-day plan because you need a comprehensive lifestyle change rather than a short-term fix. Doing any program short term and then returning to your old habits won't help you live the vibrant, healthy life you deserve. While you will likely see improvements in your health within fourteen to thirty days, we're aiming for long-term success.

Through this protocol, you will find your individual hormetic "sweet spot" for stress and shift your hormetic zone to a higher baseline where you can handle more stress and respond with greater physical, mental, and emotional resilience. In scientific terms, you will shift the inverted U that characterizes hormesis to the right and up, as shown below, because you are literally reshaping and regenerating your mind and body through repeat activation of your adaptive stress responses. Whether you are healthy and want to optimize your performance and age better or have a condition like diabetes or heart disease that you want to manage with less reliance on medication, this protocol will increase your cellular resilience and, ultimately, your mental and physical well-being.

Shifting Your Hormetic Zone

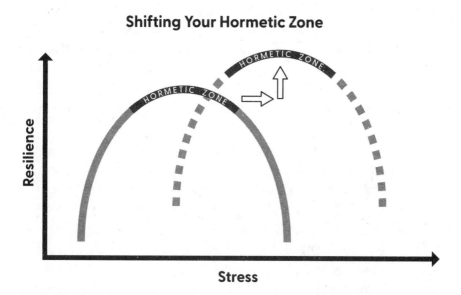

A unique aspect of this program is that it works with your body's natural rhythm by emphasizing frequency through small, repeated doses of stress that compound over time rather than intensity, pushing yourself with high doses. That's because regardless of how high the dose is, there is a limit to your biological plasticity, or the amount of growth you're capable of per challenge. Hormesis has been tested with thousands of stimulants across different organisms, including plants, microbes, and animals. These studies have concluded that a single biological stressor can improve functioning by around 20 to 25 percent. This suggests that there might be a natural ceiling to how much a single biological stress can help us grow. However, repeated exposure to the same low-dose biological stress can increase the improvements 60 to 90 percent. That means you can nearly double your human performance by making repeat cycles of stress and recovery a habit. You can build layers of fitness with rhythmic, intermittent, low-intensity stress, just like our ancestors did.

HOW TO USE THE STRESS PARADOX PROTOCOL

The Stress Paradox Protocol includes a protocol for incorporating each hormetin. Each protocol starts with assessing your current zone. If you fall in the red zone, you are living in your comfort zone, and your distressed cells need some TLC; in the yellow zone, your cells are doing all right, but there's potential to strengthen and grow; in the green zone, your cells are thriving, and these challenges will help maintain your vitality; and, in the platinum zone, your cells are at the pinnacle of health, and you are on track to be a super-ager. You will likely be in a different starting zone for each hormetin, already optimal for some and lacking in others. The latter are the ones that will help you make the biggest strides in your overall health. You want to get to the green zone (or platinum zone if you are a high achiever!) in as many protocols as possible.

Each protocol provides a framework for finding the amount of stress and recovery that is right for you. You don't want too high a dose or inadequate recovery, but you do want to challenge yourself outside your comfort zone. The protocols will guide you with parameters for getting started and increasing your stress exposure over time through internal feedback. They are designed to help you personalize the challenges to maximize your growth through iterative cycles of stress and recovery. Keep in mind that your hormetic zone can change daily based on factors like rest level and stress tolerance. Generally, more intense stress requires longer recovery time. Each protocol ends with suggestions for maintaining your new habits and a checklist to know when to move to the next challenge.

You can start with any of the protocols and do them in any order. Since the cellular stress responses work in overlapping ways, each challenge makes the subsequent ones easier. The protocols allow you the flexibility to integrate them into your daily routine without feeling overburdened. You can use them as a self-paced, guided approach with room to decide what to do each day based on your schedule and preferences. Go slow and honor your body. Every time you challenge yourself, you are doing something positive for yourself and reframing your relationship with stress.

Let's get started!

PROTOCOL #1: THE PHYTO-STRESS PROTOCOL

A good starting point is fueling yourself with phytochemicals that restore your body's balance and prime your innate resilience. In this challenge, you are going to step up your phytochemical intake. The following chapter will help you with tips and recipe templates for turning your kitchen into a hormetic kitchen. You will have over thirty delicious, phytochemical-rich recipes created by my incredibly talented friend Ashley Madden, a pharmacist turned culinary school–trained plant-based chef and certified holistic nutritionist. We developed this protocol based on our shared philosophy that food is medicine.

Assess Your Phytochemical Stress Zone

Before challenging yourself with phytochemicals, begin by assessing your current intake. The top ten list of hormetic phytochemicals in Chapter 4 includes options from all plant-based food groups, so you can estimate your phytochemical intake based on the number of plant foods you consume. It's not a perfect method because some plant foods, like blueberries and apples, contain more than one of the phytochemicals in our top ten list, but it will give you a good sense of how many plant chemicals you consume.

Assess your starting zone by tracking your meals, snacks, and beverages for a day and counting the number of different plant foods you eat. Give yourself a point for each fruit, vegetable, whole grain, legume (bean, lentil, or pea), nut, seed, herb, or spice. For example, a salad with lettuce, tomatoes, carrots, cucumbers, and olives would count as five plant foods. Beverages such as green tea, hibiscus tea, black tea, and coffee also count as one point. We are counting only whole foods, not processed foods (i.e., tomatoes but not ketchup; potatoes but not potato chips; fruit but not fruit juice).

Your 24-hour Plant Intake Log

What Did You Eat?	Number of Different						
	Fruits	Vegetables	Whole Grains	Legumes	Nuts & Seeds	Herbs & Spices	Coffee or Tea
Breakfast							
Lunch							
Dinner							
Snacks							
Beverages							

Tally your total points and find your starting zone:

Phytochemical Stress Zone

	Red Zone	Yellow Zone	Green Zone	Platinum Zone
Plant food groups per day (average)	5 or fewer	6 to 10	11 to 14	15 or more

The Phytochemical Challenge

Step 1. Stress—eating more phytochemicals!

Once you know your starting zone, the next step is to challenge yourself by increasing the quantity and diversity of phytochemicals you eat every day. The mouthwatering recipes in Chapter 14 will help you. They are organized into three levels of plant power: Go-To, Powered-Up, and Supercharged, with the number of plants included with each recipe. If you currently don't eat many plant-based foods, we recommend starting with the Go-To versions of each recipe. Then, gradually increase your plant-based intake by mixing it up from the different plant power levels and increasing the number of plant-based meals you have each day.

As you incorporate more plant-based foods, pay attention to how you feel. If you experience excessive gas, bloating, or abdominal discomfort, you may have dosed your intake too high or too fast. Reduce the amount and give yourself more time to adapt and recover. Spend two to four weeks in each zone before moving to the next. Some people will adjust faster than others, so go at your own pace. When you are in your hormetic zone, you will feel more energy, creativity, and improved mood without experiencing gastrointestinal distress.

We understand that cooking can be intimidating and overwhelming. To help increase your confidence in the kitchen, we've included ten meal and dessert templates in Chapter 14 that simplify cooking and guide you in preparing scrumptious meals with ease. We highly recommend trying each template to build your cooking skills while increasing your phytochemical intake. Think of it as combining two good stressors—mental and phytochemical!

Step 2. Recovery—building adaptations to toxins

Give your body breaks between meals or an overnight fast to allow adequate time after phytochemical stress for regeneration and growth.

Keep It Up

As you become a pro at rhythmically incorporating low-dose phytochemical stress throughout your day, you may find yourself in a pattern that is common: having the same meals in rotation. We are creatures of habit after all! I get that and I tend to do the same. It makes it so that we don't have to think about what we are going to eat at every meal. However, if you get in the pattern of eating the same breakfast, the same lunch, and the same dinner day after day—even if they are healthy meals—you aren't optimizing your dietary intake for health.

After you reach your zone goal, you should continue going outside your comfort zone with new fruits, vegetables, grains, legumes, nuts, seeds, herbs, and spices. More diversity translates to activating more stress response pathways and greater synergy in how they get amplified in your body to increase your mental, physical, and emotional resilience. Visit your local farmers' market and make it a fun adventure. Did you know that there are over ten thousand varieties of tomatoes alone? Since 90 percent of our calories are from fifteen of the fifty thousand edible plants in this world, we are missing out on 99.97 percent of plant-based variety! That's like going only to the same vacation spot, driving only one car make or model, going to only one restaurant, or watching the same movie. Life wouldn't be as colorful, and neither are our plates. Seeking variety is an integral part of a stress-enhancing mindset.

The beauty of recipe templates is that you can mix and match ingredients and make simple swaps to continually add variety. For example, you can swap out different vegetables in your sheet pan dinner or try different fruit in your smoothie. Making substitutions will also help you make recipes that are your own, that include the foods that make you feel best and fit your preferences, taking into account your culture, medical conditions, and allergies. That is important for making your new eating pattern sustainable long term. I've included a list of foods that contain high amounts of stress-enhancing hormetic phytochemicals, roughly in order of highest to lowest amount, to give you ideas for food swaps.

Phytochemicals

Resveratrol	Sulforaphane	Quercetin
Red grapes (especially skins)	Broccoli sprouts	Capers
Red wine	Broccoli	Elderberries
Dark chocolate with high cocoa content	Brussels sprouts	Onions
Peanuts	Cabbage	Kale
Pistachios	Cauliflower	Cranberries
Blueberries	Kale	Raspberries
Cranberries	Collard greens	Apples
Raspberries	Mustard greens	Dark cherries
Blackberries	Turnips	Dark plums
Strawberries	Bok choy	Red grapes
Red apples (especially skins)	Arugula	Red wine
Pomegranates	Kohlrabi	Black and green tea
Hibiscus tea	Watercress	Tomatoes
Rhubarb	Radishes	Nectarines
Red cabbage	Wasabi	Peaches
Red onions	Horseradish	Black currants
		Blueberries
		Goji berries
		Chia seeds
		Asparagus
		Spinach
		Red leaf lettuce
Allicin	**Capsaicin**	**Curcumin**
Garlic (especially fresh)	Jamaican hot peppers	Turmeric root
Shallots	Tabasco peppers	Turmeric powder
Onions	Jalapeño peppers	Curry powder
Leeks	Cayenne peppers	
Chives	Poblano peppers	
Scallions	Banana peppers	

Luteolin	Genistein	Ferulic acid
Celery	Soybeans	Bran (rice bran, wheat
Parsley	Soybean sprouts	bran, oat bran, corn
Thyme	Roasted soy nuts	bran) .
Peppermint	Fermented soy (natto,	Whole grains (brown
Artichokes	tempeh)	rice, whole wheat)
Broccoli	Soy milk	Seeds (flaxseed, sesame
Bell peppers	Tofu	seeds)
Carrots	Miso	Nuts (almonds, peanuts)
Oranges	Edamame	Vegetables (tomatoes,
Rosemary	Soy yogurt	sweet corn, carrots)
Oregano		Fruits (oranges,
Brussels sprouts		pineapples, apples,
Cabbage		peaches, bananas)
Kale		Black coffee
Spinach		Legumes (lentils, kidney
Chamomile tea		beans, black-eyed
Goji berries		peas)
Rutabagas		Herbs (parsley, dill)
Radishes		
Peanuts		
Leeks		
Cauliflower		
Apples		
Beets		
Chili peppers		
Onions		
EGCG		
Matcha green tea		
powder		
Green tea		
White tea		
Oolong tea		
Black tea		
(regular > decaf;		
loose leaf > tea bag)		

If you get derailed, keep in mind that you've built some great skills to help you get right back on track. Periodically counting your daily plant intake can help ensure that you are staying in your goal zone.

The Phyto-Stress Protocol Mastery Checklist

You are ready for the next challenge once you have:

☐ Reached your target phytochemical zone for a minimum of seven consecutive days.
☐ Found the kind, dose, and interval of phytochemical intake that make you feel best.
☐ Prepared a recipe from each of the templates.
☐ Tried food swaps that add diversity and personalize your meals.

PROTOCOL #2: THE MITOHORMESIS FITNESS PROTOCOL

The main goal in this challenge is to improve the energy production of your mitochondria through exercise stress. This training is hard, but it's crucial for powering your cells with the energy they need for repair and growth, and thus, improving your overall health and longevity. The primary exercise we'll focus on is aerobic, which is the most effective type for supporting your mitochondria. However, keep in mind that you need strong muscles to power your aerobic capacity, so in addition to this protocol, make sure to include at least two days of resistance or strength training weekly.

Assess Your Exercise Stress Zone

To optimize your mitochondrial health and cardiorespiratory fitness, you need two types of aerobic training: consistent moderate-intensity workouts and high-intensity interval training. The moderate workouts steadily increase your mitochondrial volume, laying a strong foundation. The high-intensity intervals act as a powerful boost for enhancing mitochondrial growth and function. This strategy is based on periodization, which involves alternating the intensity and volume of workouts to maximize your body's adaptations to training.

To figure out your moderate-intensity zone, count the minutes each week you spend doing activities like walking, jogging, hiking, dancing, or cycling at an effort level of five to six on a scale of one to ten. For high-intensity trainings, just track how many HIIT workouts you do weekly.

Moderate Intensity and HIIT Zone

	Red Zone	Yellow Zone	Green Zone	Platinum Zone
Average minutes per week	0 to 59 minutes	60 to 149 minutes +/- HIIT	150 to 180 minutes and at least 1 HIIT	More than 180 minutes and 2 or more HIIT

The Exercise Stress Challenge

Step 1. Exercise stress

In this challenge, we will work up to harder challenges of moderate intensity and high-intensity interval training. There are templates for each with versions for different fitness levels. Your energy level can also fluctuate daily. You should choose the workout that's challenging without overexerting yourself.

The key difference between this challenge and standard exercise guidelines is that guidelines are static—they don't change over time. This challenge is intended to be dynamic—you should continually adjust your routine to stay in your hormetic zone as your fitness level improves.

The Moderate-Intensity Challenge

During moderate-intensity workouts, you exercise at a steady and consistent effort level for a set duration, starting with a dynamic stretch to warm up. Your exercise intensity level for the session should be between five and six on a scale of one to ten, where you can talk in short sentences, but you can't sing. This type of training increases energy demand, which stimulates your muscles to produce more mitochondria to meet the higher need. It also makes mitochondria more efficient at making ATP. If carrying on a conversation is easy, you are likely at low intensity and need to push harder; if you can hardly manage more than a few words, ease up, as you are likely at a high intensity.

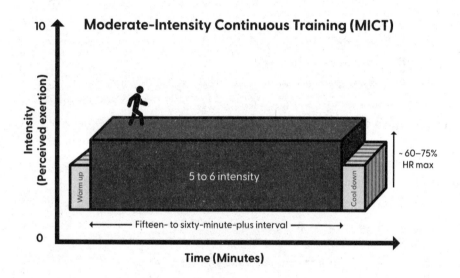

You can modify your moderate-intensity workouts based on your goals, fitness level, and time commitment.

The workout:

1. Select an aerobic activity, such as walking, cycling, swimming, hiking, Vinyasa yoga, elliptical machine, or dancing.
2. For two minutes, do your planned activity at a low intensity (two to three out of ten) to warm up.
3. Perform the aerobic activity at a continuous moderate intensity, between five and six out of ten. As your fitness improves, you will be able

to do more work, either at higher power or speed, over a given time. For example, you may start with a slow walk but gradually be able to do a brisker walk or slow jog at the same intensity level. The aim of this challenge is to gradually increase the duration of the workout.

- **Red zone**: If you are just starting out, begin with a five-to-fifteen-minute workout. Slow-paced walking or cycling are good options. If you are exercising outdoors, pick a flat route. On exercise machines, use lower speed or resistance settings. Aim to work up to a forty-five-minute session.
- **Yellow zone:** Work toward exercising at moderate intensity for forty-five to sixty minutes.
- **Green or platinum zone:** Gradually extend the duration of your workout to sixty minutes or longer. As your fitness level improves, you may be able to do activities like running, spin class, Zumba, fast swimming, stair climbing, hiking hills, or rucking while staying at a five to six intensity level.

Total duration: Will vary based on fitness level.

High-Intensity Interval Challenge

High-intensity interval protocols involve short bursts of seconds to minutes of intense exercise followed by lower intensity exercise or rest, repeated several times. There are infinite variations, but the key is alternating between pushing hard and resting, but not fully recovering between bursts, to get several cycles of rapid stress and recovery. During the high-intensity parts, you want to exercise at the intensity you can sustain for the duration of the interval. Generally, the longer the high-intensity interval, the lower the intensity level you will be able to sustain. We are aiming for HIIT that are between 80 and 95 percent of your maximum heart rate but not an "all out" 100 percent maximum effort as in sprint interval trainings (SIT). You should feel like you're working at a level above six but no more than nine during the high-intensity interval phase.

HIIT promotes rapid creation of new mitochondria and improves their function in a shorter workout than moderate-intensity exercises. It uses both of your energy systems, which leads to unique health benefits, including better mitochondrial efficiency.

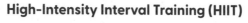

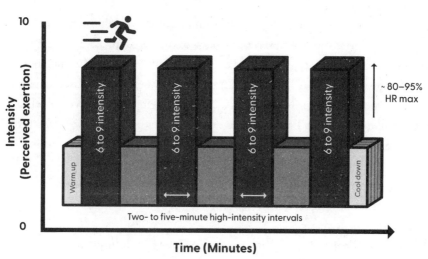

You can begin to incorporate HIIT workouts once you can comfortably do a moderate-intensity exercise for at least fifteen minutes. Otherwise, HIIT may be too strenuous. And if you can't do all the intervals at first, don't worry. Begin with as many as you can handle and gradually work your way up. You can adjust the workouts to suit your health and fitness level. In the following HIIT trainings, the intensity of the intervals starts just above a level of six and gradually increases to a level of nine.

Basic Training

This protocol is based on a Japanese study in a group of middle-aged and older adults that involved walking in intervals of fast-paced vigorous intensity for three minutes, alternating with slower-paced light intensity for three minutes, for thirty minutes four or more times a week. Compared to a group that walked thirty minutes at a continuous moderate-intensity pace, the interval walking group significantly improved their cardiorespiratory fitness (with a nearly 15 percent increase in VO_2 max) and had a much larger decrease of nearly 20 percent in chronic disease risk factors after five months.

Here we are similarly doing three-minute intervals alternating between low- and higher intensity exercise. This workout is a great way to ease into HIIT as the high intensity is a six to seven out of ten, just a bit above a moderate-intensity workout. You can choose any aerobic exercise, including one you may be currently doing, like walking, rowing, hiking, cycling, elliptical, or dancing. Instead of doing the exercise at a steady rate, switch between high and low intensity.

Maximum intensity: 6 to 7; at this intensity, speaking a full sentence should feel difficult.

The workout: 3 × 3 Alternate 3 minutes of high intensity with 3 minutes of low intensity for 3 rounds.

1. Warm up for 5 minutes at a low to moderate intensity (2 to 5 out of 10), where you can comfortably carry on a conversation.
2. For 3 minutes, increase your effort to between 6 and 7 out of 10, where you can speak in breathy sentences but talking is not enjoyable.
3. Back down to low intensity for 3 minutes to catch your breath and lower your heart rate.
4. Repeat the cycle 3 times.
5. Cool down at low intensity for 2 minutes.

Total duration: 25 minutes

The Norwegian Standard Setter

The Norwegian 4 × 4 protocol is one of the most studied interval-training protocols and has been proven to be effective in a broad range of people, including
high-risk groups like those with heart failure, cardiovascular disease, type 2
diabetes, and metabolic syndrome and in people who are sedentary. For example, a 2008 study by the Norwegian University of Science and Technology
tested this protocol in sedentary middle-aged men and women with metabolic
syndrome. After doing this workout three times a week for sixteen weeks, they
had a 35 percent increase in VO_2 max, which was over twice the improvement
of a moderate-intensity exercise group, and showed a greater reduction in metabolic syndrome risk factors. I often recommend this protocol.

Maximum intensity: 7 to 8, where you can say only a few words.

The workout: 4 × 4 Alternate 4 minutes of high-intensity
exercise with 3 minutes of rest for 4 rounds.

1. Warm up for 3 minutes, doing a low to moderate intensity activity
   like walking.
2. Exercise hard at an intensity level of 7 to 8 for 4 minutes. You can
   do various forms of exercise, such as running, cycling, rowing, or
   using a stair-stepper.
3. Slow down for 3 minutes to catch your breath and slow your heart
   rate. Keep the intensity low enough to recover and prepare for
   the next high-intensity bout but not so low that you cool down
   completely.
4. Repeat this cycle 4 times.
5. End with a 2-minute cooldown at low intensity to slowly return
   your heart rate and breathing to normal.

Total duration: 33 minutes

The Tabata Twist Super Challenge

Don't be fooled by the short duration of this workout. While it's only fifteen minutes, not including the warm-up and cooldown, it's tough and in-
tended for people at a high fitness level. This protocol is based on the Tabata
protocol developed in the 1990s by Izumi Tabata, PhD, for Japan's Olympic
speedskating team. The original Tabata protocol alternates twenty seconds of
near-maximum effort with ten seconds of rest for eight rounds. Our version is
modified with longer intervals because two-to-five-minute intervals are more
effective for improving cardiorespiratory fitness. The original workout used a
stationary bike, but you can do this modified Tabata Twist on a bicycle, treadmill, elliptical, rowing machine, with bodyweight exercises, or even dancing
in your living room!

Maximum intensity: 8 to 9, where it's hard to speak.

The workout: 5 × 2 Alternate 2 minutes of high-intensity
exercise with 1 minute of rest for 5 rounds.

1. Warm up for 3 minutes with a low- to moderate-intensity activity.
2. Exercise hard but not "all out" for 2 minutes at an 8 to 9 intensity
    level.
3. Slow down for 1 minute to catch your breath and slow your heart
    rate.
4. Repeat this cycle a total of 5 times.
5. Cool down for 2 minutes at a 1 to 2 very low intensity to gradually
    bring your heart rate and breathing back to normal.

Total duration: 20 minutes

Step 2. Recovery—post-workout growth

After exercise, your muscles need time to repair and rebuild. Different from
the rapid stress-recovery you do in HIIT, this recovery period is crucial for

being strengthened by stress and preventing overuse injuries. There are two kinds of recovery: passive and active, and both are important after intense workouts like HIIT. It's best not to do HIIT on consecutive days and to limit it to no more than three times a week.

During passive recovery, you are allowing your body the rest it needs to undergo changes to become more efficient after exercise. Even though it's called passive recovery, you should work on rehydrating your body by drinking plenty of fluids; getting adequate sleep (many restorative processes including muscle growth and tissue repair happen during sleep!); and replenishing your muscle energy stores with adequate protein to help with muscle repair, unprocessed carbohydrates, such as fruits and vegetables, to restore glycogen, and nutrients such as vitamins and minerals that help heal and prevent injuries.

Active recovery means doing light activities that help reduce muscle soreness and inflammation, such as light walking, stretching, or yoga. My favorite, which is one of the most effective, is cold therapy! Lots of research backs this up. Several reviews and meta-analyses show that cold water immersion immediately after high-intensity exercise improves muscle power and flexibility and reduces soreness to support and speed up recovery, with shorter, colder sessions being the most effective. However, be aware that if your goal is to build muscle mass, cold exposure within four hours of training can hinder muscle gains. Since both vigorous exercise and cold water immersion increase mitochondrial biogenesis, an added benefit of combining them is boosting mitochondrial volume.

Keep It Up

Your short-term goal is to reach the green or even platinum zone. But long term, it's about maintaining your routine and continuously challenging your body in new ways. Just as it takes a variety of phytochemicals to unlock your potential, varying your exercises to engage different muscle groups maximizes your mitochondrial density. Try new and fun activities like mountain climbing, trampoline workouts, or Hula-Hooping. You can also mix bodyweight resistance exercises like push-ups, squats, burpees, or pull-ups into the high-intensity intervals of your HIIT workouts.

Regularly check on how you feel and your progress. Keep track of your symptoms and health markers, like body composition and VO$_2$ max. If you're not seeing improvements, you may need to tweak your training. You can use wearables to make sure you are reaching the recommended levels of exercise intensity based on your heart rate. Tracking progress helps you understand your body's response to various exercise challenges and helps you see how much you have achieved!

Mitohormesis Fitness Protocol Mastery Checklist

You are ready for the next challenge when you have:

- ☐ Completed two weeks with at least two moderate-intensity workouts and one to two HIIT sessions each week.
- ☐ Become familiar with gauging your exercise intensity, either by rating how hard it feels, using the "talk test," or tracking your heart rate.
- ☐ Tried at least three different kinds of aerobic exercises.

PROTOCOL #3: THE THERMAL STRESS PROTOCOL

Of all the good stressors, deliberate cold and heat exposure are probably the most underutilized for their health-enhancing benefits. We are going to change that! You don't have to invest in expensive equipment like a cold plunge tub or a sauna in your home. I will share some easy DIY options. Using these methods, you will activate your body's cold shock and heat shock response, which we don't do often enough in our comfort-oriented lives. You will likely notice a boost in focus, energy, and mood. Remember, your mindset toward stress affects how your body responds. When you feel discomfort from cold and heat, think about the positive outcomes rather than resist the experience. Breathe deeply and remind yourself that you are reprogramming your body and getting better at stress. As you get more accustomed, you can even cycle back and forth between cold and heat for contrast therapy. Thermal therapy does come with risks and may not be right for you if you have any serious chronic illness, so with this, and the other protocols, check with your doctor before proceeding. But here again, we'll go slowly, finding the right dose and duration for you.

THE DELIBERATE COLD STRESS PROTOCOL

Assess Your Cold Stress Zone

How often do you deliberately expose yourself to cold? To figure out your cold stress zone, think about how many days a week you take a cold shower, sit in a cold tub, lower your thermostat below 64°F (18°C), or use a cryo-chamber.

Cold Stress Zone

	Red Zone	Yellow Zone	Green Zone	Platinum Zone
Average days per week	None, I like to stay cozy!	Periodically, less than once a week	Regularly, at least once a week	Frequently, two or more times per week

The Cold Stress Challenge

Step 1. Stress—cold exposure

Before starting the cold exposure challenge, ask yourself four questions:

1. How will you do it?
2. How cold will it be?
3. How long will you stay exposed?
4. How often will you do it?

This 4 Hows approach makes sure your exposure is effective, challenging, and safe. As you make cold exposure a regular part of your routine, keep asking these questions because your answers might change. Factors like your sleep and the time of day can affect how challenging the temperature feels. Be ready to adjust as needed.

The 4 Hows of Deliberate Cold Exposure

How to do it?	Cold air	Cold shower	Cold/ice water	Cryotherapy
How cold?	Below 64°F (18°C)	50°F to 60°F (10°C to 15°C)	Below 60°F (15°C)	-166°F to -256°F (-110°C to -160°C)
How long?	Up to 6 hours	30 seconds to 5 minutes	1 to 2 minutes	1 to 3 minutes
How often?	Up to daily	Up to daily	2 to 3 times per week max	2 to 3 times per week max

How will you do it?

There are many ways to expose yourself to cold stress. Choose a method based on your preferences, your tolerance for cold, what's available to you, cost, and how much time you can commit. If you live in a cold place like Norway, Canada, or the Great Lakes in North America, you can conveniently step outside or take a dip in an icy lake. But if you live in a tropical region, you may need to be more creative.

Water conducts heat away from the body much faster and to a greater extent than air. If you are in the red zone, begin with less conductive methods like lowering your home's thermostat in winter, spending time outdoors in the cold, or taking a cold shower. Slowly work up to fully immersing yourself in a cold bathtub. Start with lukewarm water and transition to only cold tap water. Be careful with ice baths and icy lakes—they can be dangerous if you're not used to the cold.

How cold?

You don't need to hit a specific temperature for cold stress. The aim is for a level of cold that makes you feel noticeably uncomfortable, but not unsafe. As your cold tolerance increases, you can make it more challenging, like going from a cold shower to a cold tub, and eventually, to an ice bath. You can use temperatures from clinical studies as a helpful guide, but adjust them as you need:

- **Cold air:** Below 64°F (18°C) wearing shorts and a T-shirt. Wear more layers with lower temperatures.
- **Cold water:** Below 60°F (15°C), often between 50°F to 60°F (10°C to 15°C) in studies. Cold tap water is usually 45°F to 60°F (7°C to 15°C). Icy lakes can be around 32°F (0°C). For a safer and more manageable experience, submerge up to your neck. You can keep your hands out or wear a cap for extra warmth.
- **Whole-body cryotherapy:** Typically –166°F to –256°F (–110°C to –160°C).

How long?

Just because two minutes of cold exposure is good, it doesn't mean ten minutes is better. Your body doesn't work that way. There is a biological limit to the growth you can acquire through hormesis from each exposure to stress. The goal isn't to tolerate being in cold water for ten minutes. Instead, keep the cold exposure brief and intermittent, similar to HIIT. The best results come from alternating between intense cold and recovery. Staying in the cold for too long can turn into chronic harmful stress instead of being beneficial.

The colder the temperature, the shorter you should keep the exposure. Extrapolating from clinical trials, for indoor air, aim for up to six hours with a lower thermostat setting; cold showers should last between thirty seconds and five minutes; and cold water immersion should be limited to one to two minutes. Once you are used to the cold, try colder temperatures rather than longer times. Keep track of how long you spend in the cold; it will help you set goals for the next time. Counting seconds is a good way to measure time and train your mind to think clearly during cold-induced stress.

How often?

Too much of anything, even if it's good for you, isn't beneficial. When planning how often to use cold stress, consider your recovery time. Ideally, do cold water immersion up to three sessions per week. In each session, you can alternate several times between one to two minutes in the cold and warming up, similar to HIIT. Cold showers or exposure to cold air can be done more often, even daily. But remember to take breaks occasionally to maintain the stress benefit of cold. This approach, like with muscles, prevents overtraining.

Step 2. Recovery—experiencing cold-induced adaptations

After cold exposure, let your body warm up on its own, without using a heater. This keeps brown fat activated and your metabolic rate higher for several hours. Your core temperature will go back to normal in about a half hour, but you will experience an increase in energy, focus, and mood for much longer.

Keep It Up

Even a single exposure to cold can turn on your brown fat and burn energy. However, with *repeated* stress you can significantly increase your brown fat volume, control your blood sugar and cholesterol, lower your risk of metabolic and cardiovascular disease, improve your mood and resilience, and live a healthier life. Mix up the kinds of cold challenges to keep your body stimulated. Keeping a journal is helpful to track your progress and how you feel.

THE HEAT STRESS PROTOCOL

Assess Your Heat Stress Zone

Sauna is the most researched type of heat therapy, and we know the most about its health-enhancing effects. But when assessing your heat stress zone, count other forms of deliberate heat exposure, such as taking a hot shower, relaxing in a hot tub, or spending time outside on a hot, sunny day. These can also be therapeutic.

Heat Stress Zone

	Red Zone	Yellow Zone	Green Zone	Platinum Zone
Average days per week	None, I can't stand the heat!	Periodically, less than once a week	Regularly, at least once a week	Frequently, two or more times per week

The Heat Stress Challenge

Step 1. Stress–heat exposure

We can use the 4 Hows framework for heat exposure just as we did for cold exposure.

The 4 Hows of Deliberate Heat Exposure

How to do it?	Hot air	Hot shower	Hot tub	Sauna
How hot?	Over 92°F (33°C)	102°F to 104°F (39°C to 40°C)	102°F to 104°F (39°C to 40°C)	158°F to 203°F (70°C to 95°C)
How long?	Up to hours	Less than 10 minutes	Less than 10 minutes	5 to 20 minutes
How often?	Up to daily	Up to daily	Up to daily	Up to daily

How will you do it?

If you have access to a sauna, it's a great way to get the benefits of heat exposure. If not, filling a bathtub with hot water is a practical alternative, but be careful because water heats your body faster than air. Your body's core temperature can rise quickly, possibly by 1.8°F to 2°F (1°C to 1.2°C) in just

10 minutes. Also, your body can't cool down as effectively in water because sweat can't evaporate to dissipate heat.

If you aren't accustomed to a lot of heat, you can start by spending time outside on hot days instead of always being in air-conditioning. Or, start with a hot shower to get used to the heat before taking a hot bath.

How hot?

The exact temperature isn't as important as keeping the exposure challenging but safe. Here is some guidance based on the research:

- **Sauna:** A common practice is "the rule of 200," where the sauna temperature in Fahrenheit plus humidity level equals about 200. Studies use temperatures from 158°F to 203°F (70°C to 95°C).
- **Hot tub:** Water conducts heat more efficiently than air, so hot tubs don't need to be as hot as saunas. Typical temperatures are 102°F to 104°F (39°C to 40°C). Tap water can get hotter (120°F or higher), so be careful to avoid burns.
- **Ambient air:** Since skin usually is between 92.3°F and 98.4°F (33.5°C and 36.9°C), it may be difficult to be challenged by ambient air unless you live in a climate that is consistently very warm.

How long?

Remember, the aim isn't to stay in the heat for a long time. Keep your sessions short—usually five to twenty minutes in a sauna and under ten minutes immersed in hot water. As you get more comfortable with the heat, increase the temperature instead of staying longer to get the most benefits. You're looking for a quick and intense reaction to the heat.

How often?

Using a sauna at least once a week is helpful, but two to three sessions per week gives you more benefits. Four to seven times a week can even further reduce the risk of overall mortality compared to two to three times. If you only have time or access one or two days a week, you can do several sauna sessions in a day, provided you cool down in between sessions.

Step 2. Recovery—building heat-induced adaptations

After heat exposure, let your body recover from the heat stress and cool down on its own. Don't do any strenuous activities right away. Also, make sure to drink plenty of water and fluids to replace what you lost through sweating.

Keep It Up

Treat heat exposure as a regular health habit, similar to eating a diet rich in phytochemicals and doing regular vigorous exercise. Used over the long term, deliberate heat exposure can significantly improve your general health and well-being. It has been linked with lower risks of cardiovascular-related deaths, Alzheimer's disease, and overall mortality, as well as reduced depression and psychosis.

*Pro tip: Plan to do cold exposures in the morning to help you wake up and feel more alert. Use heat exposure, like sauna, in the evening because it relaxes your muscles. Plus, the natural process of cooling down after the heat helps you sleep better.

Thermal Stress Protocol Mastery Checklist

You are ready for the next challenge when you have:

- □ Completed at least seven sessions of cold or heat therapy.
- □ Adjusted to a slightly higher or lower temperature.
- □ Found your ideal settings for 4 Hows by tracking how you feel.
- □ Tried more than one method of cold or heat therapy.

PROTOCOL #4: THE CIRCADIAN FAST PROTOCOL

Fasting isn't for everyone, particularly if you are underweight, pregnant or lactating, or have a history of disordered eating. But it's a great tool for healthy adults and those with chronic conditions such as prediabetes, diabetes, hypertension, or obesity. Whenever I start someone on time-restricted eating, I first want to know their current eating patterns. How long is your eating window? How long is your fasting window? How soon upon waking do you eat your first calorie, and how long before sleep do you eat your last? In this challenge, your goal is to fast at least twelve hours a day but ideally closer to fourteen hours a day, which means eating all of your calories in a ten-hour time frame. At the same time, you will be adjusting your mealtimes to match your body's natural clock by consuming your first calorie of the day at least an hour after you wake up and having your last calorie at least two hours before bedtime.

The challenge also involves keeping your eating window the same on both weekdays and weekends as much as possible. Think of it like this: just as we use weather forecasts to plan our day, our circadian clocks use past experiences to prepare for daily activities. If your eating times change a lot, particularly your start times, it can confuse your peripheral clocks as to when to rev up your digestive system, hormones, and enzymes, which makes your metabolism less efficient. Our goal is to combine the benefits of fasting stress with those of an optimal recovery that syncs eating with our body's natural daily cycle.

Assess Your Fasting Stress Zone

To assess your fasting stress zone, track when you consume your first and last calorie each day for a few days. Calorie-containing drinks, like coffee with cream, or juice, count as your first calorie, but noncaloric drinks like water don't break a fast (fasting purists debate this, but black coffee or plain tea are generally considered to not break a fast). Also, track when you wake up and when you go to bed. Use this information to figure out your usual eating window and how it lines up with your circadian rhythm. We can do a basic assessment to estimate your circadian alignment by looking at the number of hours between your last calorie and when you go to bed. If this gap is two hours or more, your eating is likely in sync with your circadian rhythm. You can keep track of all this by using a tracking sheet, like the sample below.

Daily Tracking Sheet

Day	Wake-Up Time	First Calorie Consumed	Last Calorie Consumed	Bedtime	Eating Window	Circadian Sync
Monday	6:30 a.m.	8:00 a.m.	8:00 p.m.	10:30 p.m.	12 hours	Yes
Tuesday	7:00 a.m.	9:00 a.m.	10:30 p.m.	11:00 p.m.	13.5 hours	No
Wednesday						
Thursday						
→						

Then use the information you just gathered to find your circadian fast zone:

Circadian Fast Zone

	Red Zone	Yellow Zone	Green Zone	Platinum Zone
Eating window	More than 12 hours	11 to 12 hours	10 to 11 hours	Less than 10 hours
Circadian sync	Inconsistent	Inconsistent	Fairly consistent	Very consistent

The Circadian Fast Challenge

When starting this part of the challenge, remember that the hormetic amount of fasting stress varies based on your health, age, and gender. We will aim for a 14:10 circadian fast as our ultimate goal, with fourteen hours of fasting and a ten-hour eating window, but you can adjust it to fit your needs. Any change from the common habit of eating throughout the day is a big step forward. Restricting your eating window is hard because food plays many roles beyond nutrition; it's also part of our social lives and emotional responses. So, as with the other challenges, we'll make changes bit by bit.

Step 1. Stress—your fasting window: start with a twelve-hour window and gradually extend to fourteen hours

When you fast, your body switches from burning glucose to burning fat for energy. Start your fast in the evening, working toward consuming your last calorie at least two hours before you go to sleep. You can still have calorie-free beverages, but no snacks. Having a regular bedtime helps keep your central and peripheral body clocks in sync. For your circadian biorhythm, aim to go to bed between 10:00 and 11:00 p.m. and get seven to nine hours of sleep. Keep fasting through the night.

Pro tip: When you travel to a different time zone, try to eat at least an hour after you wake up in the new zone and stop eating at least two hours before bedtime. This will help you metabolize food more efficiently and adjust more easily to the new day-night cycle.

The Circadian Fasting Switch

⊙	Metabolic Switches		⊙
✕	Fast	Eat	✓
Burn Fat	Burn Fat	Burn Glucose	
Break Down	Break Down	Build Up	
Repair & Recycle	Repair & Recycle	Grow & Remodel	
Aim for 14 Hours	Aim for 14 Hours	Aim for 10 Hours	
🌙	Start 2 to 3+ Hours Before Bed	Start 1+ Hour After Waking	

In the morning, wait at least an hour after waking before eating. During this time, consume only drinks without calories, like water, black coffee, or plain tea, to effectively extend your overnight fast. Staying well hydrated is important during this phase because you need to replace the fluids you're not getting from food to meet your daily needs.

If you are not yet fasting for at least twelve hours a day, gradually extend your overnight fast by shortening your eating window by an hour each week. For example, you can start eating thirty minutes later and stop eating thirty minutes earlier, or any combination that works for you. Once a twelve-hour eating window feels comfortable, work toward reducing it to ten hours by shortening your eating window by fifteen to thirty minutes each week.

Troubleshooting tips: When you narrow your eating window, it's common to feel hungry and irritable. While this is normal, it should feel manageable and not too uncomfortable. This feeling usually gets better within the first thirty days. If your symptoms are severe or persistent, make your eating window a bit longer and reduce it more slowly. You are in your hormetic zone when you're not hungry while fasting, feel mentally clearer, and have more energy as your body gets better at using fat for energy. You are likely to also notice better mood, sleep, digestion, and regularity, since fasting gives your digestive system a break. If you continue to feel hungry, try a small snack during your fasting window. If that doesn't help, the problem might be with your recovery, meaning you might not be getting enough nutrients during your eating window. We'll address this next.

Step 2. Recovery—your eating window: start with a twelve-hour window and gradually decrease to ten hours

When you eat your first calorie of the day, you switch back to burning glucose. This marks the beginning of your active eating window. You don't need to count or limit calories because you are limiting the time you eat instead. However, aim for larger meals earlier, like a big breakfast or lunch, and lighter meals later in the day.

Recovery after fasting is more than just feasting. The foods you choose when breaking your fast influence the benefit you get from fasting. Just as there is a method to fasting, there is a strategy behind recovery. You want to eat nutrient-dense foods that maximize fasting benefits, keep you feeling full and satisfied during fasting, and support your overall goal of a healthy, sustainable lifestyle.

Principle #1: Minimize processed foods

Processed foods are concentrated with calories, unhealthy fats, refined grains, and sugars, which cause a spike in insulin levels. This delays the drop in insulin and energy that signals your cells to switch to energy-conservation mode and begin internal housecleaning and recycling. Choosing whole or minimally processed foods enhances the anti-inflammatory and antioxidant benefits you get from fasting. It also supports your body with nutrients, like vitamins and minerals, phytochemicals, and fiber, that make you feel better, reduce your risk of chronic disease, and help you live longer.

Principle #2: Get enough protein

It's essential to get enough protein during your eating window. The amount of protein you eat affects how much fat or muscle you lose during intermittent fasting. Studies on time-restricted eating show that eating between 0.9 to 1.2 grams of protein per kilogram of your body weight can limit muscle loss from weight loss to about 20 percent. For someone who weighs 75 kilograms (165 pounds), that's around 68 to 90 grams of protein a day.

While protein is important for building and maintaining muscle, too much protein can have downsides. It may accelerate aging and increase the risk of chronic diseases. A 2014 study found that a high-protein diet (20 percent or more of calories from proteins) in people aged fifty to sixty-five was linked to a 75 percent increase in overall mortality and four times the risk of dying from cancer over an eighteen-year span. However, for people over sixty-five, eating more protein was actually tied to a lower risk of cancer and death. If you are sixty-five or older, aim for 1.2 to 2.0 grams of protein per kilogram of body weight each day.

Principle #3: Lean on plant protein

The source of your protein matters as well. In the 2014 study mentioned earlier, the increased risk of mortality and cancer-related death from high-protein diets diminished or disappeared when the protein was sourced from plants. This could be because of insulin-like growth factor 1 (IGF-1), a hormone with a structure similar to insulin that promotes cell growth. Diets high in protein, especially animal protein, are associated with higher IGF-1 levels. Animal proteins have all the essential amino acids in high amounts, which can lead to too much IGF-1 production, a problem not seen with plant proteins.

IGF-1 also strongly activates mTOR, the master regulator of cell growth and metabolism. Too much mTOR activity can speed up aging and increase cancer risk. Animal proteins, rich in branched-chain amino acids such as leucine, activate mTOR more than plant proteins. Even a small shift toward plant protein can aid in longevity. A comprehensive review and meta-analysis found that just a 3 percent increase in daily energy from plant proteins can reduce the risk of death from all causes by 5 percent. For these reasons, I recommend getting most of your protein from plant sources like beans, lentils, and peas.

Keep It Up

Fasting is a lifestyle that aligns with your body's natural processes. Being consistent with your mealtimes during the week and on weekends makes fasting easier and strengthens your body's circadian rhythms. However, it's okay to occasionally deviate from your schedule. Events like late dinners, social gatherings, or travel can disrupt your routine. The goal of adding good stress to your life is to enjoy a better quality of life, so be flexible. Just get back to your routine the next day. Taking a short break from fasting once in a while may even help keep the practice challenging for your body. Once you are comfortable with your fasting pattern, you can try different fasting methods or longer fasts for continued adaptation.

Pro tip: exercise while fasting

A benefit of time-restricted eating over other fasting methods is that it pairs well with exercise. It's actually better to exercise while fasting rather than after eating since it enhances the level of autophagy (cellular cleanup) and mitochondrial biogenesis (creating new mitochondria), making the most of these good stressors.

The Circadian Fast Protocol Mastery Checklist

You are ready for the next challenge when you have:

- ☐ Restricted eating to the time window that feels optimal for you for at least seven days.
- ☐ Synchronized your fasting cycle with your circadian clock by not eating at least two hours before your bedtime for at least seven days.
- ☐ Consumed enough protein for your body weight and loaded up on nutrient-rich whole foods during your eating window.

PROTOCOL #5: THE 20 PERCENT YES CHALLENGE

I recently read Shonda Rhimes's memoir, *Year of Yes*, in which she describes how challenging herself for one year to say yes to everything that scared her changed her life. I thought it was a perfect example of putting good psychological stress to work. So, consider this the challenge of "yes!"—of taking on good psychological stress so you can discover your potential.

For our purposes, though, we don't need to say yes to *everything* that scares us—we're going to focus on 20 percent. Why? Because that is the amount you need to avoid the emotional exhaustion and feeling of lack of personal accomplishment that characterize burnout from chronic stressors like certain work demands, lack of support, personal conflict, or unexpected financial hardship. Research on burnout in physicians, which is alarmingly high, has shown that spending 20 percent of your effort toward a goal that resonates with your sense of self can counter burnout from prolonged or repeated stress. For every 1 percent below this threshold, the risk of burnout increases. Other industries have also applied this 20 percent benchmark, including the 20% Project at 3M, Innovation Time Off at Google, and the Genius Hour in schools. So, for this challenge, our goal is to bring in that 20 percent of good psychological challenges to make you more resilient and empowered against depleting stressors that you may not be able to change. I certainly do encourage you to take big steps where you can or make time for relaxation and self-care, but we're not necessarily talking about lowering your "bad" stress here; we're talking about countering it by adding good stress to reach our 80/20 rule.

I do think that "no" is also a powerful word, especially when we can use it to protect ourselves from letting stress get overwhelming. And we do need some boundaries to be able to drop our shoulders and create a safe space where we can be in our thoughts, to step away, at least in our minds, even if only for a few moments—this is, in fact, an important kind of *recovery*, which we will get to. But we often say no for comfort, for avoiding even good opportunities. So, this challenge is about saying "yes!" to opportunities that expand us, and an emphatic "yes!" to the life-altering path it can lead to. Because saying yes requires confronting parts of yourself that make saying no more comfortable. By being brave, you tell yourself you are worthy. You will find that the more you say yes to good stress, the more you will recognize and naturally say no to stressors that weigh you down. That's the beautiful thing about good stress—the good gradually pushes out the bad.

Remember that good psychological stress involves choice, control, and predictability. It stimulates and excites with a degree of uncertainty but not to the point of being overwhelming. And it aligns with your sense of purpose and social good.

Assess Your Good Psychological Stress Zone

This challenge is different from the others because it is not physical or concrete. It is more subjective and emotional. We can define most of the parameters for physical stressors—do x things for y time—but emotional and psychological challenges need to be guided by your intuition and your own inner sense of being.

Be honest with yourself. How often do you say what you want to say; do what you dream; learn what you have wanted; explore where you have imagined; or pursue what personally matters? How often do you sit on the sidelines and think these opportunities are for other people—and that you don't have the skills, knowledge, talent, or experience, or you worry that you may fail or about what people may think of you? To differentiate this type of good stress from the chronic, toxic stress in your life, we are going to do an exercise.

Write down all the stresses you're facing. Then go through the list to distinguish each one from good or bad types of stress. Do they deplete you of energy or bring excitement and joy to your life? Are they obligations that you don't have time for or interest in? Are they aligned with greater meaning and purpose? Place them into two buckets. Your good stress bucket includes challenges that energize, excite, and motivate you. These are ones that make you feel you are doing something good, for yourself or for others, or that you are accomplishing or learning something meaningful. Your bad stress bucket includes stressors that you can't change or control and ones that drain you.

Then see: How much do you have in each bucket right now? How full is your bad stress bucket? How full is your good stress bucket? How close to the 80/20 benchmark of bad stress to good stress are you?

Good Psychological Stress Zone

	Red Zone	Yellow Zone	Green Zone	Platinum Zone
How full is your good stress bucket?	0 to 5%	5 to 15%	15 to 20%	More than 20%

The Good Psychological Stress Challenge

With intermittent fasting we want to fast long enough to switch from burning glucose to fat and then go back to burning glucose by breaking the fast to increase our metabolic flexibility and physical resilience. In this challenge, we will work on increasing our psychological flexibility and emotional resilience by switching our stress response on and off. Additionally, we will strengthen our cognitive flexibility and mental resilience by switching from intense mental focus to recovery. Increasing psychological and cognitive flexibility will help you navigate change with emotions, thoughts, and behaviors that are creative, innovative, and aligned with your values.

This challenge follows the two-step cycle that is central to growing from good stress: stress and recovery. We'll stress and recover, stress and recover, knowing that stress fortifies us. Through small challenges and the subsequent growth during recovery, you are preparing yourself for when bigger opportunities arise. Tiny tweaks lead to transformation. The neurochemicals you release from good psychological and mental stress, like dopamine, oxytocin, and BDNF, protect you from harm and make your stress response work for you. Keep in mind that we each react differently to the *same* psychological

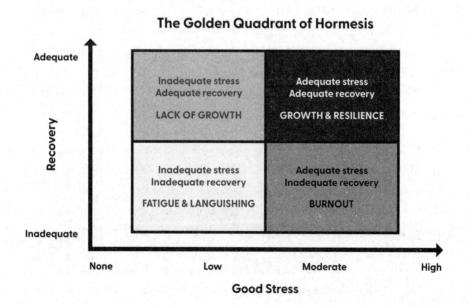

The Golden Quadrant of Hormesis

stress—the sweet spot of psychological stress for you won't look the same as it will for others. If your current stress level is high or if you have a history of trauma or mental illness, be careful not to overdo it.

Step 1: Stress—your good psychological challenge

Let's fill up your good psychological stress bucket! Pick a good stress challenge. Something that lights you up but also scares you a little. Something that feels stimulating but not overwhelming. By tuning into your gut, it will be easier to feel your way to this than think your way there. This needs to be something that you want to do, not something you think you should want to do. It should sing to your soul. The catch is that it can't be something you are already doing. It could be something that challenges your thinking or expresses your values. It can be anything from learning more about something you've always been curious about; hitting send on an email to your boss asking for a promotion; volunteering for something you believe in; posting about a personal experience; taking the first step to starting the business you have always dreamed about; or writing a book! It needs to fulfill these criteria:

1. It has to be congruent with your self-identity.
2. It must be something that deeply matters to you and possibly feels like it has meaning and purpose beyond you.
3. It gets you excited but not overwhelmed. It pushes you outside of your comfort zone but feels doable.
4. It builds your confidence and expands your belief in what's possible for you.

Write it down to help you stay accountable and then go for it! Make sure to check in with your emotions so you're staying in your hormetic zone. Don't try to suppress negative emotions. Negative emotions tell you you're either veering into bad stress or too much stress. Smothering negative feelings can cover up bad stress and keep you in situations that are counterproductive. Positive emotions tell you you're on the right track for expanding your resilience and self-belief. Ask yourself: Did the experience increase my belief in my ability to handle stress? Did it leave me feeling alert and energized? Did it encourage creativity and big-picture thinking? Or: Did I feel overwhelmed? Did the situation make me want to fight or flee? The right dose of good stress should leave you with positive emotions. The idea is to get you closer to aligning your day-to-day activities with your values and personal mission. More often, we are trapped by our own self-defeating thoughts than we are by circumstance.

Step 2: Recovery—growing from psychological stress

Recovery is critical for learning from intense stress and for bringing stress levels back to normal. Without recovery, stress hormones can stack to a harmful range. Just like there is an optimal way to recover from physiological stressors to enhance bioplasticity, there is an optimal way to recover from psychological and mental stress to enhance neuroplasticity. This recovery is more than relaxation. Reading a book; lying on a sofa; cooking a meal; catching up with friends; or watching a movie are wonderful ways to add joy to your life, but they don't calm your busy mind. What you need is a deeper kind of rest, where you are awake but your body is in a profound calm similar to what we experience during restorative slow-wave sleep. In this state of deep rest, brain waves slow in frequency and your parasympathetic nervous system dials down stress, allowing you to fully recharge. This deep rest helps your body regenerate and grow at the cellular level. It's more effective at building neuroplasticity than just relaxing, especially after periods of intense focus or learning.

How do we get to this state? There are many ways to get to deep rest. They overlap with mind-body practices, but if you struggle with meditation, know that deep rest is inherently different. I like to get to deep rest by immersing myself in nature, taking in its wonder and expansiveness, which naturally induces a sense of calm. Nature decreases cortisol, boosts our immune system, decreases heart rate and blood pressure, and reduces overall stress. You can get in sync with nature by grounding all of your senses with a 5-4-3-2-1 nature prescription. This involves finding five things you can see, four things you can hear, three things you can feel, two things you can smell, and one thing you can taste.

If you don't have access to nature, you can achieve deep rest even at home or work by doing a body scan. To do this, find a quiet place and sit comfortably or lie down. Close your eyes and take a couple of deep breaths. Bring your awareness to your body, starting from the top of your head, and work your way down to your toes, checking for any areas where you are storing tension. Once you identify these areas, focus on releasing the tension by relaxing your muscles. Beginning with your forehead, what sensations do you notice? Move to your eyes—are you squeezing them shut? If so, relax your eye muscles. Next is your nose—what is the pattern of your breathing? Are you taking shallow breaths or holding your breath? Rhythmically take a few deep breaths. Next, your mouth—are you clenching your teeth? How are you holding your shoulders? Are they shrugged? Keep working your way down to achieve deep rest.

Keep It Up

Now that you have momentum, periodically reassess what motivates you and keep reinventing yourself. Being your boldest, healthiest, smartest, and most resilient self doesn't happen all at once, but trust that when you say yes to challenges, the universe responds in kind. That's happened to me time and time again. Keep reshaping how you spend your effort and identify ways to continually create new challenges.

When my children were little, I used to love reading to them about the amazing "thinks" one can think from Dr. Seuss's book, *Oh, the Thinks You Can Think!* In it, he encourages children to imagine all the directions they can go and assures them that they can be masters of their destiny. And now, you are on your own, and with childlike imagination, keep challenging yourself to steer toward endless possibilities and dreams.

The 20 Percent Yes Challenge Mastery Checklist

You are ready for the next challenge when you have:

☐ Said yes to a think you can think.

CHAPTER 14

Creating Your Hormetic Kitchen

Recipes and Customizable Meal Templates

A hormetic kitchen is a space where you can experiment with the full spectrum of phytochemicals and learn to transform plants into delicious and powerful meals that support your health and happiness. In our home, the kitchen is the heart of the house. It's where we gather to spend time together and share meals. The kitchen's warmth and comfort make it a perfect space for creativity, self-expression, and expanding your horizons with flavors and cuisines from around the world.

In order to give you freedom and flexibility to gradually introduce an abundance of phytonutrients and simplify meal preparation, we have included ten recipe templates for popular types of meals, such as stir-fries and one-pot meals. They are designed to increase your confidence in the kitchen by providing a framework that will help you feel comfortable creating your own approach to stress and healing. Once you have the basic formula down, you can swap and add ingredients based on seasonal availability and your personal taste preferences. You can keep things simple by sticking with the base ingredients of the templates, or you can add suggested options for making endless variations. It's a way to think like a chef but prepare meals from any starting point, whether you are an experienced home cook or kitchen novice. The essential components of a hormetic kitchen are growth and versatility. We don't just want to give you a fish. We want to teach you how to fish.

HOW TO USE THE RECIPE TEMPLATES

Each template comes with three different recipes: Go-To, Powered-Up, and Supercharged. As you move from Go-To to Powered-Up and finally to Supercharged, you will see a deliberate rise in the phytotoxin content in each recipe. I encourage you to try making each dish and use these progressions as a helpful guide when preparing your own phytonutrient-rich meals.

Points

For every recipe, you will find points that are proportional to its phytotoxin power. This point system is calculated using a simple and imperfect method. We have allocated one point to each whole food item, including spices and herbs. For spice blends, we are allotting three points, as they contain three or more spices. This is not an exact science but a helpful tool to keep track of the good phytotoxin stress in your diet, especially if your baseline diet lacks plant foods. However, it is important to remember to get your points from different plant foods.

Making It Your Own

To provide flexibility with the recipes, each template includes suggestions for additional ingredients that can be combined in various amounts and ways that pair well together.

Cooking Methods

The templates use healthy and easy cooking methods that help retain maximum nutritional value without adding unnecessary or unhealthy fats. These methods include roasting, steaming, simmering, steeping, and oil-free sautéing. These techniques not only preserve the natural flavors of whole foods, but also introduce new and exciting tastes in your dishes.

Sauces

The secret sauce to any meal is, well, the sauce! We've included a variety of sauces and salad dressings that will elevate your meals to gourmet adventures. Eating for vitality doesn't have to be dull or uninspiring. You can experience healing while indulging in mouthwatering deliciousness.

Gluten-Free

If you follow a gluten-free diet, you can easily adapt all these recipes to suit your needs. Simply opt for gluten-free oats; substitute soy sauce with gluten-free tamari; choose gluten-free whole grains such as quinoa, buckwheat, millet, teff, and rice; and avoid seitan.

BUILD-YOUR-OWN RECIPE TEMPLATES

Before we begin, I want to emphasize the importance of mindset when it comes to hormesis. Keep an open mind and lighthearted approach in the kitchen. Be flexible and have fun. We often put so much pressure on ourselves to create the perfect meal. Food is important, but it doesn't need to be serious or intimidating. If a new combination you've tried is disappointing, note what you've learned, what worked and what didn't, and take those lessons into the next meal. Most importantly, congratulate yourself for trying something new.

Here is an overview of what's ahead:

Recipe Template List

1. Build-Your-Own Smoothie
2. Build-Your-Own Oatmeal
3. Build-Your-Own Muffin
4. Build-Your-Own Sheet Pan Dinner
5. Build-Your-Own One-Pot Meal

6. Build-Your-Own Stir-Fry
7. Build-Your-Own Puréed Veggie Soup
8. Build-Your-Own Salad
9. Build-Your-Own Nourish Bowl
10. Build-Your-Own Power Balls

Sauces and Dressings List

- Teriyaki Sauce
- Orange Ginger Sauce
- Balsamic and Thyme Sauce
- Green Herb Sauce
- Cashew Sour Cream
- Tahini Dill Sauce
- Miso Walnut Sauce
- Creamy Roasted Red Pepper Sauce
- Fat-Free Apple Cider Vinaigrette
- Almond Thai Dressing
- Sesame Balsamic Dressing

BUILD-YOUR-OWN SMOOTHIE

Smoothies have come to symbolize health and vitality, but all smoothies are not created equally—adding nutrient-dense whole foods and limiting added sugar is key. Leafy greens are generally underconsumed in the modern-day diet, making them an excellent addition to smoothies, as are omega-3-rich seeds and nuts, veggies, and berries. For this smoothie template we're using leafy greens and banana as our base. Choose robust greens like kale if you prefer a more intense green hue and flavor, or ease into green smoothies with baby spinach. Achieving the desired consistency will require adjusting the liquid content based on the quantity of whole foods used.

Smoothie Master Template

Makes 1 to 3 servings

- 1 to 2 cups fresh greens
- 1 large frozen banana
- ¼ to 1 cup other fresh or frozen fruit

- ½ to 1½ cups unsweetened dairy-free milk, water, or cooled brewed green or white tea, plus more as needed

Recommended greens: spinach, kale, bok choy, or a combination

Recommended fruit: mangoes, pineapple, blueberries, raspberries, strawberries, blackberries, cranberries, cherries, apples, oranges, peaches

Optional Additions

- Pinch to 1 teaspoon ground spices: cinnamon, ginger, nutmeg, turmeric, allspice
- ½ to 1 cup vegetables: raw cauliflower, raw zucchini, raw or cooked beet, raw celery, raw cucumber, raw or cooked broccoli, cooked pumpkin, cooked sweet potato
- Handful fresh herbs: basil, cilantro, mint, parsley
- 1 to 2 tablespoons super seeds: flaxseed, chia seeds, hemp seeds (or a mixture)
- 1 teaspoon to 3 tablespoons nut or seed butter or whole nuts or seeds
- 1 teaspoon to 2 tablespoons flavor additions: unsweetened cocoa or cacao powder, matcha powder, ground espresso
- ¼ to ½ avocado
- Citrus zest or juice
- 1 to 2 tablespoons wheat germ
- ¼ cup unsweetened soy or nut yogurt
- Enhancers: ¼- to ½-inch-piece fresh turmeric root or ginger root, 1 to 2 tablespoons green, veggie, or protein powders

How-To

Place the greens, banana, fruit, milk (or water or tea) in a blender, as well as any other additions you've chosen. Start blending on low and then increase the speed to high. Blend on high until the mixture is smooth and pourable. If your blender has a tamper, use it to push the whole foods into the blade as it's blending. If your blender doesn't have a tamper, you might need to add additional liquid to thin as needed and note that the more ingredients you add to your smoothie, the more liquid you will also need to add to achieve a slurp-able consistency.

SMOOTHIE RECIPES

GO-TO

Everyday Green Smoothie

Makes 1 to 2 smoothies

- 1 cup packed baby spinach
- 1 large frozen banana
- ½ cup coarsely chopped peeled apple or orange
- ½ cup unsweetened almond milk, plus more as needed
- 1 tablespoon ground flaxseed
- 1 tablespoon peanut butter or almond butter

▶ 6 points

POWERED-UP

Revved-Up Red Velvet Smoothie

Makes 2 smoothies

- 1 cup packed coarsely chopped bok choy
- 1 large frozen banana
- ½ cup frozen raspberries
- ½ cup frozen pitted dark cherries
- 1 cup unsweetened soy milk, plus more as needed
- Pinch ground nutmeg
- 1 tablespoon chia seeds
- 1 tablespoon almond butter or cashew butter
- 2 tablespoons unsweetened cocoa or cacao powder

▶ 9 points

SUPERCHARGED

Green Energy Smoothie

Makes 2 smoothies

- 1 cup packed coarsely chopped kale (stems removed)
- ½ cup baby spinach
- 1 large frozen banana
- 1 cup frozen cubed pineapple or mango
- ½ cup cooled brewed green tea
- ½ cup unsweetened soy milk, plus more as needed

- ¼ teaspoon ground cinnamon
- ½ cup coarsely chopped celery
- ½ cup coarsely chopped cucumber
- Handful fresh basil leaves
- 2 tablespoons hemp seeds
- 4 Brazil nuts

▶ 12 points

Make-Your-Own Smoothie Variations

There are many things you can throw into a smoothie to keep yourself challenged. You will find that the additions will change the satiety and consistency of your smoothie. For example, adding flaxseed or chia seeds will have a thickening effect. Less liquid can turn your smoothie into a sorbet-like frozen treat—which is a favorite in our house. However, keep the added fruit (banana included) to no more than 2 cups total (1 cup or less per serving).

Phytochemical Suggestions

Here are some smoothie combinations that work well:

- Raspberries, cauliflower, peanut butter
- Mango, orange, spinach, almond butter
- Beets, cocoa powder, soy yogurt

BUILD-YOUR-OWN OATMEAL

Oatmeal is a popular breakfast option and for good reason—it's nutritious and easy. This creamy oatmeal template is versatile and encourages you to incorporate other rolled or cooked grains—in other words, more phytotoxins—which will add more texture and flavor. It can be customized with various toppings like fruits, nuts, and seeds, catering to different tastes and dietary preferences. There are no rules with oatmeal!

Oatmeal Master Template

Makes 4 to 6 servings

- 1½ cups old-fashioned rolled oats
- ½ cup any rolled or flaked grain or 1 cup cooked grains
- ½ to 3 teaspoons ground spices
- Big pinch sea salt
- 2 cups water or cooled brewed green or white tea
- 2 cups unsweetened dairy-free milk, plus more as needed

Recommended grains: (rolled or flaked) more oats, spelt, quinoa, barley, rye, or a mixture; (cooked) quinoa, millet, teff, amaranth, buckwheat, or a mixture

Recommended spices: cinnamon, allspice, turmeric, cardamom, nutmeg, ginger, cloves, pumpkin spice mix

Recommended milks: soy, almond, oat, hazelnut, cashew, pea

Optional Additions

- 2 to 4 tablespoons nut or seed butter: peanut, almond, cashew, sunflower seed, tahini
- 1 to 2 cups fresh fruit: apples, banana, berries, cherries, mangoes, pineapple, peaches, pears, dragon fruit, pomegranate arils, grapes, oranges
- ¼ to 1 cup vegetables: grated raw carrots or zucchini; cooked pumpkin or sweet potato
- ¼ cup dried fruit: raisins, goji berries, apricots, cranberries, apples, prunes, cherries, mango
- 2 to 4 tablespoons super seeds: ground flaxseed, chia seeds, hemp seeds

- 2 to 4 tablespoons chopped raw, unsalted nuts or seeds: almonds, hazelnuts, walnuts, cashews, Brazil nuts, pecans, sunflower seeds, pumpkin seeds, sesame seeds, pistachios
- 2 to 4 tablespoons unsweetened wheat germ
- Unsweetened soy yogurt
- Maple syrup

How-To

1. Add the rolled oats and rolled or flaked or cooked grains, spices, salt, water or tea, and milk to a medium pot and bring to a boil over high heat. Lower the heat to a simmer and cook for 8 to 10 minutes, stirring often, until most of the liquid is absorbed, and the oatmeal is thick.
2. Turn off the heat and whisk in any nut or seed butters or other additions you'd like warmed, like fresh, frozen, or dried fruit, and let the oatmeal rest for 5 to 10 minutes. Add more milk to thin if needed. Divide among bowls and garnish with any chosen toppings.

OATMEAL RECIPES

GO-TO

Everyday Oatmeal

Makes 4 to 6 servings

- 2 cups old-fashioned rolled oats
- Pinch sea salt
- 2 cups water
- 2 cups unsweetened soy milk, plus more as needed
- ¾ teaspoon ground cinnamon
- 2 tablespoons peanut butter or other nut or seed butter

Toppings (Per Bowl)

- 1 tablespoon ground flaxseed
- ½ cup fresh or frozen raspberries (if frozen, stir into the oatmeal as it cooks)
- Maple syrup for drizzling, optional

▶ **6 points**

POWERED-UP

Apple Alarm Oatmeal

Makes 4 to 6 servings

- 1½ cups old-fashioned rolled oats
- ½ cup rolled spelt flakes
- Pinch sea salt
- 1 teaspoon ground cinnamon
- ½ teaspoon ground allspice
- 2 cups water
- 2 cups unsweetened soy milk, plus more as needed

- 3 tablespoons smooth almond butter
- 1 apple, peeled and grated
- ¼ cup raisins

Toppings (Per Bowl)

- 2 tablespoons raw, unsalted pumpkin seeds

* For this oatmeal it's best to stir the apples and raisins into the pot along with the almond butter so they soften a bit.

▶ 9 points

SUPERCHARGED

Stressed Out (in a Good Way!) Oatmeal

Makes 4 to 6 servings

- 1½ cups old-fashioned rolled oats
- 1 cup cooked white quinoa
- Pinch sea salt
- 4 cups unsweetened almond milk, plus more as needed
- 1 teaspoon ground cinnamon
- ½ teaspoon ground ginger
- ¼ teaspoon ground cardamom
- ¼ teaspoon ground nutmeg
- ¼ teaspoon ground turmeric

- Pinch ground black pepper
- 2 tablespoons cashew butter or sunflower seed butter

Toppings (Per Bowl)

- 1 tablespoon hemp seeds
- ¼ cup pomegranate arils
- ¼ cup fresh blueberries
- ¼ cup unsweetened soy yogurt
- Maple syrup for drizzling, optional

▶ 14 points

Make Your Own Oatmeal Variations

Ready to try your own combinations? A tip to keep in mind is that if your oatmeal is too thin, add some chia seeds or ground flaxseed and let the oatmeal rest for 5 minutes until thickened. If your oatmeal is too thick, thin it by adding more milk or water.

You can store leftovers in a sealed container in the fridge for up to 5 days. Most oatmeal will thicken significantly once cooled or after being refrigerated, but you can add more water or milk when reheating to loosen again.

Phytochemical Suggestions
Oatmeal pairings we recommend:

- Cooked sweet potato, pears, and pumpkin spice mix
- Mango, raisins, and almond butter
- Blueberries, green tea, cashew butter

BUILD-YOUR-OWN MUFFIN

Let's rethink the muffin! What was once considered a processed, carb-laden treat has been transformed into a wholesome, health-supportive meal or snack. This nutrient-dense muffin recipe template is built on whole grain and nut flours and is studded with a host of mineral-rich, vitamin-packed, antioxidant-loaded, plant-based ingredients.

Muffin Master Template

Makes 10 to 12 muffins

- 1½ cups oat flour
- 1 cup almond flour
- 2 tablespoons coconut sugar
- 1½ teaspoons baking powder
- ½ teaspoon baking soda
- ¼ teaspoon sea salt
- ½ to 2 teaspoons dried spices or herbs

- 2 tablespoons ground flaxseed
- ¾ cup puréed or mashed fruit or cooked starchy vegetable
- ¼ cup maple syrup
- ¼ cup nut or seed butter
- ½ teaspoon pure vanilla extract
- ½ cup dairy-free milk of choice, plus more if needed*

Increase milk to ¾ cup if using sweet potato, butternut squash, or pumpkin purée.

Recommended spices or herbs: cinnamon, cardamom, clove, fennel, allspice, ginger, turmeric, nutmeg, rosemary, thyme

Recommended fruit or vegetables: mashed bananas, unsweetened apple-sauce, mashed cooked sweet potato, mashed cooked winter squash, un-sweetened pumpkin purée

Recommended nut or seed butters: peanut butter, almond butter, cashew butter, sunflower seed butter, tahini

Optional Additions

- ½ to 1 cup total crunchy and/or chewy bits: nuts, seeds, dried fruit, dark chocolate chips, cacao nibs
- 1 cup fruit: berries; chopped peeled apples, pears, or peaches; chopped pitted cherries
- ½ to 1 cup grated veggies: carrot, zucchini, squeezed dry
- Flavor extras: 2 to 4 tablespoons cocoa or cacao powder, 1 to 2 tablespoons matcha powder, 1 to 3 tablespoons fresh citrus juice, citrus zest

How-To

1. Preheat the oven to 375°F. If using a traditional muffin pan, line it with paper liners.

2. In a large bowl, mix together all the dry ingredients.

3. In a medium bowl, add the puréed or mashed fruit or veggie of choice, maple syrup, nut or seed butter, and vanilla. Whisk together until smooth. Now pour in the milk and mix again.

4. Prepare any additions you're using (i.e., chop the nuts, grate the veggies) and set aside.

5. Now pour the wet mixture into the dry ingredients and mix until no dry spots remain. These muffins don't contain any glutinous flours, so you don't need to worry about overmixing. The batter should be thick, a little thicker than cake batter, but not stiff. If it is stiff, add a little more milk to loosen.

6. Fold your chosen additions (nuts, seeds, dried fruit, fresh fruit, grated veggies, et cetera) into the batter.

7. Using a spring-release scoop or spoon, portion about ⅓ cup of the batter into each muffin mold. You will get anywhere from 10 to 12 muffins, depending on your chosen additions. The more delicious bits added, the higher the yield.

8. Place the pan in the oven and bake for 18 to 25 minutes, depending on your oven and the specific combinations chosen. The looser the batter, the longer it will take. The stiffer the batter, the shorter the cooking time. Check after about 18 minutes for doneness by gently touching the middle of the muffin. The muffins are done when slightly firm to the touch and no longer wet in the middle. Remove the pan from the oven and let the muffins cool in the pan on a cooling rack for 15 to 20 minutes. They will firm up. Then, pop them out of the pan and let them cool completely on the cooling rack. Keep the muffins in a lidded container in the fridge for up to 4 days or in the freezer for up to 3 months.

Notes

If you want to reduce the added sweetener in these muffins, you can decrease the coconut sugar or maple syrup (or both). To reduce the maple syrup, simply replace what you omit with more milk. No adjustments are needed if you reduce or omit the coconut sugar.

If you add fresh citrus juice, reduce the milk by the same amount added.

You can make your own oat flour by adding rolled oats to a food processor and processing until a flour-like consistency is reached.

MUFFIN RECIPES

GO-TO

Banana Berry Walnut Muffins

Makes 10 to 11 muffins

- 1½ cups oat flour
- 1 cup almond flour
- 2 tablespoons coconut sugar
- 1½ teaspoons baking powder
- ½ teaspoon baking soda
- ¼ teaspoon sea salt
- 1 teaspoon ground cinnamon
- 2 tablespoons ground flaxseed
- ¾ cup mashed banana

- ¼ cup maple syrup
- ¼ cup almond butter
  or peanut butter
- ½ teaspoon pure vanilla extract
- ½ cup unsweetened soy milk
- ½ cup coarsely chopped walnuts
- ½ cup fresh or frozen blueberries
- ½ cup fresh or frozen raspberries

▶ 10 points

These muffins will take about 22 to 24 minutes in the oven.

POWERED-UP

Zucchini Currant and Cardamom

Makes 12 muffins

- 1½ cups oat flour
- 1 cup almond flour
- 2 tablespoons coconut sugar
- 1½ teaspoons baking powder
- ½ teaspoon baking soda
- ¼ teaspoon sea salt
- 1 teaspoon ground cinnamon

- ½ teaspoon ground cardamom
- 2 tablespoons ground flaxseed
- ¾ cup unsweetened applesauce
- ¼ cup maple syrup
- ¼ cup almond butter or
  sunflower seed butter
- ½ cup unsweetened soy milk

- ½ teaspoon pure vanilla extract
- ½ cup currants or raisins
- 1 cup diced peeled apple or pear

▶ **12 points**

These muffins will take about 23 to 25 minutes in the oven.

- 1 cup grated zucchini, squeezed dry
- Zest of 1 large orange

SUPERCHARGED

Carrot Pecan and Cranberry

Makes 12 muffins

- 1½ cups oat flour
- 1 cup almond flour
- 2 tablespoons coconut sugar
- 1½ teaspoons baking powder
- ½ teaspoon baking soda
- ¼ teaspoon sea salt
- 1 teaspoon ground cinnamon
- ½ teaspoon ground allspice
- ¼ teaspoon ground nutmeg
- ¼ teaspoon ground ginger
- 2 tablespoons ground flaxseed

- ¾ cup mashed sweet potato
- ¼ cup maple syrup
- ¼ cup almond butter or sunflower seed butter
- ½ teaspoon pure vanilla extract
- ¾ cup unsweetened soy milk
- ½ cup chopped pecans
- ¼ cup hemp seeds
- ¼ cup pumpkin seeds
- 1 cup fresh or frozen cranberries
- 1 cup grated carrot

▶ **15 points**

These muffins will take about 22 to 24 minutes in the oven.

Make Your Own Muffin Variation

A couple of things to bear in mind as you begin your muffin adventure. The more you add to the muffin batter, the denser it'll become, affecting its rise. It's not an issue, just something to note. Also, baking times will vary based on batter moisture and density. A runnier batter may take longer to cook. Last, oven temperatures can differ, affecting baking times. Some might bake quicker, others slower. Adjustments may be needed.

Phytochemical Suggestions
Great muffin pairings include:

- Pumpkin purée, chocolate chips or cacao nibs, walnuts
- Banana, cocoa powder, chopped cherries, pistachios
- Applesauce, cranberries, almonds, rosemary or thyme

BUILD-YOUR-OWN SHEET PAN DINNER

Here everything goes onto a sheet pan and into the oven. Pairing the sheet pan veggies and beans with a cooked grain is optional, as is adding a sauce, but the addition of either (or both) will bump up the nutrition, serving sizes, phytonutrient power, and flavor. Note that the size of your chopped veggies will determine the cooking time. To keep things simple in each sample recipe, we've chosen vegetables and cuts that have similar cooking times. We're also using spice mixtures (available in all grocery stores) to shorten and simplify prep.

Sheet Pan Master Template

Makes 3 to 4 servings

- 4 to 6 cups vegetables
- 1½ cups cooked or canned legumes (drained and rinsed)

  or
- 1 (14-ounce) block extra-firm tofu cut into ½-inch cubes

  or
- 1 (8-ounce) package tempeh, cut into ½-inch cubes

- 1 tablespoon fresh lemon, lime, or orange juice
- 1 tablespoon sodium-free spice mixture
- 1 tablespoon nutritional yeast
- Sea salt and black pepper to taste

Recommended vegetables: ¾-inch pieces red or yellow onion, ¾-inch pieces or sliced any color bell pepper or poblano pepper, cherry tomatoes, bite-size cauliflower florets, 2-inch broccoli florets, ½-inch pieces peeled sweet potato or winter squash, 1-inch pieces summer squash, halved or quartered brussels sprouts, ½-inch diced root veggies (white potatoes, carrots, beets)

Recommended legumes: chickpeas, black beans, navy beans, cannellini beans, pinto beans, borlotti beans

Recommended spice mixtures: herbes de Provence, Italian herbs, garam masala, mild curry powder, harissa seasoning, taco seasoning, Greek seasoning

Optional Additions

- Cooked grains: 1 to 3 cups brown rice, black rice, red rice, wild rice, quinoa, millet, buckwheat, amaranth, barley, farro, bulgur, teff
- Sauce: any sauce on pages 268–271 or a splash of tamari, more fresh citrus juice, and/or drizzle of nut or seed butter
- Garnish: fresh herbs, nuts, seeds, microgreens, sprouts, hot sauce, sliced avocados, pickled vegetables, scallions, olives, capers

How-To

1. Preheat the oven to 400°F and line a large sheet pan with parchment paper.
2. Place the veggies and drained legumes, tofu, or tempeh in a large bowl and toss with the citrus juice. Sprinkle with the chosen spice mixture and nutritional yeast and toss until all the veggies are coated. Spread everything out onto the sheet pan. Season with salt and black pepper.
3. Place the pan in the oven and roast for 20 minutes. Then flip everything and roast for another 5 to 15 minutes. The veggies are done when they're all fork-tender and starting to brown. The larger the cut and the denser the vegetable, the longer the time required in the oven.
4. While the veggies and beans are in the oven, make the sauce (if using) according to directions and reheat your grains.
5. When the veggies and beans are done, divide among bowls, serve with warm cooked grains, drizzle with sauce, and garnish as you wish.

SHEET PAN RECIPES

GO-TO

Easy Broccoli and Bean Sheet Pan

Total time in the oven: 20 to 25 minutes

- 1 cup coarsely chopped red onion (1 medium red onion)
- 3 cups 2-inch broccoli florets (1 medium head broccoli)
- 1 tablespoon fresh lemon juice
- 1 tablespoon Italian seasoning
- 1 tablespoon nutritional yeast
- 1½ cups cooked or canned cannellini beans (drained and rinsed)
- Sea salt and black pepper to taste
- 3 cups cooked brown rice
- 1 batch Sesame Balsamic Dressing (page 271)

▶ 11 points (including sauce)

POWERED-UP

Fierce Fiesta Sheet Pan

Total time in the oven: 25 to 30 minutes

- 1 cup cherry tomatoes, whole or halved
- 1 cup thickly sliced red bell pepper (1 medium pepper)
- 1 cup thickly sliced poblano pepper (1 small poblano pepper)
- 2 cups roughly chopped peeled sweet potato (½-inch pieces; 1 medium sweet potato)
- 1½ cups cooked or canned pinto beans (drained and rinsed)
- 1 tablespoon fresh lime juice

- 1 tablespoon sodium-free taco seasoning
- 1 tablespoon nutritional yeast
- Sea salt and black pepper to taste
- 3 cups cooked millet
- 1 batch Cashew Sour Cream (page 269) or sliced avocado

Garnishes (Per Plate)
- Hot sauce
- Handful sprouts

▶ **14 points (including sauce)**

SUPERCHARGED

Anti-Inflammatory Sheet Pan

Total time in the oven: 25 to 30 minutes

- 1 cup coarsely chopped red onion (1 medium red onion)
- 4 cups bite-size cauliflower florets (1 medium head cauliflower)
- 1 cup coarsely chopped yellow bell pepper (1 medium pepper)
- 1½ cups cooked or canned chickpeas (drained and rinsed)
- 1 tablespoon fresh lemon juice
- 2 teaspoons garam masala

- 2 teaspoons curry powder
- 1 tablespoon nutritional yeast
- Sea salt and black pepper to taste
- 3 cups cooked white quinoa
- 1 batch Green Herb Sauce (page 268)

Garnishes (Per Plate)
- 1 scallion, sliced
- Red pepper flakes

▶ **20 points (including sauce)**

Make Your Own Sheet Pan Variation

When pairing ingredients, choosing veggies that are similar in cooking time is key. For example, potatoes are better paired with other root veggies like beets or carrots, as opposed to quicker-cooking broccoli or asparagus. If some veggies are starting to burn and others aren't yet cooked, remove the cooked veggies from the pan and keep warm until the others are done. Be careful not to overcrowd your sheet pan; this will result in slower and uneven cooking. Use your largest sheet pan or two medium sheet pans if needed. If you are serving with whole grains, keep in mind that 1 cup dry grains yields 3 cups cooked.

Phytochemical Suggestions
Sheet pan pairings we recommend:

- Brussels sprouts, cauliflower, chickpeas, herbes de Provence, Miso Walnut Sauce (page 270)
- Beets, potatoes, sweet potatoes, borlotti beans, Italian herbs, Sesame Balsamic Dressing (page 271)
- Zucchini, tomatoes, red onion, tofu, Greek seasoning, olives, fresh lemon juice

BUILD-YOUR-OWN ONE-POT MEAL

One-pot meals save time and reduce cleanup, but their simplicity and convenience don't require any nutritional or phytochemical sacrifice. Stews, dals, rice pilafs, and curries are all delicious, health-supportive meals you can make by using a single pot.

One-Pot Meal Master Template

Makes 4 servings

- 1 medium red or yellow onion, diced
- ½ teaspoon sea salt, plus more to taste
- 3 to 6 garlic cloves, minced
- 1 to 2 tablespoons dried herbs or spice mixture
- 4 to 5 cups diced vegetables
- ½ cup split red lentils or 1½ cups cooked or canned legumes (drained and rinsed)

- 1 (15-ounce) can diced tomatoes (with or without juices)
- 3 to 4 cups vegetable broth or water
- 1 teaspoon to 2 tablespoons acid: fresh lemon or lime juice, white or red wine vinegar, rice vinegar, apple cider vinegar
- Black pepper to taste

Recommended spices: thyme, rosemary, oregano, basil, turmeric, cumin, coriander, smoked paprika, ground fennel, curry powder, garam masala, Italian mixed spices, herbes de Provence, cayenne pepper, red pepper flakes, or any others

Recommended vegetables: leeks, mushrooms, bell peppers, cauliflower, zucchini, tomatoes, carrots, celery, potatoes, sweet potatoes, winter squash, summer squash, white or green cabbage, turnips, parsnips, eggplant, fennel, celeriac, beets, okra, or others

Recommended legumes: black beans, chickpeas, navy beans, cannellini beans, borlotti beans, kidney beans, or others

Optional Additions

- 2 to 3 tablespoons nut or seed butters: almond butter, peanut butter, cashew butter, sunflower seed butter, tahini
- 1 to 2 cups coarsely chopped greens: spinach, kale, bok choy, Swiss chard, mustard greens
- 1 cup frozen green peas
- 1 cup frozen corn kernels
- 1 cup cooked grains
- 1 to 2 tablespoons tamari
- 1 to 3 teaspoons white or dark miso

How-To

1. In a soup pot, sauté the onion and salt with ¼ cup water for 7 to 10 minutes, until the onion is soft and translucent. Add water, a few tablespoons at a time, to prevent burning and stir often.
2. Add the garlic and chosen spices and cook for another 30 seconds, stirring.
3. Now add the vegetables and cook, stirring often, for another 5 minutes. Again, add water as needed to prevent burning. If using mushrooms, resist adding too much water as they'll release their own juices as they cook.
4. Next, pour the split red lentils or other cooked legumes, diced tomatoes (with or without the juices), and broth or water into the pot and bring to a boil over high heat. Once boiling, reduce the heat to a simmer, partially cover, and cook for 25 to 35 minutes. Stir occasionally and ensure the veggies are submerged in the liquid; if not, add more broth or water. Remove the cover and turn the heat off. The veggies should be cooked through and tender. If using red lentils, these should also be tender.
5. If using nut or seed butter, add it now and wait a few minutes to let it melt into the broth. Then stir vigorously until creamy.
6. Finally, add the acid, greens, and any other additions and let everything rest for 5 minutes or until the greens have wilted. If you want a looser consistency, add more water or broth. Taste and add more salt and black pepper as needed. Scoop into bowls and enjoy.

Notes

If adding miso, it's best to remove a portion of the liquid from the pot and whisk it together with the miso, then return both back to the pot.

If using frozen green peas or corn kernels, add them to the pot for the last minute of cooking.

Cooked grains can be stirred into the pot or, if your meal is already thick like a stew, served alongside.

ONE-POT MEAL RECIPES

`GO-TO`

Smoky Squash and Lentils

- 1 medium red onion, diced
- ½ teaspoon sea salt, or more to taste
- 4 garlic cloves, minced
- 2 teaspoons smoked paprika
- 2 teaspoons dried oregano
- 2 teaspoons ground cumin
- ¼ to ½ teaspoon red pepper flakes, optional
- 4 cups cubed peeled butternut or kabocha squash

- 1½ cups cooked or canned brown lentils (drained and rinsed) or ½ cup dried split red lentils
- 1 (14.5-ounce) can diced tomatoes (with the juices)
- 3½ cups vegetable broth, plus more as needed
- 1 tablespoon fresh lime juice
- Black pepper to taste

▶ 11 points

`POWERED-UP`

Moroccan Chickpeas and Rice

- 1 medium yellow onion, diced
- ½ teaspoon sea salt, or more to taste
- 5 garlic cloves, minced
- 1½ teaspoons ground cumin
- 1½ teaspoons ground coriander
- 1 teaspoon ground cinnamon
- ¼ teaspoon ground turmeric or ¾ teaspoon grated fresh turmeric root
- Pinch cayenne pepper, or more to taste

- Pinch black pepper, or more to taste
- 3 cups bite-size cauliflower florets
- 1 (14.5-ounce) can diced tomatoes (with the juices)
- 1½ cups cooked or canned chickpeas (drained and rinsed)
- 2½ to 3 cups vegetable broth
- 3 tablespoons almond butter
- 2 tablespoons fresh lemon juice
- 1 cup frozen green peas
- 3 cups cooked brown rice, for serving

▶ 15 points

SUPERCHARGED

Reinvented Root Veggie Stew

- 1 medium yellow onion, diced
- ½ teaspoon sea salt, or more to taste
- 4 garlic cloves, minced
- 1 heaping tablespoon fresh rosemary leaves, minced
- 2 teaspoons dried thyme
- Pinch black pepper or to taste
- ½ cup diced celery
- 1 cup diced carrot or parsnip
- 1 large portobello mushroom, chopped (about 1 cup)
- 1 cup diced peeled turnip or rutabaga
- 1 cup diced peeled sweet potato

- 1 cup diced peeled white potato
- 4 cups vegetable broth, plus more if needed
- 1 (14-ounce) can diced tomatoes (drained; reserve juices for your next soup)
- 1½ cups cooked or canned cannellini beans (drained and rinsed)
- 2 tablespoons cashew butter or tahini
- 1 teaspoon white wine vinegar
- 1 cup coarsely chopped Swiss chard leaves
- 1 cup baby spinach
- 1 tablespoon white miso

▶ 17 points

Make Your Own One-Pot Meal Variation

In one-pot meals, spices build flavor, beans offer protein, nut and seed butters create a creamy consistency, and greens add color and vibrancy. You also have the choice to determine the meal's thickness—whether it's thick like a stew or more brothy like a soup—by adjusting the amount of liquid used. The key is to ensure the vegetables are always submerged in liquid while cooking.

Phytochemical Suggestions

Great combinations for this template include:

- Curry powder, sweet potatoes, cauliflower, and split red lentils
- Rosemary, thyme, white beans, potatoes, and kale
- Dried basil, fennel, turnip, and Swiss chard

BUILD-YOUR-OWN STIR-FRY

Stir-frying is a quick cooking method where bite-size pieces of food are cooked over high heat in a pan or wok, while being constantly stirred around. Veggies and whole foods are added to the pan in order of density, with the denser veggies being cooked first and the more delicate leafy greens added last. A traditional stir-fry uses oil, but it can easily be done without any oil at all.

Stir-fry moves fast, so it's best to be prepped. Have all the veggies chopped and ready to go, keep a measuring cup or glass of water next to the stove, cook the grains or noodles ahead of time, and make sure the sauce and garnishes are also prepped. If you want to skip the suggested sauces, you can season the veggies with soy sauce or tamari, any vinegar, or a squeeze of fresh lemon juice. You can also use your preferred sauce.

Stir-Fry Master Template

Makes 2 to 4 servings

- Stir-fry sauce of your choice (three options follow)
- 5 to 7 cups vegetables: a mixture of firm and soft vegetables and/or leafy greens
- 3 large garlic cloves, minced
- 1½ cups thawed frozen shelled edamame or Baked Tofu (page 267)

Firm vegetables: sliced onions, sliced bell peppers, 1-inch broccoli florets, ½-inch cauliflower florets, thinly sliced carrot rounds, sliced brussels sprouts, chopped cabbage, baby corn, sliced or chopped mushrooms

Soft vegetables: sliced summer squash, chopped asparagus, snow peas, snap peas

Leafy greens: kale, collard greens, bok choy, Swiss chard, baby spinach

---

Optional Additions

- 3 cups cooked grains or cooked whole grain noodles, for serving
- Garnishes: thinly sliced scallions, julienned cucumber, julienned carrots, shredded cabbage, fresh herbs, nuts, seeds, sprouts, hot peppers, sesame seeds, hot sauce

How-To

1. Put all the sauce ingredients in a jar and shake vigorously. Set aside.
2. Warm a large skillet or wok over medium to high heat. Once hot, add the firm vegetables and a few tablespoons of water and cook, stirring, for 3 to 4 minutes, until they start to soften. Stir constantly. Add more water, a couple of tablespoons at a time, to prevent burning. The water will cook off quickly; keep cooking and stirring until the veggies start sticking then add more as needed.
3. Next, add the soft veggies and hearty greens (like kale or collard greens), garlic, and cook for another 1 to 2 minutes, stirring. If your firm veggies aren't fork-tender yet, reduce the heat to medium-low, add a couple of tablespoons of water if the pan is dry, and cover the pan. Cook for another minute, then remove the cover. This will steam the veggies. They're done when just tender and vibrant.
4. Shake the sauce again in case it has separated and pour it into the pan. Toss in any delicate greens (like baby spinach) as well as the edamame or tofu and simmer over medium heat for 30 to 60 seconds, until the sauce starts to thicken and the greens are vibrant.
5. If serving with grains or noodles, spoon those onto plates first, then top with the veggie mixture. Garnish with your favorite toppings.

STIR-FRY SAUCE RECIPES

Teriyaki Sauce

- 3 tablespoons tamari or soy sauce
- 2 tablespoons rice vinegar
- 1 tablespoon maple syrup
- 2 teaspoons finely grated fresh ginger
- 1 to 3 teaspoons vinegar-based hot sauce
- 1 tablespoon arrowroot starch
- ⅓ cup water or vegetable broth

▶ 2 points

Orange Ginger Sauce

- ½ cup fresh orange juice
- 3 tablespoons tamari or soy sauce
- 1 tablespoon rice vinegar
- 1 tablespoon maple syrup
- 1 tablespoon finely grated fresh ginger
- 1 tablespoon arrowroot starch

▶ 2 points

Balsamic and Thyme Sauce

- 3 tablespoons tamari or soy sauce
- 2 tablespoons balsamic vinegar
- 1 teaspoon red wine vinegar
- 1 tablespoon maple syrup
- 2 teaspoons finely grated fresh ginger
- 1 tablespoon smooth Dijon mustard
- 1 teaspoon nutritional yeast
- ¾ teaspoon dried thyme
- 1 tablespoon arrowroot starch
- ½ cup water or vegetable broth

▶ 2 points

STIR-FRY RECIPES

GO-TO

Cauliflower Stir-Fry

Makes 2 to 4 servings

- Teriyaki Sauce (page 245)
- 1 cup thinly sliced red onion
- 2 cups ½-inch cauliflower florets
- 2 cups thinly sliced red bell pepper
- 3 garlic cloves, minced

- 1½ cups frozen shelled edamame, thawed
- 3 cups cooked brown rice, for serving

Garnishes (Per Bowl)
- 1 tablespoon sesame seeds

▶ 9 points (including sauce)

POWERED-UP

Winter Stir-Fry

Makes 2 to 4 servings

- Balsamic and Thyme Sauce (page 245)
- 1 cup thinly sliced yellow bell pepper
- 1 cup thinly sliced fennel bulb
- 2 cups thinly sliced brussels sprouts
- 2 cups coarsely chopped portobello mushrooms

- 3 garlic cloves, minced
- 1 cup coarsely chopped kale
- 1 batch Baked Tofu (page 267)
- 3 cups cooked white quinoa, for serving

Garnishes (Per Bowl)
- 2 tablespoons chopped hazelnuts

▶ 11 points (including sauce)

SUPERCHARGED

Broccoli Stir-Fry

Makes 2 to 4 servings

- Orange Ginger Sauce (page 245)
- 1 cup thinly sliced carrot rounds
- 3 cups 1-inch broccoli florets
- 1 cup snap peas
- 3 garlic cloves, minced
- 1 cup packed coarsely chopped bok choy
- 1 cup packed baby spinach

- 1 batch Baked Tofu (page 267)
- 3 cups cooked whole grain noodles, for serving

Garnishes (Per Bowl)
- 2 tablespoons chopped cashews
- ¼ cup sprouts of your choice
- Thinly sliced scallions

▶ 13 points (including sauce)

Make Your Own Stir-Fry Variation

Here are some stir-fry tips.

- Cut the vegetables in uniform pieces and keep in mind that thinner sliced and smaller diced veggies will cook faster.
- Keep the density and cooking times of vegetables in mind. Layer them into the pan and adjust the order of addition based on the vegetables you've chosen.
- For denser vegetables like carrots or potatoes, it's best to precook them slightly by blanching or microwaving to reduce stir-fry time.
- If you're using a nonstick pan, keep the heat to medium. Avoid getting it scorching hot as this can degrade the nonstick coating.
- Mushrooms aren't considered firm, but meatier mushrooms, like portobellos, cook better when added at the beginning of an oil-free stir-fry with the harder, denser veggies.
- If using greens, it's best to avoid salad greens or tender greens as they don't stand up to heat very well.

- You can swap 1½ cups cooked beans for the edamame or the tofu.
- Arrowroot starch is a thickening agent, similar to cornstarch, but less processed.

Phytochemical Suggestions

Here are some combinations that work well in this stir-fry template:

- Bell peppers, zucchini, snow peas, cherry tomatoes, tofu
- Mixed mushrooms (button, enoki, cremini), bean sprouts, edamame
- Onions, broccoli, asparagus, spinach, tofu

A Note on Herbs and Spices

The secret to a flavorful whole food, phytotoxin-loaded diet is the liberal and intentional use of fresh and dried herbs and whole and ground spices. These seasonings are a crucial element in food preparation in every culture. Buy herbs and spices in small quantities as they become rancid and lose their flavor and antioxidant power with age and with exposure to light, heat, and oxygen. Keep them in a dark, cool, and dry place. Blended spice mixes, like curry powders and herbes de Provence, offer convenience by combining regional flavors.

Here are some herb and spice combinations from around the world:

- Basil, oregano, thyme (Mediterranean)
- Cumin, coriander, turmeric, cardamom, clove, cinnamon, nutmeg (Indian)
- Cumin, chili powder, paprika, cilantro (Mexican)
- Cumin, coriander, paprika, cinnamon, garlic, caraway (North African)
- Lemongrass, Thai basil, cilantro (Thai)
- Thyme, rosemary, marjoram, savory, bay leaf (French)
- Thyme, sumac, oregano, marjoram (Middle Eastern)
- Star anise, cloves, cinnamon, Szechuan peppercorn, fennel (Chinese)
- Paprika, saffron, dried chili pepper, oregano (Spanish)

BUILD-YOUR-OWN PURÉED VEGGIE SOUP

Puréed vegetable soups are nutritional powerhouses. They are also extremely versatile. You can include nearly any vegetable, spice, or herb. While this template draws on commonly used vegetables, you can get creative and blend pretty much anything into a soup. Similarly, you can add whatever flavors you love.

Puréed Veggie Soup Master Template

Makes 4 to 6 servings

- 2 cups diced yellow onion
- 2 to 4 garlic cloves, minced
- 1 to 3 teaspoons ground spices or dried herbs
- ½ teaspoon sea salt, plus more to taste
- Pinch black pepper, optional

- 4 to 5 cups coarsely chopped peeled vegetables
- 4 to 5 cups low-sodium vegetable broth
- 1 to 2 tablespoons fresh lemon juice

Recommended vegetables: carrots, potatoes, beets, cauliflower, sweet potatoes, winter squash, bell peppers, fennel, broccoli, turnips, rutabaga, kohlrabi, and many others

Optional Additions

- 2 to 4 tablespoons nuts or seeds: almonds, cashews, hazelnuts, sunflower seeds, Brazil nuts
- Fresh herbs and spices: 1 to 3 teaspoons finely grated fresh ginger, ¼ to ½ cup fresh herbs: cilantro, dill, parsley, mint, sage
- Flavoring agents: tamari or soy sauce, miso, vinegar
- 1 to 2 cups chopped greens: spinach, kale, Swiss chard, bok choy, mustard greens
- 1 cup cooked whole grains
- 1½ cups cooked or canned beans (drained and rinsed)
- Garnishes: fresh herbs, nuts, seeds, microgreens, pickled vegetables, capers, olives, sliced avocado, baby arugula

---

How-To

1. Add the onions to a large soup pot and simmer with ¼ cup of water over medium to high heat for 10 minutes, adding water as needed to prevent burning, stirring often. Cook until the onions are translucent.

2. Add the garlic, spices, salt, and pepper and cook for another 30 seconds.

3. Add all the vegetables (except any green veggies) and cook, stirring, for another few minutes. Next, add the broth and bring to a boil over high heat. Once boiling, reduce the heat to low, partially cover, and simmer for 25 to 30 minutes, until all the vegetables are fork-tender. If your soup includes a quicker-cooking green vegetable, like broccoli or asparagus, add it to the pot in the last 3 to 5 minutes of simmering to prevent overcooking. When the green veggies are vibrant and just tender, they're done.

4. Remove the soup from the heat and carefully transfer to a blender. Do this in batches if needed. Be sure not to fill the blender over three-quarters full.

5. Add the lemon juice, any nuts or seeds, fresh herbs, and/or any flavoring elements you want blended in. Blend until silky smooth. You can also use an immersion blender, but a high-speed blender will be better at purée-ing nuts and seeds.

6. Return the soup to the pot, add any beans and/or leafy greens and simmer for another few minutes until the greens are wilted. Note that if you're making a green soup (like the Mean Green Phytonutrient Machine Soup, page 251) you can add the greens right to the blender and blend them to brighten the color. Taste and add more salt and pepper as needed. Divide among bowls and garnish with desired toppings.

PURÉED VEGGIE SOUP RECIPES

GO-TO

Carrot Soup

Makes 4 to 6 servings

- 2 cups diced onion
- 4 garlic cloves, minced
- 1¼ teaspoons ground coriander

- ¼ teaspoon ground cinnamon
- ½ teaspoon sea salt, or more to taste

- Freshly cracked black pepper to taste
- 4 cups coarsely chopped carrots
- 4 cups vegetable broth

- 2 tablespoons fresh lemon juice
- ¼ cup cashews

Garnishes (Per Bowl)
- Handful fresh cilantro leaves

▶ **9 points**

POWERED-UP

Vitality Boost Beet Soup

Makes 4 to 6 servings

- 2 cups diced yellow onion
- 3 garlic cloves, minced
- 2 teaspoons ground fennel seed
- 1 teaspoon ground cumin
- ½ teaspoon sea salt, plus more to taste
- Freshly cracked black pepper to taste
- ½ cup diced celery
- 1 cup diced carrots

- 2 cups coarsely chopped peeled purple beets
- 4 cups vegetable broth
- 1 tablespoon fresh lemon juice
- 1 tablespoon finely minced peeled fresh ginger (2-inch knob)
- 1½ cups cooked or canned navy beans (drained and rinsed), optional (add after puréeing)

Garnishes (Per Bowl)
- Handful microgreens or sprouts

▶ **12 points**

SUPERCHARGED

Mean Green Phytonutrient Machine Soup

Makes 4 to 6 servings

- 2 cups diced yellow onion
- 4 large garlic cloves, minced
- 1 teaspoon ground cumin
- 1 teaspoon ground coriander
- ¼ teaspoon ground turmeric or ¾ teaspoon grated fresh turmeric root

- ½ teaspoon sea salt or to taste
- 1 cup diced celery
- 1 cup diced peeled russet potato
- 4 cups vegetable broth, plus as needed

continued

- 2 cups coarsely chopped broccoli florets*
- 2 tablespoons fresh lemon juice
- 1 cup packed coarsely chopped kale (stems removed)
- 4 to 6 Brazil nuts, coarsely chopped (about 2 tablespoons)

- ¼ cup packed fresh dill
- 2 teaspoons finely minced peeled fresh ginger (1-inch knob)

Garnishes (Per Bowl)
- Pinch red pepper flakes
- 1 tablespoon pumpkin seeds

▶ **15 points**

* For this soup we're going to add the broccoli to the pot for the last 5 minutes to avoid overcooking it. We're also adding the kale and dill right to the blender and puréeing them into the soup.

Make Your Own Puréed Veggie Soup Variation

When designing your own puréed soup, here are some things to remember.

Color: Consider what color whole foods and spices will blend to look appealing. Brown soups can be tasty but don't shout vitality. For example, green and yellow ingredients work well together, as do red and purple or white and orange.

Vegetables: Think about the season. What grows together? In winter, butternut squash and cauliflower pair wonderfully, as do asparagus and zucchini in the summer.

Spice: What's the dominant spice profile? Choose one or two. Consider popular pairings like thyme and rosemary, cumin and cinnamon, or fennel and oregano.

Season and brighten at the end: All meals, and especially puréed soups, are elevated by a hint of citrus and a light reseasoning with salt and pepper at the end of cooking.

Add more: You can bulk up any puréed soup by adding cooked legumes, cooked grains, or leafy greens after the soup has been puréed. These additions will bump up the phytotoxin and macronutrient profile as well as increase serving size.

Creaminess: Blending nuts and seeds or their butters into a soup will make them creamier and richer; however, you can omit these additions if you'd prefer a lighter, nut/seed-free soup.

Thick or thin: You can control the texture or consistency of your soup by reducing or adding more liquid. If you're not certain, it's best to take a conservative initial approach and start with less liquid. You can always add more, but it's much harder to take it away.

Phytochemical Suggestions

Great phytochemical combinations for a puréed soup include:

- Tomatoes, red bell peppers, and basil
- Sweet potatoes, carrots, and curry powder
- Spinach, zucchini, and basil
- Cauliflower, broccoli, and cashews

BUILD-YOUR-OWN SALAD

A salad is a blank slate—anything is possible! Adjust, add, or omit to suit your own preferences. While it's helpful to consider "what grows together, goes together," don't hesitate to pair unconventional ingredients and explore different textures and contrasting flavor combinations. This template, which is inspired by the traditional green salad, serves as a road map to craft a robust, satisfying, and phytonutrient-packed meal. When selecting your greens, prioritize freshness and opt for the finest quality available—a good rule for any recipe!

Salad Master Template

Makes 2 large or 4 small salads

- 3 to 4 cups leafy greens
- 2 to 4 cups vegetables

- 1 to 2 cups cooked plant protein

Recommended greens: any lettuce, spinach, arugula, watercress, kale, endive, frisée

Recommended vegetables: can be raw, steamed, or roasted

If using raw veggies, these are the best cuts:

- Finely chopped or cut into small florets: cauliflower, broccoli, broccolini
- Grated or shredded: beets, cabbage, brussels sprouts

- Peeled into ribbons: carrots, zucchini, cucumbers
- Diced or thinly sliced: onions, cucumbers, bell peppers, radishes, tomatoes, celery, fennel

Recommended plant proteins: lentils, chickpeas, kidney beans, black beans, black-eyed peas, white beans, pinto beans, edamame, seitan, tempeh, tofu, quinoa

Optional Additions

- ½ to 1 cup cooked grains: quinoa, teff, amaranth, bulgur, buckwheat, freekeh, any rice
- ¼ to ½ cup any nuts or seeds: almonds, walnuts, sesame seeds, pistachios, peanuts, sunflower seeds, hemp seeds, pumpkin seeds, hazelnuts
- ¼ cup dried fruit: raisins, currants, apricots, cranberries, elderberries, cherries
- ½ to 1 cup fresh fruit: grapes, peaches, pears, apples, nectarines, oranges, berries
- 2 to 4 tablespoons drained capers or sliced olives
- ¼ cup coarsely chopped sun-dried tomatoes
- ½ to 1 avocado, diced
- ¼ to ½ cup fresh herbs: dill, tarragon, chives, cilantro, mint, basil
- ¼ to ½ cup microgreens or sprouts

How-To

1. Prepare any cooked components first like roasted veggies or baked tofu. If there are no cooked components, move to the next step.
2. Make your dressing according to the directions and set aside (see page 268).
3. Add 2 to 4 tablespoons of the dressing to the bottom of a large salad bowl. Add your greens of choice and toss to coat. Alternatively, if you're using a more fibrous green like kale, add a couple of tablespoons of dressing to the bowl, add the kale, and using your hands, massage the dressing into the leaves for 30 to 60 seconds to help soften the fibers.
4. Next, add your veggies and protein and any other ingredients you've chosen. Drizzle everything with more dressing and toss again. Divide the salad among bowls and garnish with selected toppings.

SALAD RECIPES

GO-TO

Supreme Chopped Sesame Salad

Makes 2 large or 4 small salads

- Sesame Balsamic Dressing (page 271)
- 3 cups coarsely chopped romaine lettuce
- 1 cup finely chopped broccoli
- 1 cup thinly sliced red bell pepper
- 1 cup thinly sliced cucumber
- 1½ cups cooked or canned chickpeas (drained and rinsed)
- ¼ cup sliced raw or toasted almonds
- ¼ cup dried cranberries or elderberries

▶ 9 points (including dressing)

Brilliant Beet and Walnut Salad

Makes 2 large or 4 small salads

- Miso Walnut Sauce (page 270)
- 2 cups mixed lettuces
- 1 cup baby spinach
- 2 cups roasted bite-size cauliflower florets
- 1 cup grated purple beet
- 1 cup grated or shredded red cabbage

- 1 batch Pan-"Fried" Tempeh (page 268)
- ¼ cup chopped raw or toasted walnuts
- ½ cup diced apple or pear
- ½ cup halved or quartered red grapes
- ¼ cup broccoli sprouts

▶ 14 points (including sauce)

Regenerate and Repair Salad

Makes 3 large or 6 small salads

- Tahini Dill Sauce (page 269)
- 2 cups coarsely chopped or torn kale leaves
- 1 cup coarsely chopped red leaf lettuce
- 1 cup shredded brussels sprouts
- 1 cup thinly sliced yellow bell pepper
- 1 medium carrot, peeled into ribbons
- 1 cup roasted winter squash or sweet potato

- 1 cup frozen shelled edamame, thawed
- 1 cup cooked white quinoa or wild rice
- 3 tablespoons hemp seeds
- ¼ cup raw or toasted pumpkin seeds
- ¼ cup pomegranate arils
- 3 tablespoons drained capers
- ¼ cup packed fresh dill, chopped
- 1 medium avocado, thinly sliced

▶ 17 points (including sauce)

Make Your Own Salad Variation

Salads won't hold up well after they've been dressed, so feel free to cut the recipe in half for a single serving and add dressing only to what will be eaten. The key to an enjoyable and interesting salad is keeping veggies and fruit cut small and in different shapes. Using tools like mandolines, vegetable peelers, box graters, and julienne peelers can make veggie prep easier.

Pro Tips

- For best salad results, incorporate different textures like crunchy, creamy, chewy, and crispy.
- For balanced taste, try incorporating different flavor profiles like salty, sweet, sour, spicy, and bitter.

Phytochemical Suggestions

Here are some suggested pairings:

- Spinach, black beans, bell peppers, avocados, jalapeños, red onions
- Kale, quinoa, blueberries, carrots, radishes, grapefruit
- Arugula, white beans, cucumber ribbons, roasted beets, walnuts

BUILD-YOUR-OWN NOURISH BOWL

A nourish bowl, also known as a Buddha bowl, power bowl, or grain bowl, does exactly as the name suggests—nourishes. This type of meal is balanced in taste, nutrition, color, and texture, and the ingredients are usually arranged in sections. Elements typically include seasonal vegetables, greens, grains, legumes, nuts, seeds, and often, seaweed; essentially, all the plant-based food groups. The components can be cooked or raw, pickled or fermented, sprouted or soaked, or a mixture of everything. The wonderful thing about a nourish bowl is that you can tailor it exactly to your liking and to what you have on hand. You can also adjust the portion sizes to meet your hunger levels.

The anatomy of the bowl is helpful to keep in mind—a nourish bowl is usually half vegetables and leafy greens and half whole grains, starchy vegetable, and legumes. And unlike garnishes for many meals, the toppings for a nourish bowl are essential. They often add the missing piece, whether it be some needed crunch, saltiness, sweetness, or a pop of vibrant green. The final and most important piece of a nourish bowl is the sauce or dressing—it will tie everything together. For this template, we're using steaming as our primary cooking method; see the box below for more instruction if you're not familiar with this method of cooking.

Nourish Bowl Master Template

Makes 1 large bowl or 2 small bowls

- Sauce of choice (page 268), fresh citrus juice, tamari, or vinegar
- ½ to 1 cup cooked grains: quinoa, any rice, amaranth, buckwheat, teff, millet, bulgur
- ½ to 1 cup cooked plant protein: lentils, chickpeas, kidney beans, black beans, black-eyed peas, white beans, pinto beans, edamame, seitan, tempeh, tofu, quinoa
- ½ to 1 cup steamed starchy vegetable, optional: sweet potatoes, winter squash, potatoes

- 2 to 3 cups raw or steamed non-starchy vegetables: broccoli, cauliflower, brussels sprouts, radishes, cucumbers, zucchini, carrots, asparagus, beets, bell peppers, jarred artichokes (packed in water)
- ½ to 2 cups raw or steamed greens: spinach, collard greens, kale, Swiss chard, bok choy, lettuces, cabbage, mustard greens, sprouts, arugula, endive, escarole (salad greens are best used raw)

Optional Additions

- For bold flavor: sun-dried tomatoes, capers, olives, pickled vegetables, sauerkraut, kimchi, vinegar or tamari/soy sauce
- For spice: chilis, hot sauce, jalapeños

- For crunch: raw or toasted nuts or seeds, sprouted whole grains, toasted whole spices, julienned raw veggies
- For color and extra phytonutrients: microgreens, fresh herbs, sliced onions, cherry tomatoes
- For richness: sliced avocados, extra sauce, or drizzle of nut or seed butter
- To brighten: fresh citrus juice

How-To

1. First, prepare your chosen sauce and set aside until needed.
2. Next, if not using already-cooked grains, prepare those according to the directions and keep warm until needed. If not using canned or already-prepared legumes, cook those accordingly as well. If you already have these prepared, you can reheat grains or beans in a small pan, microwave, or add to the pot of steaming veggies for the last minute of cooking time.
3. Decide what vegetables will be added to the bowl raw (if any). Prepare those (slice, chop, grate) and set aside. These will be listed in our sample recipes in parentheses as "raw."
4. Choose and prepare the vegetables you're going to steam. They will be listed in the ingredient list in order of density. Fill the bottom of a large pot with a couple of inches of water or to just below the steamer basket level. Place the steamer basket in the pot and bring to a boil. Once boiling, add the starchy and densest vegetables first and cover the pot. Steam until these dense vegetables are almost tender, then add the softer or more delicate vegetables, cover again, and cook until tender. Add any leafy greens you want to cook for the final minute or two of steaming until bright green. Here you can also add any grains or legumes you'd like to reheat. Once everything is cooked, remove the cover and take the steamer basket out of the pot to halt cooking.
5. Arrange the grains, legumes, steamed vegetables and greens, and raw vegetables in the bowl in sections. Add desired toppings and drizzle with sauce.

Steaming

This nourish bowl template relies on steaming as the main cooking method. Steaming is fast, healthy, and easy. All you need is a steamer basket and a pot. The basic method of steaming is the same for all whole food ingredients, but the time required will depend on the vegetable. It's convenient to steam different vegetables together. Just start with the denser ones and gradually add the rest in decreasing density order, saving leafy greens for the end. Keeping vegetables separate is ideal. If you have a smaller basket, layer the vegetables (placing denser ones at the bottom). Layering will extend cooking times.

When steaming, keep checking to make sure there is still water in the pot, and add more if it's all cooked off before the veggies are fork-tender. Things that can affect cooking time:

- Cut the vegetables in uniform pieces and note that the smaller the cut, the quicker the cooking time.
- An overcrowded steamer basket will result in longer cooking times and some items may cook unevenly.
- Keep checking for doneness. Vegetables are done when just fork-tender and vibrant in color. Overcooking starchy veggies like sweet potato isn't an issue but try to avoid overcooking delicate and green veggies.

Steaming guide to cooking times*

Longer-Cooking Vegetables
12 to 15 minutes

Beets · White potatoes · Winter squash

Medium-Cooking Vegetables
7 to 12 minutes

Brussels sprouts · Carrots · Cauliflower · Sweet potatoes

Quick-Cooking Vegetables
2 to 5 minutes

Asparagus · Bell peppers · Broccoli · Cabbage · Snow peas · Zucchini

Leafy Greens
1 to 3 minutes (until bright green)

Bok choy (stems steam longer) · Collard greens · Kale · Spinach ·
 Swiss chard

Times vary with veggie size

NOURISH BOWL RECIPES

GO-TO

Weeknight Healing Bowl

- Tahini Dill Sauce (page 269)
- ½ cup cooked brown rice
- ½ cup cooked or canned brown lentils (drained and rinsed)
- ½ cup thinly sliced red cabbage

  ▸ 10 points (including sauce)

Veggies to Steam
- 1 cup coarsely chopped unpeeled kabocha squash
- 2 cups 1-inch broccoli florets
- 1 cup baby spinach

POWERED-UP

Revitalizing Rainbow Bowl

- Almond Thai Dressing (page 271)
- ½ cup cooked millet
- 1 cup Baked Tofu (page 267)
- ½ cup thinly sliced red bell pepper
- ½ cup grated beet

Veggies to Steam
- 1 cup cubed sweet potato (with or without peel)

- 2 cups coarsely chopped bok choy

Garnishes
- ¼ cup fresh cilantro leaves or mint leaves
- 1 to 2 scallions, thinly sliced
- Thinly sliced chili peppers

▶ 14 points (including sauce)

SUPERCHARGED

Mighty Mediterranean Bowl

- Creamy Roasted Red Pepper Sauce (page 270)
- 1 cup cooked white quinoa
- ½ cup cooked or canned borlotti beans (drained and rinsed)
- ½ cup drained water-packed canned artichokes, quartered
- 1 cup baby arugula

Veggies to Steam
- 2 cups 1-inch cauliflower florets
- ½ cup thinly sliced yellow bell pepper
- ½ cup thinly sliced zucchini

Garnishes
- ¼ cup thinly sliced black or green olives
- ¼ cup thinly sliced red onion
- ¼ cup cherry tomatoes, halved
- 2 tablespoons pine nuts

▶ 18 points (including sauce)

Make Your Own Nourish Bowl Variation

The sky is the limit on the number of nourish bowl combinations you can make from this template.

Phytochemical Suggestions

Here are nourish bowl food pairings that we recommend:

- Millet, sweet potatoes, broccoli, tempeh, avocado, cilantro, pumpkin seeds
- Wild rice, brussels sprouts, kale, cannellini beans, sun-dried tomatoes
- Quinoa, asparagus, snap peas, edamame, fresh dill, lemon juice

BUILD-YOUR-OWN POWER BALLS

Power balls are two-bite snacks that offer many essential macro- and micronutrients. Made from whole foods like nuts, seeds, and dried fruit, these delicious treats will satisfy your sweet tooth while also delivering a host of beneficial plant compounds and phytotoxins.

Power Ball Master Template

Makes 20 to 24 balls

- 1½ cups old-fashioned rolled oats
- ½ cup pitted medjool or deglet noor dates
- 1 cup other dried fruit
- 1 cup nuts or seeds
- 2 to 4 tablespoons nut or seed butter
- Pinch sea salt
- 1 to 4 tablespoons liquid

Recommended dried fruit: raisins, cranberries, apple, mango, apricots, elderberries, cherries, pineapple, or an additional cup of dates, or a mixture

Recommended nuts or seeds: almonds, walnuts, peanuts, cashews, hazelnuts, pistachios, pecans, pumpkin seeds, sunflower seeds

Recommended nut or seed butters: peanut, almond, cashew, sunflower seed, tahini

Recommended liquid: dairy-free milk, water, fresh citrus juice, cooled brewed tea, espresso, or coffee

Optional Additions

- Dry flavoring additions: 2 to 4 tablespoons unsweetened cocoa powder, 1 to 2 tablespoons matcha powder, 1 to 2 tablespoons ground espresso, ½ to 3 teaspoons ground spices
- Citrus zest: lemon, orange, lime
- Grated veggies: ½ cup finely grated carrot or beet
- Crunchy additions: ¼ to ½ cup cacao nibs or vegan dark chocolate chips, 2 to 4 tablespoons hemp seeds, ¼ to ½ cup unsweetened flaked coconut
- For rolling/coating: ⅓ cup crushed nuts, seeds, unsweetened flaked coconut, hemp seeds, or sesame seeds

How-To

1. Add the oats, dates, other dried fruit, nuts, seeds, nut or seed butters, salt, chosen liquid, and any dry powdered additions to a food processor. Process continuously until the mixture starts clumping together. If you're adding any zest, grated veggies or crunchy bits, add them now and pulse the processor a few times to combine everything.

2. Transfer the mixture to a bowl. Use a ¾-ounce spring-release scoop to scoop the dough (or scoop out about 2 tablespoons) and roll into balls.

3. If coating the power balls, spread your chosen coating out onto a small plate and gently roll the balls in the coating. Refrigerate the balls for about an hour before serving for best results. These will keep in the fridge for up to 5 days and the freezer for up to 3 months. You can enjoy them directly from the freezer as well.

POWER BALL RECIPES

GO-TO

PB&C Power Balls

Makes 20 balls

- 1½ cups old-fashioned rolled oats
- ½ cup pitted medjool or deglet noor dates
- 1 cup dried cranberries

- 1 cup almonds
- ¼ cup peanut butter
- Pinch sea salt
- ¼ cup dairy-free milk

▶ 6 points

POWERED-UP

Longevity Latte Power Balls

Makes 22 to 24 balls

- 1½ cups old-fashioned rolled oats
- ¾ cup pitted medjool or deglet noor dates
- ¾ cup raisins
- 1 cup raw cashews
- ¼ cup almond butter or sunflower seed butter

- Pinch sea salt
- ¼ cup cooled brewed strong coffee or espresso
- ½ teaspoon ground cinnamon
- ⅓ cup cacao nibs
- ⅓ cup hemp seeds, for rolling

▸ 9 points

SUPERCHARGED

Potent Carrot Cake Power Balls

Makes 22 to 24 balls

- 1½ cups old-fashioned rolled oats
- ½ cup pitted medjool or deglet noor dates
- ½ cup dried apple rings
- ½ cup dried apricots
- 1 cup pecans
- 3 tablespoons cashew butter or sunflower seed butter

- Pinch sea salt
- ¼ cup fresh orange juice
- 1 teaspoon ground cinnamon
- ½ teaspoon ground allspice
- ¼ teaspoon ground nutmeg
- Zest of 1 orange
- ½ cup finely grated carrot
- ⅓ cup unsweetened coconut, for rolling

▸ 13 points

Make Your Own Power Ball Variation

As you make power balls with different flavors and textures, here are some troubleshooting tips.

- If the mixture is too crumbly and not sticking together, add more liquid, 1 tablespoon at a time, and process again.
- If the mixture is too sticky, add more oats and process again. Chilling the mixture for 30 to 60 minutes will also make it less sticky and easier to roll.
- After rolling a few balls, it's normal for the mixture to start sticking to your hands. Rinse your hands after every third or fourth ball to reduce the stickiness.

Phytochemical Suggestions

Here are some power ball combinations that work well:

- Dried apples, cinnamon, almonds, sunflower seed butter
- Dried cranberries, lemon juice, flaked coconut, cashews
- Dried cherries, pecans, cocoa powder, orange juice

BONUS RECIPES

Baked Tofu

- 1 tablespoon brown rice flour
- 1 tablespoon nutritional yeast
- 1 (14-ounce) container extra-firm tofu
- Pinch sea salt

1. Preheat the oven to 400°F and line a large baking sheet with parchment paper. Mix the brown rice flour and nutritional yeast in a small bowl.

2. Drain the tofu, cut it into ¾-inch cubes, and place in a medium bowl. Sprinkle the brown rice mixture over the tofu and toss to coat all the tofu. Transfer the tofu to the prepared pan, season with salt, and bake for 30 to 35 minutes, flipping halfway through. The tofu is done when browned and firm.

    Notes: You have the option to press the tofu. This will help create a firmer texture, but if you're short on time, you can skip pressing altogether. To press the tofu, wrap in a clean dish towel, lay something heavy on top (like a cutting board with some cans of beans on top), and leave it for 15 to 20 minutes so that extra liquid is pressed out of the tofu.

Pan-"Fried" Tempeh

- 1 (8-ounce) package tempeh
- 1 tablespoon tamari or soy sauce
- 2 teaspoons balsamic vinegar

1. Cut the tempeh into ½-inch cubes and place in a medium bowl. Pour the tamari and balsamic over the tempeh and toss until the tempeh has absorbed all the liquid.
2. Warm a medium or large nonstick skillet over medium heat. Transfer the tempeh to the skillet and cook for 5 minutes until the tempeh is browned. Add water, a couple of tablespoons at a time if needed, to prevent burning.

SAUCES AND DRESSINGS

Keep all sauces in the fridge in a sealed container, where they'll last for up to 5 days.

Green Herb Sauce

- ¾ cup cashews, soaked in hot water for 1 to 3 hours
- 3 tablespoons fresh lemon juice
- 1 teaspoon red wine vinegar

- 1 teaspoon agave, optional
- ¾ teaspoon smooth Dijon mustard
- Pinch red pepper flakes
- ½ teaspoon sea salt or to taste
- 1 cup fresh mint leaves or dill
- 1 cup fresh cilantro (leaves and tender stems only)
- ¾ cup water

Drain the cashews, discarding the soaking liquid, and add them to a blender with all the other ingredients. Blend until smooth. Taste and add more salt as needed.

▶ 5 points

Cashew Sour Cream

- 1 cup cashews, soaked in hot water for 1 to 3 hours
- 1 teaspoon smooth Dijon mustard
- 1 tablespoon apple cider vinegar
- Pinch sea salt or to taste
- ½ cup water, plus more as needed

Drain the cashews, discarding the soaking liquid, and add them to a blender with all the other ingredients. Blend until smooth. Add more water if needed to thin. Taste and add more salt as needed.

▶ 1 point

Tahini Dill Sauce

- ⅓ cup tahini
- 1½ teaspoons dried dill
- 3 tablespoons fresh lemon juice
- 1 garlic clove, minced
- Sea salt to taste
- 3 tablespoons water, plus more as needed

In a medium bowl, add the tahini, dill, lemon juice, garlic, and salt. Mix with a fork until combined. It will be thick. Now add the water and mix again. Add more water if needed to reach the desired consistency. Taste and add more salt as needed.

▶ 4 points

Miso Walnut Sauce

- ¾ cup raw or toasted walnuts
- 1 tablespoon plus
  2 teaspoons white miso
- 1 tablespoon maple syrup
- 1 large garlic clove,
  crushed and peeled
- 2 tablespoons fresh lemon juice
- 1 teaspoon red wine vinegar
- 1 teaspoon smooth Dijon mustard
- ¾ cup water, plus
  more as needed
- Salt and black pepper to taste

Add all the ingredients to a blender. Blend until smooth. Add more water if needed to reach the desired consistency. Taste and add more salt and pepper as needed.

▶ 5 points

Creamy Roasted Red Pepper Sauce

- ½ cup sunflower seeds, soaked
  for 1 to 3 hours in hot water
- 1 medium red bell pepper,
  roasted (about ½ cup strips)
- 1 garlic clove, crushed
  and peeled
- 1 tablespoon nutritional yeast
- ½ teaspoon dried thyme
- ¼ teaspoon red pepper flakes
- ¼ teaspoon sea salt
- Pinch black pepper
- 2 tablespoons fresh lemon juice
- 1 teaspoon red wine vinegar
- ¾ cup water

Drain the sunflower seeds, discarding the soaking liquid, and add them to a blender with all the other ingredients. Blend until smooth. Taste and add more salt and black pepper as needed.

▶ 7 points

Fat-Free Apple Cider Vinaigrette

- 2 tablespoons smooth
  Dijon mustard
- 2 tablespoons apple cider
  vinegar (with the mother*)
- ¼ teaspoon dried oregano
- ¼ teaspoon onion powder
- ¼ teaspoon dried parsley
- 1 tablespoon maple syrup
- Sea salt and black
  pepper to taste

Add all the ingredients to a small bowl or jar and whisk until combined. Taste and add more salt and pepper as needed.

Unfiltered versions of apple cider vinegar are unrefined, cloudy, and have sediment at the bottom of the bottle. This sediment is known as the "mother" and is a collection or culture of bacteria. The mother is a probiotic and has a host of other health benefits.

▶ **4 points**

Almond Thai Dressing

- ⅓ cup almond butter
- ¼ cup fresh lime juice
- 1 tablespoon tamari or soy sauce
- 1 tablespoon agave or maple syrup
- 1 tablespoon minced peeled fresh ginger
- 1 large garlic clove, crushed and peeled
- 1 to 2 teaspoons vinegar-based hot sauce
- ⅓ cup water, plus more as needed

Add all the ingredients to a blender. Blend until smooth. Add more water if needed to reach desired consistency.

▶ **5 points**

Sesame Balsamic Dressing

- ¼ cup tahini
- 2 tablespoons balsamic vinegar
- 2 tablespoons tamari or soy sauce
- 2 tablespoons brown rice vinegar or regular rice vinegar
- 1 tablespoon maple syrup, optional
- 2 teaspoons smooth Dijon mustard
- Pinch black pepper
- ⅓ cup water, plus more as needed

Add all the ingredients to a medium bowl and whisk until smooth. Add more water if needed to reach desired consistency.

▶ **2 points**

Epilogue

The best way to change the world is in concentric circles: start with
yourself and work your way out from there.
                —James Clear, author of *Atomic Habits*

Several years ago, I had the privilege of interviewing Dr. William Foege, who
is a former director of the Centers for Disease Control, and the current executive director of the Carter Center and consultant to the Bill & Melinda Gates
Foundation. Throughout his career, Dr. Foege was instrumental in eradicating
smallpox in the late 1970s, and in the discovery of Legionnaires' disease, Reye's
syndrome, toxic shock syndrome, and HIV/AIDS. I asked him what lessons he
had learned from overcoming some of the biggest crises in public health. He
said he had a different take on the phrase "First, do no harm."

He explained that we usually think this portion of the oath medical professionals take refers to "errors of commission"—the idea that, above all, *what we
do* should not cause any injury or harm to our patients. Yet what he has seen is
that far more people die and suffer because of our "errors of omission"—"by
not sharing our science, by not using . . . the tools that we have," meaning the
prevention not practiced. He explained that because the price of those omis-
sions is usually not seen, it is often discounted.

I thought back to that sunny day in Boston more than two decades prior
when I, along with my classmates, stood on the lawn in front of the steps of
our medical school entrance, with our right hand raised during our gradu-
ation ceremony, taking that Hippocratic oath. Then I thought about what
I must take great care not to omit, what could potentially cause more harm
by not being shared because of its potential for preventing illness than tools
we use for treatment. Over the years since taking that oath, what I've come
to regard as the most critical aspect of health and healing is an empowering

element—one that preserves dignity when illness ravishes the mind and body and transcends even the most advanced technology: hope.

The science of good stress gives us hope. It's hope for what is possible for each of us. It's hope that wherever you are and whatever you are dealing with, you have the ability to be stronger, better, and healthier. It's hope that what you need to get there is already in you. You have innate gifts that you can stretch and recover, nudge and reshape, and push until you reach the limits of your physical, mental, and emotional potential. This is the science I must take great care to not omit; the science that needed to be shared so it could be practiced.

I am imagining you facing a challenge, but instead of having that familiar feeling of dread and overwhelm, you aren't daunted. Now, the things that seemed hard feel welcome, even necessary. You look forward to them because you know they enhance you. The challenges you traded for comfort have become your sources of strength, because you know that the rewards of stress are inseparable from its discomfort. This is what I want for you.

As I said at the beginning, this book is not about seismic challenges but, rather, "ordinary" ones. It's about leaning into daily stresses and experiencing, if only for brief moments, living outside your comfort zone. And it's trusting that those challenges will build on each other, reshaping and rewiring your body and enabling you to become a stronger, healthier, and happier version of yourself.

Don't do it just for you. Building resilience does benefit you individually, but those benefits go well beyond the self. Your internal state, your level of resilience, is highly contagious, much like a virus. Even when we aren't consciously communicating with others, our physiological systems are interacting in profound ways. Researchers Nicholas Christakis and James Fowler found that a person's happiness can ripple up to three degrees of separation through a social network. Think about that. If you are a central "node" in the network, you not only influence your friends but the friends of your friends' friends. Other health behaviors are similarly contagious. Obesity, for example, also clusters in networks up to three degrees of separation.

You also spread your influence by what you feel in your heart. Literally. Your heart actually produces a bioelectromagnetic field that transmits emotional information about your internal state to the sphere around you.

Dr. Rollin McCraty's research shows that when we are resilient, we radiate an energy that communicates cohesion and coherence. We emit a synchronous rhythm that establishes cooperation, trust, and compassion. On the other hand, when we lack resilience, we emit a dyssynchronous rhythm that lacks coherence, and transmit a flow of energy that may cause social discord and adversarial interactions. Resilience, according to Dr. McCraty, is reflected in our heart's rhythm, specifically the connection between the heart, brain, and nervous system that determines our heart's coherence and beat-to-beat heart rate variability. When we emotionally connect, we spontaneously synchronize our heart rhythm variability. Two hearts literally sync and beat as one. What we hold in our heart can communicate appreciation or frustration.

When I think of this powerful capacity we have to be sources of healing and safety for each other, I think of my father. His life was filled with challenges many of us will never come close to experiencing. Yet, in his quiet, peaceful, and loving way, he never harbored anger, fear, or frustration. He was the most genuinely kindhearted and contented person I have ever met. Our family remembers any corner of the room he occupied as harboring calm and serenity. His final words to us were "All that matters is what you hold in your heart."

One of the amazing things about how health works is what I call "good stress karma": the more you contribute to the lives of others without compromising your well-being, the healthier you become. Generosity and altruism come back around to heal you. In the act of giving, we release self-healing hormones like endorphins and oxytocin. Living a purposeful and meaningful life, being a part of something bigger than ourselves, is the most powerful way to reduce our level of (bad) stress. It makes space for more good stress, so we can contribute more and live to our fullest potential. It's a beautiful, virtuous cycle, passed down millennia to increase our odds of survival, and it does today just as it did for our ancestors.

I don't want you to let go of the understanding that stress can overwhelm and constrain, because it can. But my intent is that as you go forward, you will also hold the knowledge that stress can bring confidence and freedom. The science of good stress gives us choice. It gives us an alternative to our current way of reducing and managing stress in our lives and to current health paradigms by providing a path to accessing our innate capabilities, ones that lie dormant in our modern world of comfort. Stress can access hidden parts of you that are being stifled by comfort—strong, capable, and resilient parts of you that will ripple out to others. I believe we are each born with something to bring to the world. Stress, and as a by-product, our health and resilience, is a means to that end. It's the gateway to the freedom to live more, love more, do more, and be more, for ourselves and each other.

Acknowledgments

I have to admit that, at first, the idea of writing this book while working full time, taking care of my patients, conducting research, managing administrative responsibilities, and making time for my family seemed daunting. Yet, my belief in the importance of making good stress a part of a larger conversation made me willing to get uncomfortable, and the growth I have experienced from this good stress has exceeded anything I could have ever imagined. For that, I am grateful to many people.

This book started with a fateful meeting with my literary agent, Stephanie Tade. Even though my ideas were half-baked, from the outset she believed there was something here and encouraged me to develop them into a proposal. Throughout the process, she has championed and supported me every step of the way, with her honest advice, discerning judgment, and solid experience navigating publishing. Colleen Martell has been my copilot, coach, and friend. She patiently listened to all my ideas, helped me frame them, provided ways to improve every draft, and did it all with kindness and compassion. This book would not be nearly what it is without her brilliant skills and creativity.

I am grateful beyond words for my extraordinary editor, Sarah Pelz. Her belief in this project brought it to life. With grace and incredible skill, she deftly improved the manuscript. I am incredibly honored to work with her and the entire Team Good Stress at Harvest/HarperCollins, including Emma Effinger, Justine Gardner, David Palmer, Mumtaz Mustafa, Anwesha Basu, Katie Tull, and Megan Wilson. My heartfelt thank-you also goes to Jonathan Jacobs, Ryan Benson, Meg Cassidy, Mark Fortier, and Ann Day for their invaluable expertise, creative energy, belief in the importance of this message, and support in sharing it.

There are many mentors, colleagues, and scientists who have helped shape my views about the art and science of medicine. While there are too many to list individually, I am indebted to their camaraderie and collaboration on this journey of continual learning. I have also learned tremendously through my patients and their willingness to tweak their habits. I am thankful to be a part of their lives and for the gratification of being able to practice as close to a Marcus Welby style of medicine as possible.

A special thank-you goes out to Ashley Madden (https://riseshinecook.ca/) for taking on the challenge of creating recipe templates and testing the recipes in her kitchen, and Jonathan Bonnet for being so generous with his time and knowledge.

Last, and most importantly, I want to thank my husband, Troy, who makes everything I do possible with his love and support. I couldn't ask for a better life partner. My dearest Kate, Kara, and Dana, thank you for getting everything done while Mommy spent nights and weekends working on this book. I am so proud of you. I am also indebted to my parents, Clemance Horesh and the late Isaac Horesh, who passed away in November 2022. Their unconditional love and support and the way they have lived life are in all these pages.

Notes

Introduction

5   **don't ever truly go "back to normal"**: Lena Smirnova et al., "Cellular Resilience," *Alternatives to Animal Experimentation* 32, no. 4 (November 1, 2015): 247–60, https://doi.org/10.14573/altex.1509271.

5   **revised the entire framework of stress**: Siyu Lu, Fang Wei, and Guolin Li, "The Evolution of the Concept of Stress and the Framework of the Stress System," *Cell Stress* 5, no. 6 (April 26, 2021): 76–85, https://doi.org/10.15698/cst2021.06.250.

6   **concept of stress-induced growth**: Ross Wadey, Melissa Day, and Karen Howells, ed., "Growth Following Adversity: A Conceptual Perspective," in *Growth Following Adversity in Sport: A Mechanism to Positive Change* (New York: Routledge/Taylor & Francis, 2021), 3–18.

Part I: Hardwired for Stress: Our Body's Natural Regenerative Systems

13   **If "too much of a good thing is a bad thing"**: Xin Li, Tingting Yang, and Zheng Sun, "Hormesis in Health and Chronic Diseases," *Trends in Endocrinology & Metabolism* 30, no. 12 (December 1, 2019): 944–58, https://doi.org/10.1016/j.tem.2019.08.007.

13   **He tested nearly a dozen**: Hugo Schulz and Ted Crump, "NIH-98-134: Contemporary Medicine as Presented by Its Practitioners Themselves, Leipzig, 1923:217–250," *Nonlinearity in Biology, Toxicology, Medicine* 1, no. 3 (July 2003): 295–318, https://doi.org/10.1080/15401420390249880.

13   **Arndt-Schulz law**: Edward J. Calabrese and Evgenios Agathokleous, "Theodosius Dobzhansky's View on Biology and Evolution v.2.0: 'Nothing in Biology Makes Sense Except in Light of Evolution and Evolution's Dependence on Hormesis-Mediated Acquired Resilience That Optimizes Biological Performance and Numerous Diverse Short and Longer Term Protective Strategies,'" *Environmental Research* 186 (July 1, 2020): 109559, https://doi.org/10.1016/j.envres.2020.109559.

13   **explaining how homeopathy works**: Calabrese and Agathokleous.

14   **brought him under attack**: Calabrese and Agathokleous.

14   **academic equivalent of a death sentence**: Edward J. Calabrese, "Hormesis: A Fundamental Concept in Biology," *Microbial Cell* 1, no. 5 (n.d.): 145–49, https://doi.org/10.15698/mic2014.05.145.

15   **traditional medicine proposed this rival model**: Calabrese and Agathokleous, "Theodosius Dobzhansky's View on Biology and Evolution v.2.0."

15   **shuts out an equally valid concept**: Edward J. Calabrese, "Hormesis: Path and Progression to Significance," *International Journal of Molecular Sciences* 19, no. 10 (September 21, 2018): E2871, https://doi.org/10.3390/ijms19102871.

15   **a peculiar property of toxic red cedar heartwood extract**: C. M. Southam and J. Ehrlich, "Effects of Extract of Western Red-Cedar Heartwood on Certain Wood-Decaying Fungi in Culture," *Phytopath* 33, no. 6 (September 21, 1943): 517–24.

15   **Scientists in other fields**: Calabrese, "Hormesis," n.d.

15   **Researchers in agriculture**: T. D. Luckey et al., "Growth of Germ-Free Birds Fed Antibiotics," *Antibiotics & Chemotherapy (Northfield, Ill.)* 6, no. 1 (January 1956): 37–40.

16   **ionizing radiation**: T. D. Luckey, *Hormesis with Ionizing Radiation* (Boca Raton: CRC Press, 2019), https://doi.org/10.1201/9780429276552.

16 **toxicology:** A. R. Stebbing, "Hormesis—the Stimulation of Growth by Low Levels of Inhibitors," *The Science of the Total Environment* 22, no. 3 (February 1982): 213–34, https://doi.org/10.1016/0048-9697(82)90066-3.

16 **and pharmacology:** E. Szabadi, "A Model of Two Functionally Antagonistic Receptor Populations Activated by the Same Agonist," *Journal of Theoretical Biology* 69, no. 1 (November 7, 1977): 101–12, https://doi.org/10.1016/0022-5193(77)90390-3.

16 **The biggest leap forward:** Edward J. Calabrese and Linda A. Baldwin, "Toxicology Rethinks Its Central Belief," *Nature* 421, no. 6924 (February 2003): 691–92, https://doi.org/10.1038/421691a.

16 **In the Web of Science:** Calabrese and Agathokleous, "Theodosius Dobzhansky's View on Biology and Evolution v.2.0."

17 **Your body has sensors:** Dino Demirovic and Suresh I. S. Rattan, "Establishing Cellular Stress Response Profiles as Biomarkers of Homeodynamics, Health and Hormesis," *Experimental Gerontology*, Prevention and Intervention: From Molecular Biology to Clinical Perspectives, 48, no. 1 (January 1, 2013): 94–98, https://doi.org/10.1016/j.exger.2012.02.005.

Chapter 1: The Stress Dilemma

19 **By 2015, these rates of obesity and diabetes:** "Chronic Disease Center Data Applications," July 18, 2022, https://www.cdc.gov/chronicdisease/data/statistics.htm.

19 **a dramatic rise in prescription drugs:** "Consumer Reports Examines: Do Americans Take Too Many Prescription Medications?," August 13, 2017, https://www.consumerreports.org/media-room/press-releases/2017/08/consumer_reports_examines_do_americans_take_too_many_prescription_medications/.

19 **our life expectancy is likely to drop:** S. Jay Olshansky et al., "A Potential Decline in Life Expectancy in the United States in the 21st Century," *New England Journal of Medicine* 352, no. 11 (March 17, 2005): 1138–45, https://doi.org/10.1056/NEJMsr043743.

20 **far outpaces our ability to adapt genetically:** S. Boyd Eaton, Melvin Konner, and Marjorie Shostak, "Stone Agers in the Fast Lane: Chronic Degenerative Diseases in Evolutionary Perspective," *American Journal of Medicine* 84, no. 4 (April 1, 1988): 739–49, https://doi.org/10.1016/0002-9343(88)90113-1.

20 **industrial food processing technology:** Loren Cordain et al., "Origins and Evolution of the Western Diet: Health Implications for the 21st Century," *American Journal of Clinical Nutrition* 81, no. 2 (February 2005): 341–54, https://doi.org/10.1093/ajcn.81.2.341.

20 **about 60 percent of the calories on our plates:** Eurídice Martínez Steele et al., "Ultra-Processed Foods and Added Sugars in the US Diet: Evidence from a Nationally Representative Cross-Sectional Study," *BMJ Open* 6, no. 3 (January 1, 2016): e009892, https://doi.org/10.1136/bmjopen-2015-009892.

20 **Built into our hardwired biology:** Hans-Rudolf Berthoud, Heike Münzberg, and Christopher D. Morrison, "Blaming the Brain for Obesity: Integration of Hedonic and Homeostatic Mechanisms," *Gastroenterology* 152, no. 7 (May 2017): 1728–38, https://doi.org/10.1053/j.gastro.2016.12.050.

20 **continually activate our reward systems:** Stephan J. Guyenet and Michael W. Schwartz, "Regulation of Food Intake, Energy Balance, and Body Fat Mass: Implications for the Pathogenesis and Treatment of Obesity," *Journal of Clinical Endocrinology & Metabolism* 97, no. 3 (March 1, 2012): 745–55, https://doi.org/10.1210/jc.2011-2525.

20 **designed to overwhelm the amount of reward:** Magalie Lenoir et al., "Intense Sweetness Surpasses Cocaine Reward," *PloS One* 2, no. 8 (August 1, 2007): e698, https://doi.org/10.1371/journal.pone.0000698.

20 **adapted to match capacity to demand:** David A. Raichlen and Gene E. Alexander, "Adaptive Capacity: An Evolutionary-Neuroscience Model Linking Exercise, Cognition, and Brain Health," *Trends in Neurosciences* 40, no. 7 (July 2017): 408–21, https://doi.org/10.1016/j.tins.2017.05.001.

21 **by taxing our ancient survival genes:** Lee Goldman, *Too Much of a Good Thing: How Four Key Survival Traits Are Now Killing Us* (New York: Little, Brown and Company, 2015).

21 **all Paleolithic dietary patterns:** Eaton, Konner, and Shostak, "Stone Agers in the Fast Lane."

22 ***Homo sapiens* diet of our ancestors:** Donald S Coffey, "Similarities of Prostate and Breast Cancer: Evolution, Diet, and Estrogens," *Urology: New Clinical Trial Strategies for Prostate Cancer Prevention* 57, no. 4, Supplement 1 (April 1, 2001): 31–38, https://doi.org/10.1016/ S0090-4295(00)00938-9.

22 **sustain bursts of physical movement:** Eaton, Konner, and Shostak, "Stone Agers in the Fast Lane."

22 **evenings brought everyone together:** Polly W. Wiessner, "Embers of Society: Firelight Talk Among the Ju/'hoansi Bushmen," *Proceedings of the National Academy of Sciences* 111, no. 39 (September 30, 2014): 14027–35, https://doi.org/10.1073/pnas.1404212111.

22 **The obligatory need for episodic:** Leo Pruimboom and Frits A. J. Muskiet, "Intermittent Living; the Use of Ancient Challenges as a Vaccine Against the Deleterious Effects of Modern Life: A Hypothesis," *Medical Hypotheses* 120 (November 1, 2018): 28–42, https://doi. org/10.1016/j.mehy.2018.08.002.

22 **That all began to change:** Ewen Callaway, "Farming Invented Twice in Middle East, Genomes Study Reveals," *Nature* (June 20, 2016), https://doi.org/10.1038/nature.2016.20119.

22 **That all began to change:** Joshua J. Mark, "Fertile Crescent," World History Encyclopedia, March 28, 2018, https://www.worldhistory.org/Fertile_Crescent/.

22 **That all began to change:** Erin Blakemore, "What Was the Neolithic Revolution?," *National Geographic*, April 5, 2019, https://www.nationalgeographic.com/culture/article/ neolithic-agricultural-revolution.

23 **About two hundred years ago:** Britannica, "Industrial Revolution | Definition, History, Dates, Summary & Facts," last modified April 23, 2024, https://www.britannica.com/event/ Industrial-Revolution.

23 **We currently cultivate only:** Oren Shelef, Peter J. Weisberg, and Frederick D. Provenza, "The Value of Native Plants and Local Production in an Era of Global Agriculture," *Frontiers in Plant Science* 8 (December 5, 2017): 2069, https://doi.org/10.3389/fpls.2017.02069.

23 **Infrastructure, transportation, and communication:** Britannica, "Industrial Revolution | Definition, History, Dates, Summary & Facts."

23 **diminished the importance of family:** Amanda Penn, "3 Major Social Impacts of the Industrial Revolution," *Shortform Books* (blog), November 19, 2019, https://www.shortform. com/blog/social-impact-of-industrial-revolution/.

23 **Additionally, the Information Age:** Chris Bailey, "4 Strategies for Overcoming Distraction," *Harvard Business Review*, August 30, 2018, https://hbr.org/2018/08/4-strategies-for- overcoming-distraction.

23 **Additionally, the Information Age:** Daniel J. Levitin, "Why It's So Hard to Pay Attention, Explained by Science," *Fast Company*, September 23, 2015, https://www.fastcompany. com/3051417/why-its-so-hard-to-pay-attention-explained-by-science.

23 **As a result, average life expectancy:** Eaton, Konner, and Shostak, "Stone Agers in the Fast Lane."

Chapter 2: Cellular Resilience: Getting at the Big Picture by Understanding the Small

25 **what he saw was bewildering:** Paolo Mazzarello, "A Unifying Concept: The History of Cell Theory," *Nature Cell Biology* 1, no. 1 (May 1999): E13–15, https://doi.org/10.1038/8964.

26 **called regenerative medicine:** Angelo S. Mao and David J. Mooney, "Regenerative Medicine: Current Therapies and Future Directions," *Proceedings of the National Academy of Sciences of the United States of America* 112, no. 47 (November 24, 2015): 14452–59, https://doi. org/10.1073/pnas.1508520112.

26 **cell-based therapy called immunotherapy:** NIH National Cancer Institute, "T-Cell Transfer Therapy - Immunotherapy - NCI," last updated April 1, 2022, https://www.cancer.gov/about-cancer/treatment/types/immunotherapy/t-cell-transfer-therapy.

26 **Stem cells are now:** George Kolios and Yuben Moodley, "Introduction to Stem Cells and Regenerative Medicine," *Respiration: International Review of Thoracic Diseases* 85, no. 1 (2013): 3–10, https://doi.org/10.1159/000345615.

27 **You can think of your cellular stress responses:** Lorenzo Galluzzi, Takahiro Yamazaki, and Guido Kroemer, "Linking Cellular Stress Responses to Systemic Homeostasis," *Nature Reviews Molecular Cell Biology* 19, no. 11 (November 2018): 731–45, https://doi.org/10.1038/s41580-018-0068-0.

27 **Your army is made of seven:** Demirovic and Rattan, "Establishing Cellular Stress Response Profiles as Biomarkers of Homeodynamics, Health and Hormesis."

27 **Your army is made of seven:** Suresh Rattan, "Molecular Gerontology: From Homeodynamics to Hormesis," *Current Pharmaceutical Design* 20, no. 18 (May 31, 2014): 3036–39, https://doi.org/10.2174/1381612811319666070B.

28 **conserved for millions of years:** Vittorio Calabrese et al., "Cellular Stress Responses, Hormetic Phytochemicals and Vitagenes in Aging and Longevity," *Biochimica et Biophysica Acta (BBA)—Molecular Basis of Disease*, Antioxidants and Antioxidant Treatment in Disease, 1822, no. 5 (May 1, 2012): 753–83, https://doi.org/10.1016/j.bbadis.2011.11.002.

28 **They are part of our "vitagenes":** Vittorio Calabrese et al., "Hormesis, Cellular Stress Response and Vitagenes as Critical Determinants in Aging and Longevity," *Molecular Aspects of Medicine*, Oxidative Damage and Disease, 32, no. 4 (August 1, 2011): 279–304, https://doi.org/10.1016/j.mam.2011.10.007.

28 **activate our vitagenes in two main ways:** Andrea Rossnerova et al., "The Molecular Mechanisms of Adaptive Response Related to Environmental Stress," *International Journal of Molecular Sciences* 21, no. 19 (September 25, 2020): 7053, https://doi.org/10.3390/ijms21197053.

28 **When cells sense stress:** Edward J. Calabrese, "Hormetic Mechanisms," *Critical Reviews in Toxicology* 43, no. 7 (August 1, 2013): 580–606, https://doi.org/10.3109/10408444.2013.808172.

28 **determine what genes you express:** Alexander M. Vaiserman, "Hormesis and Epigenetics: Is There a Link?," *Ageing Research Reviews* 10, no. 4 (September 1, 2011): 413–21, https://doi.org/10.1016/j.arr.2011.01.004.

28 **This mainly happens through epigenetic changes:** Rossnerova et al., "The Molecular Mechanisms of Adaptive Response Related to Environmental Stress."

29 **Good stressors are pleiotropic:** Aurelia Santoro et al., "Inflammaging, Hormesis and the Rationale for Anti-Aging Strategies," *Ageing Research Reviews* 64 (December 2020): 101142, https://doi.org/10.1016/j.arr.2020.101142.

30 **Each day, your cells' DNA accumulates:** Matt Yousefzadeh et al., "DNA Damage—How and Why We Age?," *eLife* 10 (n.d.): e62852, https://doi.org/10.7554/eLife.62852.

30 **Your DNA damage response:** Galluzzi, Yamazaki, and Kroemer, "Linking Cellular Stress Responses to Systemic Homeostasis."

30 **twenty thousand and more than one hundred thousand different proteins:** "Protein Folding: The Good, the Bad, and the Ugly," *Science in the News* (blog), March 1, 2010, https://sitn.hms.harvard.edu/flash/2010/issue65/.

30 **Heat shock proteins (HSPs) are part:** Zihai Li and Pramod Srivastava, "Heat-Shock Proteins," *Current Protocols in Immunology* 58, no. 1 (2003): A.1T.1-A.1T.6, https://doi.org/10.1002/0471142735.ima01ts58.

30 **HSPs even act as "molecular chaperones":** J. L. Camberg et al., "Molecular Chaperones," in *Brenner's Encyclopedia of Genetics*, 2nd ed., ed. Stanley Maloy and Kelly Hughes (San Diego: Academic Press, 2013), 456–60, https://doi.org/10.1016/B978-0-12-374984-0.00221-7.

30 **Another way the cellular stress response safeguards protein:** Adam Read and Martin Schröder, "The Unfolded Protein Response: An Overview," *Biology* 10, no. 5 (April 29, 2021): 384, https://doi.org/10.3390/biology10050384.

31 **This cellular cleanup function:** Danielle Glick, Sandra Barth, and Kay F. Macleod, "Autophagy: Cellular and Molecular Mechanisms," *Journal of Pathology* 221, no. 1 (May 2010): 3–12, https://doi.org/10.1002/path.2697.

31 **Energy impairment is found:** João A. Amorim et al., "Mitochondrial and Metabolic Dysfunction in Ageing and Age-Related Diseases," *Nature Reviews Endocrinology* 18, no. 4 (April 2022): 243–58, https://doi.org/10.1038/s41574-021-00626-7.

32 **remarkable molecules that support mitochondria:** Jian-Li He, Tian-Shi Wang, and Yi-Ping Wang, "Chapter 5—Sirtuins and Mitochondrial Dysfunction," in *Sirtuin Biology in Cancer and Metabolic Disease*, ed. Kenneth Maiese (San Diego: Academic Press, 2021), 79–89, https://doi.org/10.1016/B978-0-12-822467-0.00007-3.

32 **"hormetins":** Suresh I. S. Rattan, "Molecular Gerontology: From Homeodynamics to Hormesis," *Current Pharmaceutical Design* 20, no. 18 (2014): 3036–39, https://doi.org/10.21 74/13816128113196660708.

Chapter 3: The Stress Solution: Ancient Stress as a Modern Cure

33 **It was formulated in 1926:** Kelvin J. A. Davies, "Adaptive Homeostasis," *Molecular Aspects of Medicine*, Hormetic and Regulatory Effects of Lipid Oxidation Products, 49 (June 1, 2016): 1–7, https://doi.org/10.1016/j.mam.2016.04.007.

34 **we adapt to stress by establishing a new equilibrium:** Davies.

34 **causes internal "wear and tear":** Bruce S. McEwen, "Stress, Adaptation, and Disease: Allostasis and Allostatic Load," *Annals of the New York Academy of Sciences* 840, no. 1 (1998): 33–44, https://doi.org/10.1111/j.1749-6632.1998.tb09546.x.

34 **Good stress also prompts our body:** Galluzzi, Yamazaki, and Kroemer, "Linking Cellular Stress Responses to Systemic Homeostasis."

34 **stress changes us:** Megan M. Niedzwiecki et al., "The Exposome: Molecules to Populations," *Annual Review of Pharmacology and Toxicology* 59 (January 6, 2019): 107–27, https://doi.org/10.1146/annurev-pharmtox-010818-021315.

34 **the idea of a "homeodynamic space":** Rattan, "Molecular Gerontology," 2014.

35 **It's a real-time narrative:** Suresh I. S. Rattan, "Biological Health and Homeodynamic Space," in *Explaining Health Across the Sciences*, ed. Jonathan Sholl and Suresh I. S. Rattan, Healthy Ageing and Longevity (Cham: Springer International Publishing, 2020), 43–51, https://doi.org/10.1007/978-3-030-52663-4_4.

37 **two main ways to prevent noxious chemicals:** Mark P. Mattson, "Challenging Oneself Intermittently to Improve Health," *Dose-Response* 12, no. 4 (October 20, 2014): 600–618, https://doi.org/10.2203/dose-response.14-028.Mattson.

37 **A prototypic challenge:** Mattson.

37 **One of the primary adaptations:** Glenn C. Rowe, Adeel Safdar, and Zolt Arany, "Running Forward: New Frontiers in Endurance Exercise Biology," *Circulation* 129, no. 7 (February 18, 2014): 798–810, https://doi.org/10.1161/CIRCULATIONAHA.113.001590.

38 **preagricultural humans had more strength and muscularity:** Eaton, Konner, and Shostak, "Stone Agers in the Fast Lane."

38 **heat stress activates a master regulator:** Feng He, Xiaoli Ru, and Tao Wen, "NRF2, a Transcription Factor for Stress Response and Beyond," *International Journal of Molecular Sciences* 21, no. 13 (July 6, 2020): 4777, https://doi.org/10.3390/ijms21134777.

38 **heat stress activates a master regulator:** Sandra Vomund et al., "Nrf2, the Master Regulator of Anti-Oxidative Responses," *International Journal of Molecular Sciences* 18, no. 12 (December 20, 2017): 2772, https://doi.org/10.3390/ijms18122772.

38   **Deliberate cold stress:** Beat Knechtle et al., "Cold Water Swimming—Benefits and Risks: A Narrative Review," *International Journal of Environmental Research and Public Health* 17, no. 23 (January 2020): 8984, https://doi.org/10.3390/ijerph17238984.

38   **Deliberate cold stress:** W. G. Siems et al., "Improved Antioxidative Protection in Winter Swimmers," *QJM: An International Journal of Medicine* 92, no. 4 (April 1, 1999): 193–98, https://doi.org/10.1093/qjmed/92.4.193.

39   **Once their stores of carbohydrates:** Valter D. Longo and Mark P. Mattson, "Fasting: Molecular Mechanisms and Clinical Applications," *Cell Metabolism* 19, no. 2 (February 4, 2014): 181–92, https://doi.org/10.1016/j.cmet.2013.12.008.

39   **ketones have downstream effects:** Hubert Kolb et al., "Ketone Bodies: From Enemy to Friend and Guardian Angel," *BMC Medicine* 19, no. 1 (December 9, 2021): 313, https://doi.org/10.1186/s12916-021-02185-0.

39   **human brain doubled:** Smithsonian Institute, "Bigger Brains: Complex Brains for a Complex World," January 3, 2024, http://humanorigins.si.edu/human-characteristics/brains.

39   **We developed the neocortex:** Michel A. Hofman, "Evolution of the Human Brain: When Bigger Is Better," *Frontiers in Neuroanatomy* 8 (March 27, 2014): 15, https://doi.org/10.3389/fnana.2014.00015.

Part II: Good Hormetic Stressors: The Right Kind, Dose, and Duration

43   **change this common misconception:** Siyu Lu, Fang Wei, and Guolin Li, "The Evolution of the Concept of Stress and the Framework of the Stress System," *Cell Stress* 5, no. 6 (April 26, 2021): 76–85, https://doi.org/10.15698/cst2021.06.250.

44   **phenomenon called "cross-adaptation":** Eitika Chauhan et al., "Cross Stress Adaptation: Phenomenon of Interactions Between Homotypic and Heterotypic Stressors," *Life Sciences* 137 (September 15, 2015): 98–104, https://doi.org/10.1016/j.lfs.2015.07.018.

44   **"hormetic zone":** Carolin Cornelius et al., "Stress Responses, Vitagenes and Hormesis as Critical Determinants in Aging and Longevity: Mitochondria as a 'Chi,'" *Immunity & Ageing* 10 (April 25, 2013): 15, https://doi.org/10.1186/1742-4933-10-15.

45   **Prolonged stress causes a very different outcome:** Xin Li, Tingting Yang, and Zheng Sun, "Hormesis in Health and Chronic Diseases," *Trends in Endocrinology and Metabolism* 30, no. 12 (December 2019): 944–58, https://doi.org/10.1016/j.tem.2019.08.007.

45   **It sets you up so that when you recover:** Mark P. Mattson et al., "Intermittent Metabolic Switching, Neuroplasticity and Brain Health," *Nature Reviews Neuroscience* 19, no. 2 (February 2018): 63–80, https://doi.org/10.1038/nrn.2017.156.

Chapter 4: Food "Toxins" as Medicine

47   **More than five thousand phytochemicals:** Rui Hai Liu, "Health-Promoting Components of Fruits and Vegetables in the Diet," *Advances in Nutrition* 4, no. 3 (May 1, 2013): 384S-92S, https://doi.org/10.3945/an.112.003517.

47   **Thousands of studies show:** Donato F. Romagnolo and Ornella I. Selmin, "Mediterranean Diet and Prevention of Chronic Diseases," *Nutrition Today* 52, no. 5 (September 2017): 208–22, https://doi.org/10.1097/NT.0000000000000228.

47   **Thousands of studies show:** Dagfinn Aune et al., "Fruit and Vegetable Intake and the Risk of Cardiovascular Disease, Total Cancer and All-Cause Mortality—a Systematic Review and Dose-Response Meta-Analysis of Prospective Studies," *International Journal of Epidemiology* 46, no. 3 (June 1, 2017): 1029–56, https://doi.org/10.1093/ije/dyw319.

48   **Most of the thinking in phytochemical research:** Jaewon Lee et al., "Adaptive Cellular Stress Pathways as Therapeutic Targets of Dietary Phytochemicals: Focus on the Nervous System," ed. David R. Sibley, *Pharmacological Reviews* 66, no. 3 (July 1, 2014): 815–68, https://doi.org/10.1124/pr.113.007757.

48   **doesn't come close to the amount of antioxidants:** Lee et al.

48   **Even megadose antioxidant supplements:** Goran Bjelakovic, Dimitrinka Nikolova, and Christian Gluud, "Antioxidant Supplements and Mortality," *Current Opinion in Clinical Nutrition and Metabolic Care* 17, no. 1 (January 2014): 40–44, https://doi.org/10.1097/MCO.0000000000000009.

48   **Around two decades ago:** Mark P. Mattson and Aiwu Cheng, "Neurohormetic Phytochemicals: Low-Dose Toxins That Induce Adaptive Neuronal Stress Responses," *Trends in Neurosciences* 29, no. 11 (November 1, 2006): 632–39, https://doi.org/10.1016/j.tins.2006.09.001.

48   **While we absorb only tiny amounts:** Sawan Alì et al., "Healthy Ageing and Mediterranean Diet: A Focus on Hormetic Phytochemicals," *Mechanisms of Ageing and Development* 200 (December 1, 2021): 111592, https://doi.org/10.1016/j.mad.2021.111592.

48   **They also stimulate other maintenance and repair:** Mark P. Mattson and Edward J. Calabrese, "Hormesis: What It Is and Why It Matters," in *Hormesis: A Revolution in Biology, Toxicology and Medicine*, ed. Mark P. Mattson and Edward J. Calabrese (Totowa, NJ: Humana Press, 2010): 1–13, https://doi.org/10.1007/978-1-60761-495-1_1.

49   **why plants have phytochemicals:** Lee et al., "Adaptive Cellular Stress Pathways as Therapeutic Targets of Dietary Phytochemicals," July 1, 2014.

49   **Because our ancestors' survival depended:** Lee et al.

49   **another way our ancestors adapted:** Lee et al.

50   **coevolved not only with plants but also the microorganisms:** Lee et al.

50   **for nearly a billion years:** Philip L. Hooper et al., "Xenohormesis: Health Benefits from an Eon of Plant Stress Response Evolution," *Cell Stress & Chaperones* 15, no. 6 (November 2010): 761–70, https://doi.org/10.1007/s12192-010-0206-x.

50   **complexity of their stress responses rivals:** Sachin Kotak et al., "Complexity of the Heat Stress Response in Plants," *Current Opinion in Plant Biology: Physiology and Metabolism* 10, no. 3 (June 1, 2007): 310–16, https://doi.org/10.1016/j.pbi.2007.04.011.

50   **their theory proposes that when we eat a stressed plant:** Konrad T. Howitz and David A. Sinclair, "Xenohormesis: Sensing the Chemical Cues of Other Species," *Cell* 133, no. 3 (May 2, 2008): 387–91, https://doi.org/10.1016/j.cell.2008.04.019.

51   **communicate an impending downturn:** Howitz and Sinclair.

53   **The connection between phytochemicals and hormesis:** Edward J. Calabrese, "Hormesis Mediates Acquired Resilience: Using Plant-Derived Chemicals to Enhance Health," *Annual Review of Food Science and Technology* 12 (March 25, 2021): 355–81, https://doi.org/10.1146/annurev-food-062420-124437.

53   **It ignited interest in resveratrol:** "Resveratrol Commonly Displays Hormesis: Occurrence and Biomedical Significance," accessed April 30, 2023, https://doi.org/10.1177/0960327110383625.

54   **Only nanomolar amounts:** Morena Martucci et al., "Mediterranean Diet and Inflammaging Within the Hormesis Paradigm," *Nutrition Reviews* 75, no. 6 (June 1, 2017): 442–55, https://doi.org/10.1093/nutrit/nux013.

54   **resveratrol is a natural fungicide and antibiotic:** Kuzhuvelil B. Harikumar and Bharat B. Aggarwal, "Resveratrol: A Multitargeted Agent for Age-Associated Chronic Diseases," *Cell Cycle (Georgetown, Tex.)* 7, no. 8 (April 15, 2008): 1020–35, https://doi.org/10.4161/cc.7.8.5740.

54   **Resveratrol activates sirtuin 1 (SIRT1):** Mattson and Calabrese, "Hormesis."

54   **Resveratrol also stimulates:** Harikumar and Aggarwal, "Resveratrol."

54   **Resveratrol also stimulates:** Jan Martel et al., "Hormetic Effects of Phytochemicals on Health and Longevity," *Trends in Endocrinology & Metabolism* 30, no. 6 (June 1, 2019): 335–46, https://doi.org/10.1016/j.tem.2019.04.001.

54   **Resveratrol also stimulates:** Jan Martel et al., "Phytochemicals as Prebiotics and Biological Stress Inducers," *Trends in Biochemical Sciences* 45, no. 6 (June 2020): 462–71, https://doi.org/10.1016/j.tibs.2020.02.008.

54   **It was the impetus:** Calabrese, "Hormesis Mediates Acquired Resilience."

55 **It activates a master regulator:** Edward J. Calabrese and Walter J. Kozumbo, "The Phytoprotective Agent Sulforaphane Prevents Inflammatory Degenerative Diseases and Age-Related Pathologies via Nrf2-Mediated Hormesis," *Pharmacological Research* 163 (January 2021): 105283, https://doi.org/10.1016/j.phrs.2020.105283.

55 **Nrf2 is a transcription factor:** Martucci et al., "Mediterranean Diet and Inflammaging Within the Hormesis Paradigm."

55 **These enzymes ramp up our antioxidant:** Brooks M. Hybertson et al., "Oxidative Stress in Health and Disease: The Therapeutic Potential of Nrf2 Activation," *Molecular Aspects of Medicine* 32, no. 4–6 (August 2011): 234–46, https://doi.org/10.1016/j.mam.2011.10.006.

55 **Many plant "toxins" activate:** Sawan Alì et al., "Healthy Ageing and Mediterranean Diet."

55 **Many plant "toxins" activate:** Jan Martel et al., "Hormetic Effects of Phytochemicals on Health and Longevity."

55 **stresses cells by opening pores in their membrane:** Mattson and Calabrese, "Hormesis."

56 **Allicin also upregulates:** Elena Catanzaro et al., "Anticancer Potential of Allicin: A Review," *Pharmacological Research* 177 (March 1, 2022): 106118, https://doi.org/10.1016/j.phrs.2022.106118.

56 **Quercetin is another phytochemical:** Ashley J. Vargas and Randy Burd, "Hormesis and Synergy: Pathways and Mechanisms of Quercetin in Cancer Prevention and Management," *Nutrition Reviews* 68, no. 7 (July 1, 2010): 418–28, https://doi.org/10.1111/j.1753-4887.2010.00301.x.

56 **And like resveratrol, quercetin:** Alì et al., "Healthy Ageing and Mediterranean Diet."

57 **This toxin mainly builds:** Lee et al., "Adaptive Cellular Stress Pathways as Therapeutic Targets of Dietary Phytochemicals," July 1, 2014.

57 **Capsaicin can also open pores:** Mattson and Calabrese, "Hormesis."

57 **the benefit of making curcumin:** Limin Yin et al., "Induced Resistance Mechanism of Novel Curcumin Analogs Bearing a Quinazoline Moiety to Plant Virus," *International Journal of Molecular Sciences* 19, no. 12 (December 15, 2018): 4065, https://doi.org/10.3390/ijms19124065.

57 **it doubles as our defense:** Nazanin Moghaddam et al., "Hormetic Effects of Curcumin: What Is the Evidence?," *Journal of Cellular Physiology* 234 (December 4, 2018), https://doi.org/10.1002/jcp.27880.

57 **In lab studies, curcumin:** Nathan Earl Rainey, Aoula Moustapha, and Patrice Xavier Petit, "Curcumin, a Multifaceted Hormetic Agent, Mediates an Intricate Crosstalk Between Mitochondrial Turnover, Autophagy, and Apoptosis," *Oxidative Medicine and Cellular Longevity* 2020 (July 20, 2020): e3656419, https://doi.org/10.1155/2020/3656419.

57 **In lab studies, curcumin:** Abolfazl Shakeri et al., "Curcumin: A Naturally Occurring Autophagy Modulator," *Journal of Cellular Physiology* 234, no. 5 (May 2019): 5643–54, https://doi.org/10.1002/jcp.27404.

57 **It's another protective chemical:** Lee et al., "Adaptive Cellular Stress Pathways as Therapeutic Targets of Dietary Phytochemicals," July 1, 2014.

57 **reduce neuroinflammation in mice:** Ya-Min Liu et al., "Ferulic Acid Inhibits Neuro-Inflammation in Mice Exposed to Chronic Unpredictable Mild Stress," *International Immunopharmacology* 45 (April 2017): 128–34, https://doi.org/10.1016/j.intimp.2017.02.007.

58 **it can raise serotonin and norepinephrine:** Jianliang Chen et al., "Antidepressant-like Effects of Ferulic Acid: Involvement of Serotonergic and Norepinergic Systems," *Metabolic Brain Disease* 30, no. 1 (February 2015): 129–36, https://doi.org/10.1007/s11011-014-9635-z.

58 **have antidepressant-like effects:** Xingxing Zheng et al., "Ferulic Acid Improves Depressive-like Behavior in Prenatally-Stressed Offspring Rats via Anti-inflammatory Activity and HPA Axis," *International Journal of Molecular Sciences* 20, no. 3 (January 24, 2019): 493, https://doi.org/10.3390/ijms20030493.

58 **A review of twenty-one studies:** Edele Mancini et al., "Green Tea Effects on Cognition, Mood and Human Brain Function: A Systematic Review," *Phytomedicine: International*

Journal of Phytotherapy and Phytopharmacology 34 (October 15, 2017): 26–37, https://doi. org/10.1016/j.phymed.2017.07.008.

58 **EGCG works by activating multiple:** Tae Gen Son, Simonetta Camandola, and Mark P. Mattson, "Hormetic Dietary Phytochemicals," *Neuromolecular Medicine* 10, no. 4 (2008): 236–46, https://doi.org/10.1007/s12017-008-8037-y.

58 **EGCG works by activating multiple:** Martel et al., "Hormetic Effects of Phytochemicals on Health and Longevity."

58 **Genistein was originally found:** Javad Sharifi-Rad et al., "Genistein: An Integrative Overview of Its Mode of Action, Pharmacological Properties, and Health Benefits," *Oxidative Medicine and Cellular Longevity* 2021 (July 20, 2021): e3268136, https://doi. org/10.1155/2021/3268136.

58 **genistein acts as an anti-estrogen:** Fazlul H. Sarkar and Yiwei Li, "Soy Isoflavones and Cancer Prevention," *Cancer Investigation* 21, no. 5 (2003): 744–57, https://doi.org/10.1081/ cnv-120023773.

58 **genistein also activates stress responses:** Jaewon Lee et al., "Adaptive Cellular Stress Pathways as Therapeutic Targets of Dietary Phytochemicals: Focus on the Nervous System," ed. David R. Sibley, *Pharmacological Reviews* 66, no. 3 (July 1, 2014): 815–68, https:// doi.org/10.1124/pr.113.007757.

59 **luteolin's anti-inflammatory, antioxidant, and sirtuin:** Lee et al., "Adaptive Cellular Stress Pathways as Therapeutic Targets of Dietary Phytochemicals."

61 **Of the more than fifty thousand edible plants:** "Food Staple," *National Geographic*, last modified January 3, 2024, https://education.nationalgeographic.org/resource/food-staple.

61 **The order goes like this:** Kirsten Brandt and Jens Peter Mølgaard, "Organic Agriculture: Does It Enhance or Reduce the Nutritional Value of Plant Foods?," *Journal of the Science of Food and Agriculture* 81, no. 9 (2001): 924–31, https://doi.org/10.1002/jsfa.903.

61 **only about one out of ten Americans:** Seung Hee Lee, "Adults Meeting Fruit and Vegetable Intake Recommendations—United States, 2019," *MMWR. Morbidity and Mortality Weekly Report* 71 (2022), https://doi.org/10.15585/mmwr.mm7101a1.

61 **One of the largest epidemiological studies:** GBD 2017 Diet Collaborators, "Health Effects of Dietary Risks in 195 Countries, 1990–2017: A Systematic Analysis for the Global Burden of Disease Study 2017," *Lancet* 393, no. 10184 (May 11, 2019): 1958–72, https://doi. org/10.1016/S0140-6736(19)30041-8.

62 **However, consuming six cups per day:** Joshua D. Lambert and Ryan J. Elias, "The Antioxidant and Pro-Oxidant Activities of Green Tea Polyphenols: A Role in Cancer Prevention," *Archives of Biochemistry and Biophysics*, Polyphenols and Health, 501, no. 1 (September 1, 2010): 65–72, https://doi.org/10.1016/j.abb.2010.06.013.

62 **For example, only 16 percent of resveratrol:** David M. Goldberg, Joseph Yan, and George J. Soleas, "Absorption of Three Wine-Related Polyphenols in Three Different Matrices by Healthy Subjects," *Clinical Biochemistry* 36, no. 1 (January 1, 2003): 79–87, https:// doi.org/10.1016/S0009-9120(02)00397-1.

63 **These factors affect the distribution:** Liu, "Health-Promoting Components of Fruits and Vegetables in the Diet."

63 **Whole foods contain multiple:** Martucci et al., "Mediterranean Diet and Inflammaging Within the Hormesis Paradigm."

63 **For example, certain antioxidant supplements:** Soroush Seifirad, Alireza Ghaffari, and Mahsa M. Amoli, "The Antioxidants Dilemma: Are They Potentially Immunosuppressants and Carcinogens?," *Frontiers in Physiology* 5 (July 14, 2014): 245, https://doi.org/10.3389/fphys.2014.00245.

64 **In fact, beta-carotene:** Bjelakovic, Nikolova, and Gluud, "Antioxidant Supplements and Mortality."

64 **spend $12.8 billion:** "Americans Spend $30 Billion a Year Out-of-Pocket on Complementary Health Approaches," NCCIH, June 22, 2016, https://www.nccih.nih.gov/research/ research-results/americans-spend-30-billion-a-year-outofpocket-on-complementary- health-approaches.

64 **In a groundbreaking study:** Michael Ristow et al., "Antioxidants Prevent Health-Promoting Effects of Physical Exercise in Humans," *Proceedings of the National Academy of Sciences of the United States of America* 106, no. 21 (May 26, 2009): 8665–70, https://doi.org/10.1073/pnas.0903485106.

64 **However, your gut microbiome composition:** Martel et al., "Phytochemicals as Prebiotics and Biological Stress Inducers."

Chapter 5: Exercise Stress for Cellular Fitness

67 **Referred to as exerkines:** Lisa S. Chow et al., "Exerkines in Health, Resilience and Disease," *Nature Reviews Endocrinology* 18, no. 5 (May 2022): 273–89, https://doi.org/10.1038/s41574-022-00641-2.

67 **The discovery that exercise:** Scott K. Powers, Zsolt Radak, and Li Li Ji, "Exercise-Induced Oxidative Stress: Past, Present and Future," *Journal of Physiology* 594, no. 18 (September 15, 2016): 5081–92, https://doi.org/10.1113/JP270646.

67 **the type and amount of reactive oxygen species:** Scott K. Powers et al., "Exercise-Induced Oxidative Stress: Friend or Foe?," *Journal of Sport and Health Science* 9, no. 5 (September 2020): 415–25, https://doi.org/10.1016/j.jshs.2020.04.001.

67 **primarily serve as signals:** Michele Bevere et al., "Redox-Based Disruption of Cellular Hormesis and Promotion of Degenerative Pathways: Perspectives on Aging Processes," *Journals of Gerontology: Series A* 77, no. 11 (November 1, 2022): 2195–2206, https://doi.org/10.1093/gerona/glac167.

67 **As a result, the mild to moderate oxidative stress:** Li Li Ji, Zsolt Radak, and Sataro Goto, "Hormesis and Exercise: How the Cell Copes with Oxidative Stress," *American Journal of Pharmacology and Toxicology* 3, no. 1 (2008): 41–55, https://doi.org/10.3844/ajptsp.2008.44.58.

68 **The health-promoting power:** M. Fogelholm, "Physical Activity, Fitness and Fatness: Relations to Mortality, Morbidity and Disease Risk Factors. A Systematic Review," *Obesity Reviews: An Official Journal of the International Association for the Study of Obesity* 11, no. 3 (March 2010): 202–21, https://doi.org/10.1111/j.1467-789X.2009.00653.x.

68 **The health-promoting power:** Carl J. Lavie et al., "Sedentary Behavior, Exercise, and Cardiovascular Health," *Circulation Research* 124, no. 5 (March 2019): 799–815, https://doi.org/10.1161/CIRCRESAHA.118.312669.

68 **Mitochondria actually do far more:** Jonathan M. Memme et al., "Exercise and Mitochondrial Health," *Journal of Physiology* 599, no. 3 (2021): 803–17, https://doi.org/10.1113/JP278853.

68 **that converge on mitochondria:** Ashley N. Oliveira and David A. Hood, "Exercise Is Mitochondrial Medicine for Muscle," *Sports Medicine and Health Science* 1, no. 1 (December 1, 2019): 11–18, https://doi.org/10.1016/j.smhs.2019.08.008.

68 **Mitochondrial dysfunction:** Iñigo San-Millán, "The Key Role of Mitochondrial Function in Health and Disease," *Antioxidants (Basel, Switzerland)* 12, no. 4 (March 23, 2023): 782, https://doi.org/10.3390/antiox12040782.

69 **Bad stressors like a high-calorie:** Amaloha Casanova et al., "Mitochondria: It Is All About Energy," *Frontiers in Physiology* 14 (2023): 1114231, https://doi.org/10.3389/fphys.2023.1114231.

69 **Our tiny little cellular engines:** Casanova et al.

69 **"metabolic flexibility":** San-Millán, "The Key Role of Mitochondrial Function in Health and Disease."

70 **Mitochondrial dysfunction makes our metabolism:** Pankaj Prasun, "Mitochondrial Dysfunction in Metabolic Syndrome," *Biochimica et Biophysica Acta. Molecular Basis of Disease* 1866, no. 10 (October 1, 2020): 165838, https://doi.org/10.1016/j.bbadis.2020.165838.

70 **The communication between neurons:** Memme et al., "Exercise and Mitochondrial Health."

70 **neuroscientists have started to advocate:** Johannes Burtscher et al., "Boosting Mitochondrial Health to Counteract Neurodegeneration," *Progress in Neurobiology* 215 (August 1, 2022): 102289, https://doi.org/10.1016/j.pneurobio.2022.102289.

71 **They do this by cleaving:** Daniela Sorriento, Eugenio Di Vaia, and Guido Iaccarino, "Physical Exercise: A Novel Tool to Protect Mitochondrial Health," *Frontiers in Physiology* 12 (April 27, 2021): 660068, https://doi.org/10.3389/fphys.2021.660068.

71 **They form a network:** Douglas C. Wallace, "Mitochondria as Chi," *Genetics* 179, no. 2 (June 2008): 727–35, https://doi.org/10.1534/genetics.104.91769.

71 **mitochondria communicate with multiple bodily systems:** Casanova et al., "Mitochondria."

71 **mitochondria also produce hormones and essential neurotransmitters:** Casanova et al.

72 **more tailored than the standard physical activity guidelines:** Claude Bouchard, Steven N. Blair, and Peter T. Katzmarzyk, "Less Sitting, More Physical Activity, or Higher Fitness?," *Mayo Clinic Proceedings* 90, no. 11 (November 2015): 1533–40, https://doi.org/10.1016/j.mayocp.2015.08.005.

73 **cardiorespiratory fitness:** Robert Ross et al., "Importance of Assessing Cardiorespiratory Fitness in Clinical Practice: A Case for Fitness as a Clinical Vital Sign: A Scientific Statement from the American Heart Association," *Circulation* 134, no. 24 (December 13, 2016): e653–99, https://doi.org/10.1161/CIR.0000000000000461.

74 **endurance exercise raises antioxidant capacity:** Elisa Couto Gomes, Albená Nunes Silva, and Marta Rubino de Oliveira, "Oxidants, Antioxidants, and the Beneficial Roles of Exercise-Induced Production of Reactive Species," *Oxidative Medicine and Cellular Longevity* 2012 (June 3, 2012): e756132, https://doi.org/10.1155/2012/756132.

74 **can expand by as much as 40 to 50 percent:** K. M. Baldwin et al., "Respiratory Capacity of White, Red, and Intermediate Muscle: Adaptative Response to Exercise," *American Journal of Physiology* 222, no. 2 (February 1, 1972): 373–78, https://doi.org/10.1152/ajplegacy.1972.222.2.373.

74 **double the amount of antioxidant enzymes:** Oliveira and Hood, "Exercise Is Mitochondrial Medicine for Muscle."

74 **Different exercises engage different muscle groups:** Glenn C. Rowe, Adeel Safdar, and Zolt Arany, "Running Forward: New Frontiers in Endurance Exercise Biology," *Circulation* 129, no. 7 (February 18, 2014): 798–810, https://doi.org/10.1161/CIRCULATIONAHA.113.001590.

74 **the effort that you put into it:** J. Viña et al., "Free Radicals in Exhaustive Physical Exercise: Mechanism of Production, and Protection by Antioxidants," *IUBMB Life* 50, no. 4–5 (2000): 271–77, https://doi.org/10.1080/713803729.

74 **Simply moving at a leisurely pace:** Powers et al., "Exercise-Induced Oxidative Stress."

75 **train at a combination of intensities:** David J. Bishop, Cesare Granata, and Nir Eynon, "Can We Optimise the Exercise Training Prescription to Maximise Improvements in Mitochondria Function and Content?," *Biochimica et Biophysica Acta* 1840, no. 4 (April 2014): 1266–75, https://doi.org/10.1016/j.bbagen.2013.10.012.

75 **more muscle fiber types:** Memme et al., "Exercise and Mitochondrial Health."

75 **Intensity is key:** Martin J. MacInnis et al., "Superior Mitochondrial Adaptations in Human Skeletal Muscle After Interval Compared to Continuous Single-Leg Cycling Matched for Total Work," *Journal of Physiology* 595, no. 9 (May 1, 2017): 2955–68, https://doi.org/10.1113/JP272570.

75 **perceived exertion, or RPE:** Ardalan Shariat et al., "Borg CR-10 Scale as a New Approach to Monitoring Office Exercise Training," *Work (Reading, Mass.)* 60, no. 4 (2018): 549–54, https://doi.org/10.3233/WOR-182762.

75 **"talk test":** "Measuring Physical Activity Intensity | Physical Activity | CDC," October 20, 2022, https://www.cdc.gov/physicalactivity/basics/measuring/index.html.

75 **heart rate during exercise:** "Target Heart Rate and Estimated Maximum Heart Rate | Physical Activity | CDC," October 20, 2022, https://www.cdc.gov/physicalactivity/basics/measuring/heartrate.htm.

75 **Our body's built-in way:** Powers et al., "Exercise-Induced Oxidative Stress."

76 **"breaking point":** Li Li Ji, Chounghun Kang, and Yong Zhang, "Exercise-Induced Hormesis and Skeletal Muscle Health," *Free Radical Biology and Medicine*, Human Performance and Redox Signaling in Health and Disease, 98 (September 1, 2016): 113–22, https://doi.org/10.1016/j.freeradbiomed.2016.02.025.

77 **Phytochemicals, particularly polyphenols:** David C. Nieman and Laurel M. Wentz, "The Compelling Link Between Physical Activity and the Body's Defense System," *Journal of Sport and Health Science* 8, no. 3 (May 1, 2019): 201–17, https://doi.org/10.1016/j.jshs.2018.09.009.

77 **resveratrol, quercetin, and epigallocatechin gallate (EGCG):** Alistair V Nunn et al., "Inflammatory Modulation of Exercise Salience: Using Hormesis to Return to a Healthy Lifestyle," *Nutrition & Metabolism* 7 (December 9, 2010): 87, https://doi.org/10.1186/1743-7075-7-87.

Chapter 6: Cold and Heat Therapy for Activating Thermogenesis

79 **Hippocrates, believed cold water:** Knechtle et al., "Cold Water Swimming—Benefits and Risks."

79 **noradrenaline up to five times:** P. Šrámek et al., "Human Physiological Responses to Immersion into Water of Different Temperatures," *European Journal of Applied Physiology* 81, no. 5 (February 1, 2000): 436–42, https://doi.org/10.1007/s004210050065.

79 **increases dopamine levels by 250 percent:** Šrámek et al.

79 **train elite military forces:** Karen R. Kelly et al., "Prolonged Extreme Cold Water Diving and the Acute Stress Response During Military Dive Training," *Frontiers in Physiology* 13 (2022), https://doi.org/10.3389/fphys.2022.842612.

80 **adrenaline and cortisol don't change:** Šrámek et al., "Human Physiological Responses to Immersion into Water of Different Temperatures."

80 **adrenaline and cortisol don't change:** J. Leppäluoto et al., "Effects of Long-Term Whole-Body Cold Exposures on Plasma Concentrations of ACTH, Beta-endorphin, Cortisol, Catecholamines and Cytokines in Healthy Females," *Scandinavian Journal of Clinical and Laboratory Investigation* 68, no. 2 (January 1, 2008): 145–53, https://doi.org/10.108%0365510701516350.

80 **lead to *lower* baseline cortisol:** Leppäluoto et al.

80 **production of beta-endorphins:** Nikolai A. Shevchuk, "Adapted Cold Shower as a Potential Treatment for Depression," *Medical Hypotheses* 70, no. 5 (January 1, 2008): 995–1001, https://doi.org/10.1016/j.mehy.2007.04.052.

80 **opioid called dynorphin:** Rhonda P. Patrick and Teresa L. Johnson, "Sauna Use as a Lifestyle Practice to Extend Healthspan," *Experimental Gerontology* 154 (October 15, 2021): 111509, https://doi.org/10.1016/j.exger.2021.111509.

82 **adults have brown fat, too:** Aaron M. Cypess et al., "Identification and Importance of Brown Adipose Tissue in Adult Humans," *New England Journal of Medicine* 360, no. 15 (April 9, 2009): 1509–17, https://doi.org/10.1056/NEJMoa0810780.

82 **could potentially combat obesity:** Aaron M. Cypess and C. Ronald Kahn, "Brown Fat as a Therapy for Obesity and Diabetes," *Current Opinion in Endocrinology, Diabetes, and Obesity* 17, no. 2 (April 2010): 143–49, https://doi.org/10.1097/MED.0b013e328337a81f.

82 **associated with reduced visceral fat:** Andreas G. Wibmer et al., "Brown Adipose Tissue Is Associated with Healthier Body Fat Distribution and Metabolic Benefits Independent of Regional Adiposity," *Cell Reports Medicine* 2, no. 7 (July 20, 2021): 100332, https://doi.org/10.1016/j.xcrm.2021.100332.

83 **lower the risk of diabetes:** Yoanna M. Ivanova and Denis P. Blondin, "Examining the Benefits of Cold Exposure as a Therapeutic Strategy for Obesity and Type 2 Diabetes," *Journal of Applied Physiology* 130, no. 5 (May 1, 2021): 1448–59, https://doi.org/10.1152/japplphysiol.00934.2020.

83   **brown fat also clears triglycerides:** Geerte Hoeke et al., "Role of Brown Fat in Lipo-protein Metabolism and Atherosclerosis," *Circulation Research* 118, no. 1 (January 8, 2016): 173–82, https://doi.org/10.1161/CIRCRESAHA.115.306647.

83   **people who spent six hours a day:** Anouk A. J. J. van der Lans et al., "Cold Acclimation Recruits Human Brown Fat and Increases Nonshivering Thermogenesis," *Journal of Clinical Investigation* 123, no. 8 (August 1, 2013): 3395–3403, https://doi.org/10.1172/JCI68993.

83   **"beige fat":** Vivian Peirce, Stefania Carobbio, and Antonio Vidal-Puig, "The Different Shades of Fat," *Nature* 510, no. 7503 (June 2014): 76–83, https://doi.org/10.1038/nature13477.

84   **increasing mitochondrial density:** Nana Chung, Jonghoon Park, and Kiwon Lim, "The Effects of Exercise and Cold Exposure on Mitochondrial Biogenesis in Skeletal Muscle and White Adipose Tissue," *Journal of Exercise Nutrition & Biochemistry* 21, no. 2 (June 30, 2017): 39–47, https://doi.org/10.20463/jenb.2017.0020.

84   **a switch, called uncoupling protein 1 (UCP1):** Peirce, Carobbio, and Vidal-Puig, "The Different Shades of Fat."

84   **activates antioxidant and anti-inflammatory:** W. G. Siems et al., "Improved Antioxidative Protection in Winter Swimmers," *QJM: An International Journal of Medicine* 92, no. 4 (April 1, 1999): 193–98, https://doi.org/10.1093/qjmed/92.4.193.

84   **stimulates AMPK and SIRT1:** Patrick Schrauwen and Wouter D. van Marken Lichtenbelt, "Combatting Type 2 Diabetes by Turning Up the Heat," *Diabetologia* 59, no. 11 (2016): 2269–79, https://doi.org/10.1007/s00125-016-4068-3.

84   **what happens during moderate or high-intensity exercise:** Jari A. Laukkanen, Tanjaniina Laukkanen, and Setor K. Kunutsor, "Cardiovascular and Other Health Benefits of Sauna Bathing: A Review of the Evidence," *Mayo Clinic Proceedings* 93, no. 8 (August 1, 2018): 1111–21, https://doi.org/10.1016/j.mayocp.2018.04.008.

84   **range of a low-grade fever:** Katriina Kukkonen-Harjula and Kyllikki Kauppinen, "Health Effects and Risks of Sauna Bathing," *International Journal of Circumpolar Health* 65, no. 3 (June 2006): 195–205, https://doi.org/10.3402/ijch.v65i3.18102.

85   **health of the lining of your blood vessels:** Andreas J. Flammer and Thomas F. Lüscher, "Three Decades of Endothelium Research," *Swiss Medical Weekly* 140, no. 4748 (November 22, 2010): w13122–w13122, https://doi.org/10.4414/smw.2010.13122.

85   **a magical molecule called nitric oxide (NO):** Vienna E. Brunt and Christopher T. Minson, "Heat Therapy: Mechanistic Underpinnings and Applications to Cardiovascular Health," *Journal of Applied Physiology* 130, no. 6 (June 1, 2021): 1684–1704, https://doi.org/10.1152/japplphysiol.00141.2020.

85   **Nobel Prize in 1998:** Flammer and Lüscher, "Three Decades of Endothelium Research."

86   **levels of heat shock proteins can increase:** Patrick and Johnson, "Sauna Use as a Lifestyle Practice to Extend Healthspan."

86   **improve our cardiovascular and metabolic health:** Brett R. Ely et al., "Meta-Inflammation and Cardiometabolic Disease in Obesity: Can Heat Therapy Help?," *Temperature* 5, no. 1 (January 2, 2018): 9–21, https://doi.org/10.1080/23328940.2017.1384089.

86   **heat stress reduces low-grade chronic inflammation:** Sven P. Hoekstra, Nicolette C. Bishop, and Christof A. Leicht, "Elevating Body Temperature to Reduce Chronic Low-Grade Inflammation: A Welcome Strategy for Those Unable to Exercise?," *Exercise Immunology Review* 26 (2020): 42–55.

86   **gene regulator called FOXO3:** Brian J. Morris et al., "FOXO3: A Major Gene for Human Longevity—A Mini-Review," *Gerontology* 61, no. 6 (March 28, 2015): 515–25, https://doi.org/10.1159/000375235.

87   **Studies have shown that hot tubs:** Sadatoshi Biro et al., "Clinical Implications of Thermal Therapy in Lifestyle-Related Diseases," *Experimental Biology and Medicine* 228, no. 10 (November 1, 2003): 1245–49, https://doi.org/10.1177/153537020322801023.

87   **Studies have shown that hot tubs:** Patrick and Johnson, "Sauna Use as a Lifestyle Practice to Extend Healthspan."

87   **Studies have shown that hot tubs:** S. P. Hoekstra et al., "Acute and Chronic Effects of Hot Water Immersion on Inflammation and Metabolism in Sedentary, Overweight Adults," *Journal of Applied Physiology (Bethesda, Md.: 1985)* 125, no. 6 (December 1, 2018): 2008–18, https://doi.org/10.1152/japplphysiol.00407.2018.

88   **heat transfer rate of water:** Lynne Mccullough and Sanjay Arora, "Diagnosis and Treatment of Hypothermia," *American Family Physician* 70, no. 12 (December 15, 2004): 2325–32.

88   **Cold air exposure protocols:** Peirce, Carobbio, and Vidal-Puig, "The Different Shades of Fat."

88   **Studies that incorporate dry saunas:** Kaemmer N. Henderson et al., "The Cardiometabolic Health Benefits of Sauna Exposure in Individuals with High-Stress Occupations. A Mechanistic Review," *International Journal of Environmental Research and Public Health* 18, no. 3 (January 2021): 1105, https://doi.org/10.3390/ijerph18031105.

88   **Infrared saunas:** Richard Beever, "Far-Infrared Saunas for Treatment of Cardiovascular Risk Factors: Summary of Published Evidence," *Canadian Family Physician Medecin de Famille Canadien* 55, no. 7 (July 2009): 691–96.

88   **Hot baths:** Patrick and Johnson, "Sauna Use as a Lifestyle Practice to Extend Healthspan."

88   **Hot baths:** Hoekstra et al., "Acute and Chronic Effects of Hot Water Immersion on Inflammation and Metabolism in Sedentary, Overweight Adults."

89   **studies using cold air exposure:** Peirce, Carobbio, and Vidal-Puig, "The Different Shades of Fat."

89   **a water immersion study:** Šrámek et al., "Human Physiological Responses to Immersion into Water of Different Temperatures."

89   **protocol using gasping cold water:** Leppäluoto et al., "Effects of Long-Term Whole-Body Cold Exposures on Plasma Concentrations of ACTH, Beta-endorphin, Cortisol, Catecholamines and Cytokines in Healthy Females."

89   **A noteworthy 2021 study:** Susanna Søberg et al., "Altered Brown Fat Thermoregulation and Enhanced Cold-Induced Thermogenesis in Young, Healthy, Winter-Swimming Men," *Cell Reports Medicine* 2, no. 10 (October 19, 2021): 100408, https://doi.org/10.1016/j.xcrm.2021.100408.

89   **It's more beneficial to end:** Kukkonen-Harjula and Kauppinen, "Health Effects and Risks of Sauna Bathing."

Chapter 7: Cycles of Fasting, Eating, and Our Circadian Biology

91   **eats for fifteen hours:** Shubhroz Gill and Satchidananda Panda, "A Smartphone App Reveals Erratic Diurnal Eating Patterns in Humans That Can Be Modulated for Health Benefits," *Cell Metabolism* 22, no. 5 (November 3, 2015): 789–98, https://doi.org/10.1016/j.cmet.2015.09.005.

91   **metabolic switch:** Rafael de Cabo and Mark P. Mattson, "Effects of Intermittent Fasting on Health, Aging, and Disease," *New England Journal of Medicine* 381, no. 26 (2019): 2541–51, https://doi.org/10.1056/NEJMra1905136.

91   **fat is converted into ketones:** Kolb et al., "Ketone Bodies."

91   **Excess fat can spread:** Dilek Yazıcı and Havva Sezer, "Insulin Resistance, Obesity and Lipotoxicity," in *Obesity and Lipotoxicity*, ed. Ayse Basak Engin and Atilla Engin, (Cham, Switzerland: Springer International Publishing, 2017), 277–304, https://doi.org/10.1007/978-3-319-48382-5_12.

92   **roller coaster of poor metabolic health:** Meghan O'Hearn et al., "Trends and Disparities in Cardiometabolic Health Among U.S. Adults, 1999–2018," *Journal of the American College of Cardiology* 80, no. 2 (July 12, 2022): 138–51, https://doi.org/10.1016/j.jacc.2022.04.046.

92   **can even increase the risk of death:** Karlee J. Ausk, Edward J. Boyko, and George N. Ioannou, "Insulin Resistance Predicts Mortality in Nondiabetic Individuals in the U.S.," *Diabetes Care* 33, no. 6 (June 1, 2010): 1179–85, https://doi.org/10.2337/dc09-2110.

92 **a wide range of chronic diseases:** de Cabo and Mattson, "Effects of Intermittent Fasting on Health, Aging, and Disease."

94 **go beyond continuously cutting back on calories:** Mark P. Mattson et al., "Intermittent Metabolic Switching, Neuroplasticity and Brain Health," *Nature Reviews Neuroscience* 19, no. 2 (February 2018): 63–80, https://doi.org/10.1038/nrn.2017.156.

94 **the master controller:** M. N. Hall, "mTOR—What Does It Do?," *Transplantation Proceedings* 40, no. 10 Suppl. (December 2008): S5-8, https://doi.org/10.1016/j.transproceed.2008.10.009.

94 **The other two sensors:** Shinji Kume, Merlin C. Thomas, and Daisuke Koya, "Nutrient Sensing, Autophagy, and Diabetic Nephropathy," *Diabetes* 61, no. 1 (January 2012): 23–29, https://doi.org/10.2337/db11-0555.

95 **overstimulating the mTOR pathway:** Roberto Zoncu, Alejo Efeyan, and David M. Sabatini, "mTOR: From Growth Signal Integration to Cancer, Diabetes and Ageing," *Nature Reviews Molecular Cell Biology* 12, no. 1 (January 2011): 21–35, https://doi.org/10.1038/nrm3025.

95 **The buildup of cellular junk:** Tadashi Ichimiya et al., "Autophagy and Autophagy-Related Diseases: A Review," *International Journal of Molecular Sciences* 21, no. 23 (November 26, 2020): 8974, https://doi.org/10.3390/ijms21238974.

95 **Autophagy can also be turned on:** Jan Martel et al., "Hormetic Effects of Phytochemicals on Health and Longevity," *Trends in Endocrinology & Metabolism* 30, no. 6 (June 1, 2019): 335–46, https://doi.org/10.1016/j.tem.2019.04.001.

95 **Autophagy can also be turned on:** Valter D. Longo et al., "Intermittent and Periodic Fasting, Longevity and Disease," *Nature Aging* 1, no. 1 (January 2021): 47–59, https://doi.org/10.1038/s43587-020-00013-3.

96 **the level of autophagy:** Daniela Liśkiewicz et al., "Upregulation of Hepatic Autophagy Under Nutritional Ketosis," *Journal of Nutritional Biochemistry* 93 (July 1, 2021): 108620, https://doi.org/10.1016/j.jnutbio.2021.108620.

96 **more like a dimmer switch:** Zoncu, Efeyan, and Sabatini, "mTOR."

97 **no studies have compared them:** Krista A. Varady et al., "Clinical Application of Intermittent Fasting for Weight Loss: Progress and Future Directions," *Nature Reviews Endocrinology* 18, no. 5 (May 2022): 309–21, https://doi.org/10.1038/s41574-022-00638-x.

97 **repeated switching back and forth from:** de Cabo and Mattson, "Effects of Intermittent Fasting on Health, Aging, and Disease."

97 **The first study to show:** Megumi Hatori et al., "Time-Restricted Feeding Without Reducing Caloric Intake Prevents Metabolic Diseases in Mice Fed a High-Fat Diet," *Cell Metabolism* 15, no. 6 (June 6, 2012): 848–60, https://doi.org/10.1016/j.cmet.2012.04.019.

97 **we don't have just one internal clock:** Emily N. C. Manoogian et al., "Time-Restricted Eating for the Prevention and Management of Metabolic Diseases," *Endocrine Reviews* 43, no. 2 (April 1, 2022): 405–36, https://doi.org/10.1210/endrev/bnab027.

98 **Our circadian rhythm is very adaptable:** Valter D. Longo and Satchidananda Panda, "Fasting, Circadian Rhythms, and Time-Restricted Feeding in Healthy Lifespan," *Cell Metabolism* 23, no. 6 (June 14, 2016): 1048–59, https://doi.org/10.1016/j.cmet.2016.06.001.

98 **Melatonin also makes:** Heitor O. Santos et al., "A Scoping Review of Intermittent Fasting, Chronobiology, and Metabolism," *American Journal of Clinical Nutrition* 115, no. 4 (April 1, 2022): 991–1004, https://doi.org/10.1093/ajcn/nqab433.

98 **the genes regulating fat burning:** Jun Yoshino et al., "Diurnal Variation in Insulin Sensitivity of Glucose Metabolism Is Associated with Diurnal Variations in Whole-Body and Cellular Fatty Acid Metabolism in Metabolically Normal Women," *Journal of Clinical Endocrinology and Metabolism* 99, no. 9 (September 2014): E1666-1670, https://doi.org/10.1210/jc.2014-1579.

98 **men who ate dinner before bed:** Junko Yoshida et al., "Association of Night Eating Habits with Metabolic Syndrome and Its Components: A Longitudinal Study," *BMC Public Health* 18, no. 1 (December 11, 2018): 1366, https://doi.org/10.1186/s12889-018-6262-3.

98 **This cycle is partly controlled:** Longo and Panda, "Fasting, Circadian Rhythms, and Time-Restricted Feeding in Healthy Lifespan."

98 **This cycle is partly controlled:** Victoria A. Acosta-Rodríguez et al., "Importance of Circadian Timing for Aging and Longevity," *Nature Communications* 12, no. 1 (May 17, 2021): 2862, https://doi.org/10.1038/s41467-021-22922-6.

99 **A study showed that eating:** Humaira Jamshed et al., "Early Time-Restricted Feeding Improves 24-Hour Glucose Levels and Affects Markers of the Circadian Clock, Aging, and Autophagy in Humans," *Nutrients* 11, no. 6 (May 30, 2019): 1234, https://doi.org/10.3390/nu11061234.

99 **choose eating windows in the afternoon or evening:** Luisa Torres et al., "Retention, Fasting Patterns, and Weight Loss with an Intermittent Fasting App: Large-Scale, 52-Week Observational Study," *JMIR mHealth and uHealth* 10, no. 10 (October 4, 2022): e35896, https://doi.org/10.2196/35896.

99 **a rigorous controlled trial with prediabetic men:** Elizabeth F. Sutton et al., "Early Time-Restricted Feeding Improves Insulin Sensitivity, Blood Pressure, and Oxidative Stress Even Without Weight Loss in Men with Prediabetes," *Cell Metabolism* 27, no. 6 (June 5, 2018): 1212-1221.e3, https://doi.org/10.1016/j.cmet.2018.04.010.

99 **late afternoon or evening eating windows:** Sutton et al.

99 **notion that we need to start the morning with breakfast:** Alex Mayyasi, "How Breakfast Became Known as 'the Most Important Meal of the Day,'" *Business Insider*, June 21, 2016, https://www.businessinsider.com/how-breakfast-became-known-as-the-most-important-meal-of-the-day-2016-6.

100 **"the most important meal of the day":** Mayyasi.

100 **a 2023 study published:** Shuhao Lin et al., "Time-Restricted Eating Without Calorie Counting for Weight Loss in a Racially Diverse Population," *Annals of Internal Medicine*, June 27, 2023, https://doi.org/10.7326/M23-0052.

101 **Ketones, which form:** de Cabo and Mattson, "Effects of Intermittent Fasting on Health, Aging, and Disease."

101 **they go up even more:** John C. Newman and Eric Verdin, "Ketone Bodies as Signaling Metabolites," *Trends in Endocrinology and Metabolism: TEM* 25, no. 1 (January 2014): 42–52, https://doi.org/10.1016/j.tem.2013.09.002.

101 **from over fourteen hours to ten to eleven hours:** Gill and Panda, "A Smartphone App Reveals Erratic Diurnal Eating Patterns in Humans That Can Be Modulated for Health Benefits."

102 **However, the idea of 16:8:** Manoogian et al., "Time-Restricted Eating for the Prevention and Management of Metabolic Diseases."

102 **A ten-hour window:** Manoogian et al.

103 **A yearlong study using an app:** Torres et al., "Retention, Fasting Patterns, and Weight Loss with an Intermittent Fasting App."

103 **change from your baseline:** Emily N. C. Manoogian and Blandine Laferrère, "Time-Restricted Eating: What We Know and Where the Field Is Going," *Obesity* 31, no. S1 (2023): 7–8, https://doi.org/10.1002/oby.23672.

103 **Losing muscle can:** Dong Hoon Lee and Edward L Giovannucci, "Body Composition and Mortality in the General Population: A Review of Epidemiologic Studies," *Experimental Biology and Medicine* 243, no. 17–18 (December 2018): 1275–85, https://doi.org/10.1177/1535370218818161.

103 **In one study, most weight:** Dylan A. Lowe et al., "Effects of Time-Restricted Eating on Weight Loss and Other Metabolic Parameters in Women and Men with Overweight and Obesity: The TREAT Randomized Clinical Trial," *JAMA Internal Medicine* 180, no. 11 (November 1, 2020): 1491–99, https://doi.org/10.1001/jamainternmed.2020.4153.

104 **Fasting and recovery work together:** de Cabo and Mattson, "Effects of Intermittent Fasting on Health, Aging, and Disease."

104 **stick to it about 70 to 93 percent:** Manoogian et al., "Time-Restricted Eating for the Prevention and Management of Metabolic Diseases."

105 **different protective responses in the brain:** Jip Gudden, Alejandro Arias Vasquez, and Mirjam Bloemendaal, "The Effects of Intermittent Fasting on Brain and Cognitive Function," *Nutrients* 13, no. 9 (September 10, 2021): 3166, https://doi.org/10.3390/nu13093166.

105 **mentally alert and calm:** Guillaume Fond et al., "Fasting in Mood Disorders: Neurobiology and Effectiveness. A Review of the Literature," *Psychiatry Research* 209, no. 3 (October 30, 2013): 253–58, https://doi.org/10.1016/j.psychres.2012.12.018.

105 **widely prescribed antidepressant class:** Mattson et al., "Intermittent Metabolic Switching, Neuroplasticity and Brain Health," February 2018.

105 **forestalling the most common health conditions:** Varady et al., "Clinical Application of Intermittent Fasting for Weight Loss."

Chapter 8: Finding the Golden Mean in Emotional and Mental Stress

106 **Hungarian endocrinologist Hans Selye:** Michael Breitenbach, Elisabeth Kapferer, and Clemens Sedmak, "Hans Selye and the Origins of Stress Research," in *Stress and Poverty: A Cross-Disciplinary Investigation of Stress in Cells, Individuals, and Society*, ed. Michael Breitenbach, Elisabeth Kapferer, and Clemens Sedmak (Cham, Switzerland: Springer International Publishing, 2021), 21–28, https://doi.org/10.1007/978-3-030 -77738-8_2.

107 **"general adaptation syndrome":** Hans Selye, "A Syndrome Produced by Diverse Nocuous Agents," *Nature* 138, no. 3479 (July 1936): 32–32, https://doi.org/10.1038/138032a0.

107 **different kinds of stress responses:** K. Pacak et al., "Heterogeneous Neurochemical Responses to Different Stressors: A Test of Selye's Doctrine of Nonspecificity," *American Journal of Physiology* 275, no. 4 (October 1998): R1247-1255, https://doi.org/10.1152 /ajpregu.1998.275.4.R1247.

107 **Some of the ones involved:** Agorastos Agorastos and George P. Chrousos, "The Neuroendocrinology of Stress: The Stress-Related Continuum of Chronic Disease Development," *Molecular Psychiatry* 27, no. 1 (January 2022): 502–13, https://doi.org/10.1038/s41380-021-01224-9.

107 **Selye's theories have persisted:** David S. Goldstein and Irwin J. Kopin, "Evolution of Concepts of Stress," *Stress* 10, no. 2 (January 1, 2007): 109–20, https://doi. org/10.1080/10253890701288935.

108 **"anything, pleasant or unpleasant":** Hans Selye, "Stress Without Distress," in *Psychopathology of Human Adaptation* (Springer, 1974), 137–46.

108 **In 1908, Robert M. Yerkes and John Dillingham Dodson:** Robert M. Yerkes and John D. Dodson, "The Relation of Strength of Stimulus to Rapidity of Habit-Formation," *Journal of Comparative Neurology and Psychology* 18, no. 5 (November 1908): 459–82, https://doi. org/10.1002/cne.920180503.

108 **The inverted U-shaped curve:** Robert M. Sapolsky, "Stress and the Brain: Individual Variability and the Inverted-U," *Nature Neuroscience* 18, no. 10 (October 2015): 1344–46, https:// doi.org/10.1038/nn.4109.

108 **Human Connectome Project:** David C. Van Essen et al., "The WU-Minn Human Connectome Project: An Overview," *NeuroImage*, Mapping the Connectome, 80 (October 15, 2013): 62–79, https://doi.org/10.1016/j.neuroimage.2013.05.041.

109 **Assaf Oshri, PhD, and his team:** Assaf Oshri et al., "Is Perceived Stress Linked to Enhanced Cognitive Functioning and Reduced Risk for Psychopathology? Testing the Hormesis Hypothesis," *Psychiatry Research* 314 (August 2022): 114644, https://doi.org/10.1016/j .psychres.2022.114644.

112 **he redefined it as a system that helps us adapt:** Bruce S. McEwen and Huda Akil, "Revisiting the Stress Concept: Implications for Affective Disorders," *Journal of Neuroscience* 40, no. 1 (January 2, 2020): 12–21, https://doi.org/10.1523/JNEUROSCI.0733-19.2019.

112 **recalibrates our psychological stress set point:** Bruce S. McEwen, "Stressed or Stressed Out: What Is the Difference?," *Journal of Psychiatry and Neuroscience* 30, no. 5 (September 2005): 315–18.

112 **brain has receptors for hormones:** McEwen and Akil, "Revisiting the Stress Concept."

112 **stress affects the brain:** Bruce S. McEwen, Jason D. Gray, and Carla Nasca, "Recognizing Resilience: Learning from the Effects of Stress on the Brain," *Neurobiology of Stress*, Stress Resilience, 1 (January 1, 2015): 1–11, https://doi.org/10.1016/j.ynstr.2014.09.001.

112 **mold our brain through neuroplasticity:** McEwen and Akil, "Revisiting the Stress Concept."

112 **same hormone, cortisol, can have opposite effects:** Sapolsky, "Stress and the Brain."

112 **hippocampus have two distinct receptors:** McEwen and Akil, "Revisiting the Stress Concept."

113 **rapidly activating and then efficiently turning off:** E. Ronald de Kloet and Marian Joëls, "The Cortisol Switch Between Vulnerability and Resilience," *Molecular Psychiatry*, January 4, 2023, 1–15, https://doi.org/10.1038/s41380-022-01934-8.

113 **new neurons to mature from stem cells:** Elizabeth D, Kirby et al., "Acute Stress Enhances Adult Rat Hippocampal Neurogenesis and Activation of Newborn Neurons via Secreted Astrocytic FGF2," ed. Russ Fernald, *eLife* 2 (April 16, 2013): e00362, https://doi.org/10.7554/eLife.00362.

114 **changing the neuron's branches (dendrites):** McEwen and Akil, "Revisiting the Stress Concept."

114 **how we become resilient:** McEwen, Gray, and Nasca, "Recognizing Resilience."

114 **psychological stress reduced oxidative damage:** Kirstin Aschbacher et al., "Good Stress, Bad Stress and Oxidative Stress: Insights from Anticipatory Cortisol Reactivity," *Psychoneuroendocrinology* 38, no. 9 (September 2013): 1698–1708, https://doi.org/10.1016/j.psyneuen.2013.02.004.

115 **might improve our mitochondrial health:** Jing Du et al., "Dynamic Regulation of Mitochondrial Function by Glucocorticoids," *Proceedings of the National Academy of Sciences of the United States of America* 106, no. 9 (March 3, 2009): 3543–48, https://doi.org/10.1073/pnas.0812671106.

115 **actively build your resilience:** Scott J. Russo et al., "Neurobiology of Resilience," *Nature Neuroscience* 15, no. 11 (November 2012): 1475–84, https://doi.org/10.1038/nn.3234.

115 **clear picture of "bad" psychological stress:** J. M. Koolhaas et al., "Stress Revisited: A Critical Evaluation of the Stress Concept," *Neuroscience and Biobehavioral Reviews* 35, no. 5 (April 2011): 1291–1301, https://doi.org/10.1016/j.neubiorev.2011.02.003.

115 **a motivating amount of doubt:** Sapolsky, "Stress and the Brain."

116 **Examples of good stress:** Agorastos and Chrousos, "The Neuroendocrinology of Stress."

116 **Cole then went on to show:** Barbara L. Fredrickson et al., "A Functional Genomic Perspective on Human Well-Being," *Proceedings of the National Academy of Sciences of the United States of America* 110, no. 33 (August 13, 2013): 13684–89, https://doi.org/10.1073/pnas.1305419110.

116 **Those who were flourishing:** Jennifer S. Mascaro et al., "Flourishing in Healthcare Trainees: Psychological Well-Being and the Conserved Transcriptional Response to Adversity," *International Journal of Environmental Research and Public Health* 19, no. 4 (February 16, 2022): 2255, https://doi.org/10.3390/ijerph19042255.

117 **When they were nine months old:** Karen J. Parker et al., "Prospective Investigation of Stress Inoculation in Young Monkeys," *Archives of General Psychiatry* 61, no. 9 (September 2004): 933–41, https://doi.org/10.1001/archpsyc.61.9.933.

117 **In preadolescence:** Karen J. Parker et al., "Mild Early Life Stress Enhances Prefrontal-Dependent Response Inhibition in Monkeys," *Biological Psychiatry* 57, no. 8 (April 15, 2005): 848–55, https://doi.org/10.1016/j.biopsych.2004.12.024.

117 **as they got older:** Karen J. Parker et al., "Early Life Stress and Novelty Seeking Behavior in Adolescent Monkeys," *Psychoneuroendocrinology* 32, no. 7 (August 2007): 785–92, https://doi.org/10.1016/j.psyneuen.2007.05.008.

117 **Their prefrontal cortex:** Maor Katz et al., "Prefrontal Plasticity and Stress Inoculation-Induced Resilience," *Developmental Neuroscience* 31, no. 4 (June 2009): 293–99, https://doi.org/10.1159/000216540.

117 **"stress inoculation":** Russo et al., "Neurobiology of Resilience."

117 **we each react differently to the *same*:** Sapolsky, "Stress and the Brain."

118 **A higher HRV:** Janice K. Kiecolt-Glaser et al., "Stress Reactivity: What Pushes Us Higher, Faster, and Longer—and Why It Matters," *Current Directions in Psychological Science* 29, no. 5 (October 1, 2020): 492–98, https://doi.org/10.1177/0963721420949521.

119 **During this period, purposeful rumination:** Anna S. Ord et al., "Stress-Related Growth: Building a More Resilient Brain," *Journal of Neuropsychiatry and Clinical Neurosciences* 32, no. 3 (July 2020): A4-212, https://doi.org/10.1176/appi.neuropsych.20050111.

Chapter 9: The Hallmarks of Aging: When Good Cells Go Bad

123 **"successful aging":** John W. Rowe and Dawn C. Carr, "Successful Aging: History and Prospects," in *Oxford Research Encyclopedia of Psychology*, 2018, https://doi.org/10.1093/acrefore/9780190236557.013.342.

123 **Baltimore Longitudinal Study on Aging:** "About the Baltimore Longitudinal Study of Aging," National Institute on Aging, accessed April 21, 2024, https://www.nia.nih.gov/research/labs/blsa/about.

123 **the Blue Zones:** Dan Buettner, "Micro Nudges: A Systems Approach to Health," *American Journal of Health Promotion* 35, no. 4 (May 1, 2021): 593–96, https://doi.org/10.1177/08901171211002328d.

123 **"hallmarks of aging":** Carlos López-Otín et al., "The Hallmarks of Aging," *Cell* 153, no. 6 (June 6, 2013): 1194–1217, https://doi.org/10.1016/j.cell.2013.05.039.

124 **connection between our aging biology and our stress biology:** Elissa S. Epel and Gordon J. Lithgow, "Stress Biology and Aging Mechanisms: Toward Understanding the Deep Connection Between Adaptation to Stress and Longevity," *Journals of Gerontology Series A, Biological Sciences and Medical Sciences* 69 Suppl. 1 (June 1, 2014): S10-6, https://doi.org/10.1093/gerona/glu055.

124 **A landmark study on Danish twins:** A. M. Herskind et al., "The Heritability of Human Longevity: A Population-Based Study of 2872 Danish Twin Pairs Born 1870-1900," *Human Genetics* 97, no. 3 (March 1996): 319–23, https://doi.org/10.1007/BF02185763.

124 **The average life expectancy in the United States:** "Life Expectancy in the U.S. Dropped for the Second Year in a Row in 2021," August 31, 2022, https://www.cdc.gov/nchs/pressroom/nchs_press_releases/2022/20220831.htm.

125 **The concept of "compression of morbidity":** James F. Fries, "Aging, Natural Death, and the Compression of Morbidity," *New England Journal of Medicine* 303, no. 3 (July 17, 1980): 130–35, https://doi.org/10.1056/NEJM198007173030304.

126 **Hormesis is a holistic process:** Suresh I. S. Rattan, "Hormesis in Aging," *Ageing Research Reviews*, Hormesis, 7, no. 1 (January 1, 2008): 63–78, https://doi.org/10.1016/j.arr.2007.03.002.

126 **the stress we experience and how we age:** Elissa S. Epel, "The Geroscience Agenda: Toxic Stress, Hormetic Stress, and the Rate of Aging," *Ageing Research Reviews* 63 (November 1, 2020): 101167, https://doi.org/10.1016/j.arr.2020.101167.

126 **our most effective natural antiaging strategies:** Aurelia Santoro et al., "Inflammaging, Hormesis and the Rationale for Anti-Aging Strategies," *Ageing Research Reviews* 64 (December 1, 2020): 101142, https://doi.org/10.1016/j.arr.2020.101142.

127 **gut dysbiosis and inflammation were added:** Tomas Schmauck-Medina et al., "New Hallmarks of Ageing: A 2022 Copenhagen Ageing Meeting Summary," *Aging* 14, no. 16 (August 29, 2022): 6829–39, https://doi.org/10.18632/aging.204248.

128 **phytochemicals have been found to delay seven:** Anna Leonov et al., "Longevity Extension by Phytochemicals," *Molecules* 20, no. 4 (April 13, 2015): 6544–72, https://doi.org/10.3390/molecules20046544.

128   **regular chili pepper consumers:** Marialaura Bonaccio et al., "Chili Pepper Consumption and Mortality in Italian Adults," *Journal of the American College of Cardiology* 74, no. 25 (December 2019): 3139–49, https://doi.org/10.1016/j.jacc.2019.09.068.

128   **Similarly, a United States study:** Mustafa Chopan and Benjamin Littenberg, "The Association of Hot Red Chili Pepper Consumption and Mortality: A Large Population-Based Cohort Study," *PloS One* 12, no. 1 (2017): e0169876, https://doi.org/10.1371/journal.pone.0169876.

128   **combat the buildup of senescent cells:** Matthew J. Yousefzadeh et al., "Fisetin Is a Senotherapeutic That Extends Health and Lifespan," *EBioMedicine* 36 (October 2018): 18–28, https://doi.org/10.1016/j.ebiom.2018.09.015.

128   **Pomegranate contains another:** Jie Shen et al., "Dietary Phytochemicals That Can Extend Longevity by Regulation of Metabolism," *Plant Foods for Human Nutrition* 77, no. 1 (March 1, 2022): 12–19, https://doi.org/10.1007/s11130-021-00946-z.

128   **urolithin A enhanced mitochondrial health:** Pénélope A. Andreux et al., "The Mitophagy Activator Urolithin A Is Safe and Induces a Molecular Signature of Improved Mitochondrial and Cellular Health in Humans," *Nature Metabolism* 1, no. 6 (June 2019): 595–603, https://doi.org/10.1038/s42255-019-0073-4.

129   **The primary reason exercise is so effective:** Nuria Garatachea et al., "Exercise Attenuates the Major Hallmarks of Aging," *Rejuvenation Research* 18, no. 1 (February 1, 2015): 57–89, https://doi.org/10.1089/rej.2014.1623.

129   **exercise and telomere length:** Larry A. Tucker, "Physical Activity and Telomere Length in U.S. Men and Women: An NHANES Investigation," *Preventive Medicine* 100 (July 2017): 145–51, https://doi.org/10.1016/j.ypmed.2017.04.027.

129   **our natural, stem cell-based, regenerative capacity:** Chang Liu et al., "Exercise Promotes Tissue Regeneration: Mechanisms Involved and Therapeutic Scope," *Sports Medicine - Open* 9, no. 1 (May 6, 2023): 27, https://doi.org/10.1186/s40798-023-00573-9.

130   **to activate the heat shock protein response:** Patrick and Johnson, "Sauna Use as a Lifestyle Practice to Extend Healthspan."

130   **These proteins activate the proteasome:** Hyun Ju Lee et al., "Cold Temperature Extends Longevity and Prevents Disease-Related Protein Aggregation Through PA28γ-Induced Proteasomes," *Nature Aging* 3, no. 5 (May 2023): 546–66, https://doi.org/10.1038/s43587-023-00383-4.

130   **Guinness World Record:** "Most Saunas per Capita," Guinness World Records, July 1, 2013, https://www.guinnessworldrecords.com/world-records/111853-most-saunas-per-capita.

130   **men who used the sauna:** Tanjaniina Laukkanen et al., "Association Between Sauna Bathing and Fatal Cardiovascular and All-Cause Mortality Events," *JAMA Internal Medicine* 175, no. 4 (April 1, 2015): 542–48, https://doi.org/10.1001/jamainternmed.2014.8187.

131   **In the 1930s, nutrition researcher Clive McCay:** Roger B. McDonald and Jon J. Ramsey, "Honoring Clive McCay and 75 Years of Calorie Restriction Research," *Journal of Nutrition* 140, no. 7 (July 1, 2010): 1205–10, https://doi.org/10.3945/jn.110.122804.

131   **Studies consistently showed that starving:** Luigi Fontana, Linda Partridge, and Valter D. Longo, "Dietary Restriction, Growth Factors and Aging: From Yeast to Humans," *Science* 328, no. 5976 (April 16, 2010): 321–26, https://doi.org/10.1126/science.1172539.

131   **these animals also became more susceptible:** Longo et al., "Intermittent and Periodic Fasting, Longevity and Disease."

131   **Certain genetic modifications in these pathways:** Fontana, Partridge, and Longo, "Dietary Restriction, Growth Factors and Aging."

132   **intermittent fasting improves healthspan:** de Cabo and Mattson, "Effects of Intermittent Fasting on Health, Aging, and Disease."

132   **presents a unique benefit:** Longo et al., "Intermittent and Periodic Fasting, Longevity and Disease."

133   **key hallmarks connecting psychological stress and aging:** Martin Picard and Bruce S. McEwen, "Psychological Stress and Mitochondria: A Conceptual Framework," *Psychosomatic Medicine* 80, no. 2 (2018): 126–40, https://doi.org/10.1097/PSY.0000000000000544.

133 **A study on the influence of caregiving stress:** Martin Picard et al., "A Mitochondrial Health Index Sensitive to Mood and Caregiving Stress," *Biological Psychiatry* 84, no. 1 (July 1, 2018): 9–17, https://doi.org/10.1016/j.biopsych.2018.01.012.

133 **A groundbreaking study found:** Elissa S. Epel et al., "Accelerated Telomere Shortening in Response to Life Stress," *Proceedings of the National Academy of Sciences* 101, no. 49 (December 7, 2004): 17312–15, https://doi.org/10.1073/pnas.0407162101.

134 **perceived stress is hormetically associated with biological aging:** Sharon H. Bergquist et al., "Hormetic Association Between Perceived Stress and Human Epigenetic Aging Based on Resilience Capacity," *Biogerontology* 23, no. 5 (October 2022): 615–27, https://doi.org/10.1007/s10522-022-09985-8.

Chapter 10: Turning Bad Cells to Good: New Ways to Combat the Most Common Killers

136 **overloading your body's fat storage capacity:** Jakub Gołacki, Małgorzata Matuszek, and Beata Matyjaszek-Matuszek, "Link Between Insulin Resistance and Obesity—From Diagnosis to Treatment," *Diagnostics* 12, no. 7 (July 10, 2022): 1681, https://doi.org/10.3390/diagnostics12071681.

136 **nearly half of young adults with insulin resistance:** Vibhu Parcha et al., "Insulin Resistance and Cardiometabolic Risk Profile Among Nondiabetic American Young Adults: Insights from NHANES," *Journal of Clinical Endocrinology & Metabolism* 107, no. 1 (January 1, 2022): e25–37, https://doi.org/10.1210/clinem/dgab645.

137 **Breaking down excess fat:** Michael Albosta and Jesse Bakke, "Intermittent Fasting: Is There a Role in the Treatment of Diabetes? A Review of the Literature and Guide for Primary Care Physicians," *Clinical Diabetes and Endocrinology* 7 (February 3, 2021): 3, https://doi.org/10.1186/s40842-020-00116-1.

137 **triggers adaptations in hormones:** Albosta and Bakke.

137 **In one twelve-month study:** Kelsey Gabel et al., "Differential Effects of Alternate Day Fasting Versus Daily Calorie Restriction on Insulin Resistance," *Obesity (Silver Spring, Md.)* 27, no. 9 (September 2019): 1443–50, https://doi.org/10.1002/oby.22564.

138 **just one forty-five-minute session:** Rasmus Rabøl et al., "Reversal of Muscle Insulin Resistance with Exercise Reduces Postprandial Hepatic de Novo Lipogenesis in Insulin Resistant Individuals," *Proceedings of the National Academy of Sciences* 108, no. 33 (August 16, 2011): 13705–9, https://doi.org/10.1073/pnas.1110105108.

138 **Exercise disrupts this harmful loop:** Huiyun Liang and Walter F. Ward, "PGC-1α: A Key Regulator of Energy Metabolism," *Advances in Physiology Education* 30, no. 4 (December 2006): 145–51, https://doi.org/10.1152/advan.00052.2006.

138 **living in a mildly cold environment:** Paul Lee et al., "Temperature-Acclimated Brown Adipose Tissue Modulates Insulin Sensitivity in Humans," *Diabetes* 63, no. 11 (October 13, 2014): 3686–98, https://doi.org/10.2337/db14-0513.

139 **Similarly, heat therapy:** Ely et al., "Meta-Inflammation and Cardiometabolic Disease in Obesity."

139 **Plant phytochemicals improve metabolic health:** Manuela Leri et al., "Healthy Effects of Plant Polyphenols: Molecular Mechanisms," *International Journal of Molecular Sciences* 21, no. 4 (February 13, 2020): 1250, https://doi.org/10.3390/ijms21041250.

139 **the metabolic effects of psychological stress are different:** Cristina Rabasa and Suzanne L. Dickson, "Impact of Stress on Metabolism and Energy Balance," *Current Opinion in Behavioral Sciences*, Diet, Behavior and Brain Function, 9 (June 1, 2016): 71–77, https://doi.org/10.1016/j.cobeha.2016.01.011.

140 **the endothelium is an organ:** Flammer and Lüscher, "Three Decades of Endothelium Research."

140 **Intermittent fasting can help reduce the risk factors:** Bartosz Malinowski et al., "Intermittent Fasting in Cardiovascular Disorders—An Overview," *Nutrients* 11, no. 3 (March 20, 2019): 673, https://doi.org/10.3390/nu11030673.

140 **increased the production of nitric oxide:** B. Yousefi et al., "The Effects of Ramadan Fasting on Endothelial Function in Patients with Cardiovascular Diseases," *European Journal of Clinical Nutrition* 68, no. 7 (July 2014): 835–39, https://doi.org/10.1038/ejcn.2014.61.

141 **reflected in lower levels of inflammatory markers:** Malinowski et al., "Intermittent Fasting in Cardiovascular Disorders—An Overview."

141 **reduces oxidative stress:** Varady et al., "Clinical Application of Intermittent Fasting for Weight Loss."

141 **Moreover, intermittent fasting helps prevent:** Malinowski et al., "Intermittent Fasting in Cardiovascular Disorders—An Overview."

141 **heart and blood vessels adapt to cycles of exercise:** Matthew A. Nystoriak and Aruni Bhatnagar, "Cardiovascular Effects and Benefits of Exercise," *Frontiers in Cardiovascular Medicine* 5 (September 28, 2018): 135, https://doi.org/10.3389/fcvm.2018.00135.

141 **shear stress:** Samuel R. C. Weaver et al., "Non-Pharmacological Interventions for Vascular Health and the Role of the Endothelium," *European Journal of Applied Physiology* 122, no. 12 (2022): 2493–2514, https://doi.org/10.1007/s00421-022-05041-y.

141 **increase in endothelial progenitor cells:** Panagiotis Ferentinos et al., "The Impact of Different Forms of Exercise on Endothelial Progenitor Cells in Healthy Populations," *European Journal of Applied Physiology* 122, no. 7 (2022): 1589–1625, https://doi.org/10.1007/s00421-022-04921-7.

142 **Flavonoids, including quercetin, EGCG:** Amy Rees, Georgina F. Dodd, and Jeremy P. E. Spencer, "The Effects of Flavonoids on Cardiovascular Health: A Review of Human Intervention Trials and Implications for Cerebrovascular Function," *Nutrients* 10, no. 12 (December 1, 2018): 1852, https://doi.org/10.3390/nu10121852.

142 **treat cardiovascular disease by scavenging:** Rakesh Kumar Bachheti et al., "Prevention and Treatment of Cardiovascular Diseases with Plant Phytochemicals: A Review," *Evidence-Based Complementary and Alternative Medicine : eCAM* 2022 (July 4, 2022): 5741198, https://doi.org/10.1155/2022/5741198.

142 **Allicin:** Bachheti et al.

142 **Curcumin, found in turmeric, reduces blood pressure:** Bachheti et al.

142 **Kuopio Ischemic Heart Disease Risk Factor (KIHD) Study:** Laukkanen et al., "Association Between Sauna Bathing and Fatal Cardiovascular and All-Cause Mortality Events."

142 **Regular sauna use can decrease:** Brunt and Minson, "Heat Therapy."

143 **resilience is a strong protector:** Sharon H. Bergquist et al., "Hair Cortisol, Perceived Stress, and Resilience as Predictors of Coronary Arterial Disease," *Stress and Health: Journal of the International Society for the Investigation of Stress* 38, no. 3 (August 2022): 453–62, https://doi.org/10.1002/smi.3106.

143 **positive psychological well-being:** Julia K. Boehm and Laura D. Kubzansky, "The Heart's Content: The Association Between Positive Psychological Well-Being and Cardiovascular Health," *Psychological Bulletin* 138, no. 4 (July 2012): 655–91, https://doi.org/10.1037/a0027448.

143 **These natural opioids help improve:** Noboru Toda and Megumi Nakanishi-Toda, "How Mental Stress Affects Endothelial Function," *Pflügers Archiv—European Journal of Physiology* 462, no. 6 (December 1, 2011): 779–94, https://doi.org/10.1007/s00424-011-1022-6.

143 **Nearly two million cases:** "Cancer Statistics—NCI," cgvArticle, April 2, 2015, https://www.cancer.gov/about-cancer/understanding/statistics.

143 **lifestyle choices impact our cancer risk:** P. Lichtenstein et al., "Environmental and Heritable Factors in the Causation of Cancer—Analyses of Cohorts of Twins from Sweden, Denmark, and Finland," *The New England Journal of Medicine* 343, no. 2 (July 13, 2000): 78–85, https://doi.org/10.1056/NEJM200007133430201.

143 **lifestyle choices impact our cancer risk:** Farhad Islami et al., "Proportion and Number of Cancer Cases and Deaths Attributable to Potentially Modifiable Risk Factors in the United States," *CA: A Cancer Journal for Clinicians* 68, no. 1 (January 2018): 31–54, https://doi.org/10.3322/caac.21440.

144 **reprogram their metabolism to use a unique energy system:** Faiza Kalam et al., "Intermittent Fasting Interventions to Leverage Metabolic and Circadian Mechanisms for Cancer Treatment and Supportive Care Outcomes," *JNCI Monographs* 2023, no. 61 (June 1, 2023): 84–103, https://doi.org/10.1093/jncimonographs/lgad008.

144 **women who fasted less than thirteen hours:** Catherine R. Marinac et al., "Prolonged Nightly Fasting and Breast Cancer Prognosis," *JAMA Oncology* 2, no. 8 (August 1, 2016): 1049–55, https://doi.org/10.1001/jamaoncol.2016.0164.

145 **Meal timing:** Bernard Srour et al., "Circadian Nutritional Behaviours and Cancer Risk: New Insights from the NutriNet-Santé Prospective Cohort Study: Disclaimers," *International Journal of Cancer* 143, no. 10 (November 15, 2018): 2369–79, https://doi.org/10.1002/ijc.31584.

145 **as a probable carcinogen:** *IARC Monographs* Volume 124: Night Shift Work," June 2, 2020, https://www.iarc.who.int/news-events/iarc-monographs-volume-124-night-shift-work.

145 **So during exercise, they have to compete:** Pernille Hojman et al., "Molecular Mechanisms Linking Exercise to Cancer Prevention and Treatment," *Cell Metabolism* 27, no. 1 (January 9, 2018): 10–21, https://doi.org/10.1016/j.cmet.2017.09.015.

145 **Exercise can also activate immune system cells:** Hojman et al.

145 **A 2023 study on newly diagnosed breast cancer:** Tiia Koivula et al., "The Effect of Acute Exercise on Circulating Immune Cells in Newly Diagnosed Breast Cancer Patients," *Scientific Reports* 13, no. 1 (April 21, 2023): 6561, https://doi.org/10.1038/s41598-023-33432-4.

145 **The unique glucose-using metabolism:** Casanova et al., "Mitochondria."

145 **making cancer cells more "visible":** Hojman et al., "Molecular Mechanisms Linking Exercise to Cancer Prevention and Treatment."

146 **more than one thousand phytochemicals:** Young-Joon Surh, "Cancer Chemoprevention with Dietary Phytochemicals," *Nature Reviews Cancer* 3, no. 10 (December 2003): 768–80, https://doi.org/10.1038/nrc1189.

146 **phytochemicals can intervene at each stage:** Surh.

146 **phytochemicals can intervene at each stage:** Anna Rudzińska et al., "Phytochemicals in Cancer Treatment and Cancer Prevention—Review on Epidemiological Data and Clinical Trials," *Nutrients* 15, no. 8 (April 14, 2023): 1896, https://doi.org/10.3390/nu15081896.

146 **More than 250 population-based studies:** Surh, "Cancer Chemoprevention with Dietary Phytochemicals."

146 **Improving your ability to cope:** Bonnie A. McGregor and Michael H. Antoni, "Psychological Intervention and Health Outcomes Among Women Treated for Breast Cancer: A Review of Stress Pathways and Biological Mediators," *Brain, Behavior, and Immunity* 23, no. 2 (February 2009): 159–66, https://doi.org/10.1016/j.bbi.2008.08.002.

146 **unlike consuming a Western diet, is linked to increased psychological resilience:** M. Bonaccio et al., "Mediterranean-Type Diet Is Associated with Higher Psychological Resilience in a General Adult Population: Findings from the Moli-Sani Study," *European Journal of Clinical Nutrition* 72, no. 1 (January 2018): 154–60, https://doi.org/10.1038/ejcn.2017.150.

146 **cold exposure could markedly hinder:** Takahiro Seki et al., "Brown-Fat-Mediated Tumour Suppression by Cold-Altered Global Metabolism," *Nature* 608, no. 7922 (August 2022): 421–28, https://doi.org/10.1038/s41586-022-05030-3.

147 **The human brain has eighty-six billion:** Michael J. Caire, Vamsi Reddy, and Matthew Varacallo, "Physiology, Synapse," in *StatPearls* (Treasure Island, FL: StatPearls Publishing, 2023), http://www.ncbi.nlm.nih.gov/books/NBK526047/.

147 **Conditions like insulin resistance:** Olivia Sheppard and Michael Coleman, "Alzheimer's Disease: Etiology, Neuropathology and Pathogenesis," in *Alzheimer's Disease: Drug Discovery*, ed. Xudong Huang (Brisbane, Australia: Exon Publications, 2020), http://www.ncbi.nlm.nih.gov/books/NBK566126/.

147 **they make neurons more resistant to cellular injury:** Mark P. Mattson, "Lifelong Brain Health Is a Lifelong Challenge: From Evolutionary Principles to Empirical Evidence," *Ageing Research Reviews* 0 (March 2015): 37–45, https://doi.org/10.1016/j.arr.2014.12.011.

148 **up to a third of people who have a high amount:** Teresa Gómez-Isla and Matthew P. Frosch, "Lesions Without Symptoms: Understanding Resilience to Alzheimer Disease Neuropathological Changes," *Nature Reviews Neurology* 18, no. 6 (June 2022): 323–32, https://doi.org/10.1038/s41582-022-00642-9.

148 **Such activities help build a buffer:** Mattson, "Lifelong Brain Health Is a Lifelong Challenge."

148 **cognitive reserve reduced the risk:** Michael J. Valenzuela and Perminder Sachdev, "Brain Reserve and Dementia: A Systematic Review," *Psychological Medicine* 36, no. 4 (April 2006): 441–54, https://doi.org/10.1017/S0033291705006264.

149 **whether a person had a purpose in life:** Aliza P. Wingo et al., "Purpose in Life Is a Robust Protective Factor of Reported Cognitive Decline Among Late Middle-Aged Adults: The Emory Healthy Aging Study," *Journal of Affective Disorders* 263 (February 15, 2020): 310–17, https://doi.org/10.1016/j.jad.2019.11.124.

149 **Glucose is delivered to the brain:** Aleksandra Kaliszewska et al., "The Interaction of Diet and Mitochondrial Dysfunction in Aging and Cognition," *International Journal of Molecular Sciences* 22, no. 7 (March 30, 2021): 3574, https://doi.org/10.3390/ijms22073574.

149 **Besides serving as an energy source:** Nicole Jacqueline Jensen et al., "Effects of Ketone Bodies on Brain Metabolism and Function in Neurodegenerative Diseases," *International Journal of Molecular Sciences* 21, no. 22 (November 20, 2020): 8767, https://doi.org/10.3390/ijms21228767.

149 **Fasting also upregulates brain growth factors:** Mark P. Mattson et al., "Intermittent Metabolic Switching, Neuroplasticity and Brain Health," *Nature Reviews Neuroscience* 19, no. 2 (February 2018): 63–80, https://doi.org/10.1038/nrn.2017.156.

149 **In a 2018 study, Martha Clare Morris:** Martha Clare Morris et al., "Nutrients and Bioactives in Green Leafy Vegetables and Cognitive Decline," *Neurology* 90, no. 3 (January 16, 2018): e214–22, https://doi.org/10.1212/WNL.0000000000004815.

150 **Berries, particularly blueberries:** Anna Laura Cremonini et al., "Nutrients in the Prevention of Alzheimer's Disease," *Oxidative Medicine and Cellular Longevity* 2019 (2019): 9874159, https://doi.org/10.1155/2019/9874159.

150 **Other phytochemicals, such as sulforaphane:** Cremonini et al.

150 **Other phytochemicals, such as sulforaphane:** Eric A. Klomparens and Yuchuan Ding, "The Neuroprotective Mechanisms and Effects of Sulforaphane," *Brain Circulation* 5, no. 2 (2019): 74–83, https://doi.org/10.4103/bc.bc_7_19.

150 **brain's production of brain-derived neurotrophic factor:** Peter Rasmussen et al., "Evidence for a Release of Brain-Derived Neurotrophic Factor from the Brain During Exercise," *Experimental Physiology* 94, no. 10 (2009): 1062–69, https://doi.org/10.1113/expphysiol.2009.048512.

150 **While aerobic workouts:** Adrian De la Rosa et al., "Physical Exercise in the Prevention and Treatment of Alzheimer's Disease," *Journal of Sport and Health Science* 9, no. 5 (September 2020): 394–404, https://doi.org/10.1016/j.jshs.2020.01.004.

150 **While aerobic workouts:** Jane Alty, Maree Farrow, and Katherine Lawler, "Exercise and Dementia Prevention," *Practical Neurology* 20, no. 3 (May 2020): 234–40, https://doi.org/10.1136/practneurol-2019-002335.

150 **those with the highest level of exercise:** M. Hamer and Y. Chida, "Physical Activity and Risk of Neurodegenerative Disease: A Systematic Review of Prospective Evidence," *Psychological Medicine* 39, no. 1 (January 2009): 3–11, https://doi.org/10.1017/S0033291708003681.

150 **adults with mild cognitive impairment:** De la Rosa et al., "Physical Exercise in the Prevention and Treatment of Alzheimer's Disease."

150 **and Alzheimer's dementia:** Rui-Xia Jia et al., "Effects of Physical Activity and Exercise on the Cognitive Function of Patients with Alzheimer's Disease: A Meta-Analysis," *BMC Geriatrics* 19, no. 1 (July 2, 2019): 181, https://doi.org/10.1186/s12877-019-1175-2.

151 **Using a dry sauna:** Tanjaniina Laukkanen et al., "Sauna Bathing Is Inversely Associated with Dementia and Alzheimer's Disease in Middle-Aged Finnish Men," *Age and Ageing* 46, no. 2 (March 1, 2017): 245–49, https://doi.org/10.1093/ageing/afw212.

151 **Heat shock proteins act like helpers:** Andrew P. Hunt et al., "Could Heat Therapy Be an Effective Treatment for Alzheimer's and Parkinson's Diseases? A Narrative Review," *Frontiers in Physiology* 10 (2019): 1556, https://doi.org/10.3389/fphys.2019.01556.

151 **Heat therapy also:** Sven P. Hoekstra, Nicolette C. Bishop, and Christof A. Leicht, "Elevating Body Temperature to Reduce Low-Grade Inflammation: A Welcome Strategy for Those Unable to Exercise?," *Exercise Immunology Review* 26 (2020): 42–55.

Chapter 11: Living in Balance: The Cellular Connection to a Better Life

154 **The first endocannabinoid discovered:** William A. Devane et al., "Isolation and Structure of a Brain Constituent That Binds to the Cannabinoid Receptor," *Science* 258, no. 5090 (December 18, 1992): 1946–50.

154 **Cannabinoid receptors are on cells:** Daniela Matei et al., "The Endocannabinoid System and Physical Exercise," *International Journal of Molecular Sciences* 24, no. 3 (January 19, 2023): 1989, https://doi.org/10.3390/ijms24031989.

154 **lessen the effects of autoimmune conditions:** Venkatesh L. Hegde et al., "Attenuation of Experimental Autoimmune Hepatitis by Exogenous and Endogenous Cannabinoids: Involvement of Regulatory T Cells," *Molecular Pharmacology* 74, no. 1 (July 1, 2008): 20–33, https://doi.org/10.1124/mol.108.047035.

154 **adjust intestinal inflammation, motility, and pain:** K. L. Wright, M. Duncan, and K. A. Sharkey, "Cannabinoid CB2 Receptors in the Gastrointestinal Tract: A Regulatory System in States of Inflammation," *British Journal of Pharmacology* 153, no. 2 (2008): 263–70, https://doi.org/10.1038/sj.bjp.0707486.

154 **The endocannabinoid system has likely evolved:** Amit Kumar et al., "Cannabimimetic Plants: Are They New Cannabinoidergic Modulators?," *Planta* 249, no. 6 (June 2019): 1681–94, https://doi.org/10.1007/s00425-019-03138-x.

154 **For example, chronic pain conditions:** Ethan B. Russo, "Clinical Endocannabinoid Deficiency Reconsidered: Current Research Supports the Theory in Migraine, Fibromyalgia, Irritable Bowel, and Other Treatment-Resistant Syndromes," *Cannabis and Cannabinoid Research* 1, no. 1 (July 1, 2016): 154–65, https://doi.org/10.1089/can.2016.0009.

154 **researchers found that his Wim Hof Method:** Otto Muzik, Kaice T. Reilly, and Vaibhav A. Diwadkar, "'Brain over Body'-A Study on the Willful Regulation of Autonomic Function During Cold Exposure," *NeuroImage* 172 (May 15, 2018): 632–41, https://doi.org/10.1016/j.neuroimage.2018.01.067.

155 **role in the good feeling and reduced anxiety:** Otto Muzik and Vaibhav A. Diwadkar, "Hierarchical Control Systems for the Regulation of Physiological Homeostasis and Affect: Can Their Interactions Modulate Mood and Anhedonia?," *Neuroscience and Biobehavioral Reviews* 105 (October 2019): 251–61, https://doi.org/10.1016/j.neubiorev.2019.08.015.

155 **cold exposure increases endocannabinoid levels:** Lucia M. Krott et al., "Endocannabinoid Regulation in White and Brown Adipose Tissue Following Thermogenic Activation," *Journal of Lipid Research* 57, no. 3 (March 1, 2016): 464–73, https://doi.org/10.1194/jlr.M065227.

155 **and the density of CB1 receptors:** E. Dzhambazova et al., "Increase in the Number of Cb1 Immunopositive Neurons in the Amygdaloid Body After Acute Cold Stress Exposure," 2014, https://www.semanticscholar.org/paper/INCREASE-IN-THE-NUMBER-OF-CB1-IMMUNOPOSITIVE-IN-THE-Dzhambazova-Landzhov/cf7b55c59d962a1077fcb621c1c09928626609b4.

155 **called cannabimimetics:** Kumar et al., "Cannabimimetic Plants."

156 **Curcumin, resveratrol:** Kumar et al.

156 **Curcumin, resveratrol:** Jürg Gertsch, Roger G. Pertwee, and Vincenzo Di Marzo, "Phytocannabinoids Beyond the Cannabis Plant—Do They Exist?," *British Journal of Pharmacology* 160, no. 3 (June 2010): 523–29, https://doi.org/10.1111/j.1476-5381.2010.00745.x.

156 **Genistein inhibits the enzyme:** Gertsch, Pertwee, and Di Marzo.

156 **dark chocolate and cocoa powder:** Emmanuelle di Tomaso, Massimiliano Beltramo, and Daniele Piomelli, "Brain Cannabinoids in Chocolate," *Nature* 382, no. 6593 (August 1, 1996): 677–78, https://doi.org/10.1038/382677a0.

156 **The sweet spot:** Matei et al., "The Endocannabinoid System and Physical Exercise."

156 **short-term "circuit breakers":** Matei et al.

157 **We now know that endocannabinoids:** Matei et al.

157 **Short-term good stress:** Cecilia J. Hillard, "Stress Regulates Endocannabinoid-CB1 Receptor Signaling," *Seminars in Immunology* 26, no. 5 (October 2014): 380–88, https://doi.org/10.1016/j.smim.2014.04.001.

157 **In other words, the stress-endocannabinoid connection:** Maria Morena et al., "Neurobiological Interactions Between Stress and the Endocannabinoid System," *Neuropsychopharmacology* 41, no. 1 (January 2016): 80–102, https://doi.org/10.1038/npp.2015.166.

158 **how fasting affects the endocannabinoid system:** Tim C. Kirkham et al., "Endocannabinoid Levels in Rat Limbic Forebrain and Hypothalamus in Relation to Fasting, Feeding and Satiation: Stimulation of Eating by 2-Arachidonoyl Glycerol," *British Journal of Pharmacology* 136, no. 4 (June 2002): 550–57, https://doi.org/10.1038/sj.bjp.0704767.

158 **made from polyunsaturated fatty acids:** Yongsoon Park and Bruce A. Watkins, "Dietary PUFAs and Exercise Dynamic Actions on Endocannabinoids in Brain: Consequences for Neural Plasticity and Neuroinflammation," *Advances in Nutrition* 13, no. 5 (June 8, 2022): 1989–2001, https://doi.org/10.1093/advances/nmac064.

159 **Phytochemicals promote the growth:** Sarusha Santhiravel et al., "The Impact of Plant Phytochemicals on the Gut Microbiota of Humans for a Balanced Life," *International Journal of Molecular Sciences* 23, no. 15 (July 23, 2022): 8124, https://doi.org/10.3390/ijms23158124.

159 **A 2018 study found this amount of exercise:** Jacob M. Allen et al., "Exercise Alters Gut Microbiota Composition and Function in Lean and Obese Humans," *Medicine & Science in Sports & Exercise* 50, no. 4 (April 2018): 747, https://doi.org/10.1249/MSS.0000000000001495.

160 **Athletes have more beneficial bacteria:** Alex E. Mohr et al., "The Athletic Gut Microbiota," *Journal of the International Society of Sports Nutrition* 17, no. 1 (May 12, 2020): 24, https://doi.org/10.1186/s12970-020-00353-w.

160 **Cardiorespiratory fitness (VO$_2$ max) can account:** Ryan P. Durk et al., "Gut Microbiota Composition Is Related to Cardiorespiratory Fitness in Healthy Young Adults," *International Journal of Sport Nutrition and Exercise Metabolism* 29, no. 3 (May 1, 2019): 249–53, https://doi.org/10.1123/ijsnem.2018-0024.

160 **excessive or prolonged high-intensity exercise:** Mohr et al., "The Athletic Gut Microbiota."

160 **healthy men who followed a sixteen-hour fasting:** Falak Zeb et al., "Effect of Time-Restricted Feeding on Metabolic Risk and Circadian Rhythm Associated with Gut Microbiome in Healthy Males," *British Journal of Nutrition* 123, no. 11 (June 2020): 1216–26, https://doi.org/10.1017/S0007114519003428.

160 **Other studies link intermittent fasting:** Junhong Su et al., "Remodeling of the Gut Microbiome During Ramadan-Associated Intermittent Fasting," *American Journal of Clinical Nutrition* 113, no. 5 (May 8, 2021): 1332–42, https://doi.org/10.1093/ajcn/nqaa388.

160 **Furthermore, by improving the gut microbial ecosystem:** Ruth E. Patterson and Dorothy D. Sears, "Metabolic Effects of Intermittent Fasting," *Annual Review of Nutrition* 37, no. 1 (2017): 371–93, https://doi.org/10.1146/annurev-nutr-071816-064634.

160 **gut bacteria are a common pathway:** Bohan Rong et al., "Gut Microbiota—a Positive Contributor in the Process of Intermittent Fasting-Mediated Obesity Control," *Animal Nutrition* 7, no. 4 (December 1, 2021): 1283–95, https://doi.org/10.1016/j.aninu.2021.09.009.

160 **the migrating motor complex:** Eveline Deloose et al., "The Migrating Motor Complex: Control Mechanisms and Its Role in Health and Disease," *Nature Reviews Gastroenterology & Hepatology* 9, no. 5 (March 27, 2012): 271–85, https://doi.org/10.1038/nrgastro.2012.57.

161 **The brain and gut are connected:** Jane A. Foster, Linda Rinaman, and John F. Cryan, "Stress & the Gut-Brain Axis: Regulation by the Microbiome," *Neurobiology of Stress* 7 (December 2017): 124–36, https://doi.org/10.1016/j.ynstr.2017.03.001.

161 **Psychological stress can change the composition:** Lu Ma et al., "Psychological Stress and Gut Microbiota Composition: A Systematic Review of Human Studies," *Neuropsychobiology* 82, no. 5 (September 6, 2023): 247–62, https://doi.org/10.1159/000533131.

161 **gut bacteria play an important role in thermogenesis:** Claire Chevalier et al., "Gut Microbiota Orchestrates Energy Homeostasis During Cold," *Cell* 163, no. 6 (December 3, 2015): 1360–74, https://doi.org/10.1016/j.cell.2015.11.004.

161 **Both heat and cold stress:** J. Philip Karl et al., "Effects of Psychological, Environmental and Physical Stressors on the Gut Microbiota," *Frontiers in Microbiology* 9 (2018), https://www.frontiersin.org/articles/10.3389/fmicb.2018.02013.

Chapter 12: Getting Out of Your Comfort Zone

166 **brief, simple, one-time "wise interventions":** Gregory M. Walton, "The New Science of Wise Psychological Interventions," *Current Directions in Psychological Science* 23, no. 1 (February 1, 2014): 73–82, https://doi.org/10.1177/0963721413512856.

166 **people with an internal locus of control:** Dusanee Kesavayuth, Dai Binh Tran, and Vasileios Zikos, "Locus of Control and Subjective Well-Being: Panel Evidence from Australia," *PLoS ONE* 17, no. 8 (August 31, 2022): e0272714, https://doi.org/10.1371/journal.pone.0272714.

166 **more likely to adopt healthier habits:** A. Steptoe and J. Wardle, "Locus of Control and Health Behaviour Revisited: A Multivariate Analysis of Young Adults from 18 Countries," *British Journal of Psychology (London, England: 1953)* 92, no. Pt. 4 (November 2001): 659–72, https://doi.org/10.1348/000712601162400.

166 **people with an external locus of control:** Henning Krampe et al., "Locus of Control Moderates the Association of COVID-19 Stress and General Mental Distress: Results of a Norwegian and a German-Speaking Cross-Sectional Survey," *BMC Psychiatry* 21, no. 1 (September 6, 2021): 437, https://doi.org/10.1186/s12888-021-03418-5.

167 **"narrative identity":** Dan P. McAdams and Kate C. McLean, "Narrative Identity," *Current Directions in Psychological Science* 22, no. 3 (January 1, 2013): 233–38, https://doi.org/10.1177/0963721413475622.

167 **This sense of empowerment:** Douglas J. R. Kerr, Frank P. Deane, and Trevor P. Crowe, "Narrative Identity Reconstruction as Adaptive Growth During Mental Health Recovery: A Narrative Coaching Boardgame Approach," *Frontiers in Psychology* 10 (2019): 994, https://doi.org/10.3389/fpsyg.2019.00994.

167 **one study had forty-seven adults write their life stories:** Jonathan M. Adler, "Living into the Story: Agency and Coherence in a Longitudinal Study of Narrative Identity Development and Mental Health over the Course of Psychotherapy," *Journal of Personality and Social Psychology* 102, no. 2 (February 2012): 367–89, https://doi.org/10.1037/a0025289.

170 **waist should be less than half your height:** Margaret Ashwell and Sigrid Gibson, "Waist-to-Height Ratio as an Indicator of 'Early Health Risk': Simpler and More Predictive Than Using a 'Matrix' Based on BMI and Waist Circumference," *BMJ Open* 6, no. 3 (March 14, 2016): e010159, https://doi.org/10.1136/bmjopen-2015-010159.

170 **those with muscle mass index:** Preethi Srikanthan and Arun S. Karlamangla, "Muscle Mass Index as a Predictor of Longevity in Older-Adults," *American Journal of Medicine* 127, no. 6 (June 2014): 547–53, https://doi.org/10.1016/j.amjmed.2014.02.007.

170 **top range in skeletal muscle mass percentage:** Ian Janssen et al., "Skeletal Muscle Mass and Distribution in 468 Men and Women Aged 18–88 Yr," *Journal of Applied Physiology* 89, no. 1 (July 2000): 81–88, https://doi.org/10.1152/jappl.2000.89.1.81.

170 **Grip strength:** Richard W. Bohannon, "Grip Strength: An Indispensable Biomarker for Older Adults," *Clinical Interventions in Aging* 14 (October 1, 2019): 1681–91, https://doi.org/10.2147/CIA.S194543.

170 **individuals with higher grip strength:** Antonio García-Hermoso et al., "Muscular Strength as a Predictor of All-Cause Mortality in an Apparently Healthy Population: A Systematic Review and Meta-Analysis of Data from Approximately 2 Million Men and Women," *Archives of Physical Medicine and Rehabilitation* 99, no. 10 (October 2018): 2100–2113.e5, https://doi.org/10.1016/j.apmr.2018.01.008.

171 **The Rockport Walk Test:** Laura Weiglein et al., "The 1-Mile Walk Test Is a Valid Predictor of VO_2 max and Is a Reliable Alternative Fitness Test to the 1.5-Mile Run in U.S. Air Force Males," *Military Medicine* 176, no. 6 (June 1, 2011): 669–73, https://doi.org/10.7205/MILMED-D-10-00444.

171 **Then use this formula:** Kyoung Kim et al., "Changes in Cardiopulmonary Function in Normal Adults After the Rockport 1 Mile Walking Test: A Preliminary Study," *Journal of Physical Therapy Science* 27, no. 8 (2015): 2559–61, https://doi.org/10.1589/jpts.27.2559.

171 **the Cooper 12-Minute Run Test:** Kenneth H. Cooper, "A Means of Assessing Maximal Oxygen Intake: Correlation Between Field and Treadmill Testing," *JAMA* 203, no. 3 (January 15, 1968): 201–4, https://doi.org/10.1001/jama.1968.03140030033008.

172 **substantially reduce cardiovascular disease risk:** Ross et al., "Importance of Assessing Cardiorespiratory Fitness in Clinical Practice."

172 **mortality by half:** Kyle Mandsager et al., "Association of Cardiorespiratory Fitness with Long-Term Mortality Among Adults Undergoing Exercise Treadmill Testing," *JAMA Network Open* 1, no. 6 (October 5, 2018): e183605, https://doi.org/10.1001/jamanetworkopen.2018.3605.

172 **A reliable way to check for insulin resistance:** Jakub Gołacki, Małgorzata Matuszek, and Beata Matyjaszek-Matuszek, "Link Between Insulin Resistance and Obesity—From Diagnosis to Treatment," *Diagnostics* 12, no. 7 (July 10, 2022): 1681, https://doi.org/10.3390/diagnostics12071681.

172 **This method correlates well:** D. R. Matthews et al., "Homeostasis Model Assessment: Insulin Resistance and Beta-Cell Function from Fasting Plasma Glucose and Insulin Concentrations in Man," *Diabetologia* 28, no. 7 (July 1985): 412–19, https://doi.org/10.1007/BF00280883.

173 **Calculating your triglyceride-to-HDL ratio:** Cosimo Giannini et al., "The Triglyceride-to-HDL Cholesterol Ratio: Association with Insulin Resistance in Obese Youths of Different Ethnic Backgrounds," *Diabetes Care* 34, no. 8 (August 2011): 1869–74, https://doi.org/10.2337/dc10-2234.

173 **strong predictor of cardiovascular disease:** Bizhong Che et al., "Triglyceride-Glucose Index and Triglyceride to High-Density Lipoprotein Cholesterol Ratio as Potential Cardiovascular Disease Risk Factors: An Analysis of UK Biobank Data," *Cardiovascular Diabetology* 22 (February 16, 2023): 34, https://doi.org/10.1186/s12933-023-01762-2.

174 **ApoB is a more accurate marker for cardiovascular risk:** Jennifer Behbodikhah et al., "Apolipoprotein B and Cardiovascular Disease: Biomarker and Potential Therapeutic Target," *Metabolites* 11, no. 10 (October 8, 2021): 690, https://doi.org/10.3390/metabo11100690.

175 **persistent low-grade inflammation:** Shari S. Bassuk, Nader Rifai, and Paul M. Ridker, "High-Sensitivity C-Reactive Protein: Clinical Importance," *Current Problems in Cardiology* 29, no. 8 (August 1, 2004): 439–93, https://doi.org/10.1016/j.cpcardiol.2004.03.004.

175 **ideally as close to 115/75:** Sarah Lewington et al., "Age-Specific Relevance of Usual Blood Pressure to Vascular Mortality: A Meta-Analysis of Individual Data for One Million Adults in 61 Prospective Studies," *Lancet (London, England)* 360, no. 9349 (December 14, 2002): 1903–13, https://doi.org/10.1016/s0140-6736(02)11911-8.

176 **Brief Resilient Coping Scale:** Vaughn G. Sinclair and Kenneth A. Wallston, "The Development and Psychometric Evaluation of the Brief Resilient Coping Scale," *Assessment* 11, no. 1 (March 2004): 94–101, https://doi.org/10.1177/1073191103258144.

179 **ApoB and lipid goals:** Charles R. Harper and Terry A. Jacobson, "Using Apolipoprotein B to Manage Dyslipidemic Patients: Time for a Change?," *Mayo Clinic Proceedings* 85, no. 5 (May 1, 2010): 440–45, https://doi.org/10.4065/mcp.2009.0517.

Chapter 13: The Stress Paradox Protocol

181 **a single biological stressor can improve functioning:** Edward J. Calabrese et al., "Estimating the Range of the Maximum Hormetic Stimulatory Response," *Environmental Research* 170 (March 2019): 337–43, https://doi.org/10.1016/j.envres.2018.12.020.

181 **repeated exposure to the same low-dose biological stress:** Calabrese et al.

193 **This protocol is based on a Japanese study:** M. Morikawa et al., "Physical Fitness and Indices of Lifestyle-Related Diseases Before and After Interval Walking Training in Middle-Aged and Older Males and Females," *British Journal of Sports Medicine* 45, no. 3 (March 2011): 216, https://doi.org/10.1136/bjsm.2009.064816.

195 **a 2008 study by the Norwegian University:** Arnt Erik Tjønna et al., "Aerobic Interval Training Versus Continuous Moderate Exercise as a Treatment for the Metabolic Syndrome: A Pilot Study," *Circulation* 118, no. 4 (July 22, 2008): 346–54, https://doi.org/10.1161/CIRCULATIONAHA.108.772822.

196 **Tabata protocol developed in the 1990s:** I. Tabata et al., "Effects of Moderate-Intensity Endurance and High-Intensity Intermittent Training on Anaerobic Capacity and VO_{2max}," *Medicine and Science in Sports and Exercise* 28, no. 10 (October 1996): 1327–30, https://doi.org/10.1097/00005768-199610000-00018.

197 **cold water immersion immediately after high-intensity exercise:** Emma Moore et al., "Impact of Cold-Water Immersion Compared with Passive Recovery Following a Single Bout of Strenuous Exercise on Athletic Performance in Physically Active Participants: A Systematic Review with Meta-Analysis and Meta-Regression," *Sports Medicine (Auckland, N.Z.)* 52, no. 7 (July 2022): 1667–88, https://doi.org/10.1007/s40279-022-01644-9.

197 **cold water immersion immediately after high-intensity exercise:** Emma Moore et al., "Effects of Cold-Water Immersion Compared with Other Recovery Modalities on Athletic Performance Following Acute Strenuous Exercise in Physically Active Participants: A Systematic Review, Meta-Analysis, and Meta-Regression," *Sports Medicine (Auckland, N.Z.)* 53, no. 3 (March 2023): 687–705, https://doi.org/10.1007/s40279-022-01800-1.

197 **cold exposure within four hours:** Llion A. Roberts et al., "Post-Exercise Cold Water Immersion Attenuates Acute Anabolic Signalling and Long-Term Adaptations in Muscle to Strength Training," *Journal of Physiology* 593, no. 18 (September 15, 2015): 4285–4301, https://doi.org/10.1113/JP270570.

197 **an added benefit of combining:** Mohammed Ihsan et al., "Regular Postexercise Cooling Enhances Mitochondrial Biogenesis Through AMPK and P38 MAPK in Human Skeletal Muscle," *American Journal of Physiology. Regulatory, Integrative and Comparative Physiology* 309, no. 3 (August 1, 2015): R286–294, https://doi.org/10.1152/ajpregu.00031.2015.

203 **Your body's core temperature can rise:** Chuwa Tei et al., "Acute Hemodynamic Improvement by Thermal Vasodilation in Congestive Heart Failure," *Circulation* 91, no. 10 (May 15, 1995): 2582–90, https://doi.org/10.1161/01.CIR.91.10.2582.

204 **"the rule of 200":** Brunt and Minson, "Heat Therapy."

206 **adjusting your mealtimes to match your body's natural clock:** Manoogian et al., "Time-Restricted Eating for the Prevention and Management of Metabolic Diseases."

210 **The amount of protein you eat:** Mark P. Mattson, Valter D. Longo, and Michelle Harvie, "Impact of Intermittent Fasting on Health and Disease Processes," *Ageing Research Reviews* 39 (October 2017): 46–58, https://doi.org/10.1016/j.arr.2016.10.005.

210 **0.9 to 1.2 grams of protein per kilogram:** M. N. Harvie et al., "The Effects of Intermittent or Continuous Energy Restriction on Weight Loss and Metabolic Disease Risk Markers: A Randomized Trial in Young Overweight Women," *International Journal of Obesity* 35, no. 5 (May 2011): 714–27, https://doi.org/10.1038/ijo.2010.171.

210 **0.9 to 1.2 grams of protein per kilogram:** Michelle Harvie et al., "The Effect of Intermittent Energy and Carbohydrate Restriction v. Daily Energy Restriction on Weight Loss and Metabolic Disease Risk Markers in Overweight Women," *The British Journal of Nutrition* 110, no. 8 (October 2013): 1534–47, https://doi.org/10.1017/S0007114513000792.

211 **A 2014 study found that a high-protein diet:** Morgan E. Levine et al., "Low Protein Intake Is Associated with a Major Reduction in IGF-1, Cancer, and Overall Mortality in the 65 and Younger but Not Older Population," *Cell Metabolism* 19, no. 3 (March 4, 2014): 407–17, https://doi.org/10.1016/j.cmet.2014.02.006.

211 **when the protein was sourced from plants:** Levine et al.

211 **IGF-1 production:** J. P. Thissen, J. M. Ketelslegers, and L. E. Underwood, "Nutritional Regulation of the Insulin-like Growth Factors," *Endocrine Reviews* 15, no. 1 (February 1994): 80–101, https://doi.org/10.1210/edrv-15-1-80.

211 **IGF-1 production:** D. R. Clemmons, M. M. Seek, and L. E. Underwood, "Supplemental Essential Amino Acids Augment the Somatomedin-C/Insulin-like Growth Factor I Response to Refeeding After Fasting," *Metabolism: Clinical and Experimental* 34, no. 4 (April 1985): 391–95, https://doi.org/10.1016/0026-0495(85)90230-6.

211 **Animal proteins, rich in branched-chain amino acids:** Micah J. Drummond and Blake B. Rasmussen, "Leucine-Enriched Nutrients and the Regulation of mTOR Signalling and Human Skeletal Muscle Protein Synthesis," *Current Opinion in Clinical Nutrition and Metabolic Care* 11, no. 3 (May 2008): 222–26, https://doi.org/10.1097/MCO.0b013e3282fa17fb.

211 **just a 3 percent increase in daily energy from plant proteins:** Sina Naghshi et al., "Dietary Intake of Total, Animal, and Plant Proteins and Risk of All Cause, Cardiovascular, and Cancer Mortality: Systematic Review and Dose-Response Meta-Analysis of Prospective Cohort Studies," *BMJ*, July 22, 2020, m2412, https://doi.org/10.1136/bmj.m2412.

213 **spending 20 percent of your effort:** Tait D. Shanafelt and John H. Noseworthy, "Executive Leadership and Physician Well-Being: Nine Organizational Strategies to Promote Engagement and Reduce Burnout," *Mayo Clinic Proceedings* 92, no. 1 (January 1, 2017): 129–46, https://doi.org/10.1016/j.mayocp.2016.10.004.

Epilogue

272 **a different take on the phrase "First, do no harm":** "'Philosophy of Public Health' with William H. Foege, MD, MPH (Part 1 of 2) | The Whole Health Cure," September 21, 2019, https://thewholehealthcure.simplecast.com/episodes/a90bc50a.

273 **happiness can ripple:** James H. Fowler and Nicholas A. Christakis, "Dynamic Spread of Happiness in a Large Social Network: Longitudinal Analysis over 20 Years in the Framingham Heart Study," *BMJ* 337 (December 5, 2008), https://doi.org/10.1136/bmj.a2338.

273 **Obesity, for example, also clusters:** Nicholas A. Christakis and James H. Fowler, "The Spread of Obesity in a Large Social Network over 32 Years," *New England Journal of Medicine* 357, no. 4 (July 26, 2007): 370–79, https://doi.org/10.1056/NEJMsa066082.

274 **Dr. Rollin McCraty's research shows:** Rollin McCraty, "New Frontiers in Heart Rate Variability and Social Coherence Research: Techniques, Technologies, and Implications for Improving Group Dynamics and Outcomes," *Frontiers in Public Health* 5 (2017): 267, https://doi.org/10.3389/fpubh.2017.00267.

Index

About the Author

Dr. Sharon Horesh Bergquist is a physician, scientist, and internationally recognized pioneer in lifestyle medicine, a rapidly growing field that uses evidence-based lifestyle interventions for the prevention and management of disease and the optimization of health and longevity. She has been the lead investigator or coinvestigator in more than a dozen clinical trials that have received $61 million in funding for evaluating lifestyle interventions and finding early biomarkers for chronic disease, including ongoing studies for early detection of Alzheimer's disease and cancer. Her work is at the forefront of how we understand the role of stress and resilience in our health and longevity. She codirects the Emory Healthy Aging Study, one of the largest studies conducted in Atlanta, and is a coinvestigator in the National Institutes of Health (NIH) funded Emory Healthy Brain Study.

At the heart of her work is using the insights from the research to take the best possible care of her patients and building relationships that heal. Dr. Bergquist is a highly sought-after practicing internal medicine physician with more than twenty-five years of clinical experience in patient-centered care. She has a large, diverse general medicine practice and an executive health practice with longtime patients across the world, including CEOs and senior executives of Fortune 500 companies and professional sports teams, entrepreneurs, philanthropists, and societal and industry leaders. Using her approach of addressing upstream contributing pathways to fight disease and extend longevity, she has received more than forty patient care awards, including being nationally recognized in the top 1 percent of her specialty by Press Ganey, based on patient feedback, for more than a decade, and being peer-voted by her physician colleagues as one of Atlanta's Top Doctors consecutively for the past nine years.

Dr. Bergquist has appeared on or been interviewed for more than 200 news segments, including for *Good Morning America*, CNN, ABC News, the *Wall Street Journal*, NPR, and *Women's Health* magazine. Her writing has appeared on CNN.com and Huffington Post, among other sites; and her popular TED-Ed video on how stress affects the body has been viewed more than eight million times. More than 150,000 people have enrolled in her online course on nutrition and weight loss, which is available in twenty-two languages. She also hosts *The Whole Health Cure* podcast, where she interviews physicians, scientists, and health experts to share scientifically validated ways that empower prevention, disease management, and healthy aging.

Dr. Bergquist has authored more than fifty-five peer-reviewed scientific articles and abstracts and presented at national and international conferences. A leader in her field, she contributed to an upcoming book of case stories in lifestyle medicine that will be used in medical education curricula. She serves on advisory boards and global committees advancing nutrition, stress management, and other pillars of lifestyle as medicine, including the True Health Initiative and the Teaching Kitchen Collaborative. In 2012, she was invited to the White House as one of the country's top 150 primary care clinician leaders to work with presidential advisers on healthcare reform. She firmly believes in collaborating with like-minded leaders and innovators endeavoring to create a healthier world.

Dr. Bergquist is the Pam R. Rollins Professor of Medicine at Emory University School of Medicine. At her home institution, she is the medical director of Emory Executive Health and founded Emory Lifestyle Medicine & Wellness, in support of her belief that academic medicine and health systems need to lead in prevention as well as high-tech treatment of disease. A signature program developed through this initiative is the Emory Healthy Kitchen Collaborative, a twelve-month evidence-based multidisciplinary worksite wellness program and clinical trial with proven health improvement outcomes that has won scientific awards at national presentations. Through this work, the American College of Lifestyle Medicine (ACLM) has recognized Emory as one of the pioneering institutions in ACLM's health system council. Recently, the Emory School of Medicine has supported Dr. Bergquist's vision of building a top-tier "clinic of the future" with a large grant to integrate biomarker measures of health and digital therapeutics into clinical care to optimize health, well-being, and longevity.

She holds a degree in molecular biophysics and biochemistry from Yale College, received her medical degree from Harvard Medical School, and completed her internship and residency in internal medicine at the Brigham and Women's Hospital in Boston. She lives in Atlanta with her husband and three daughters.